Ischemic Heart Disease: Causes, Symptoms and Treatment

Ischemic Heart Disease: Causes, Symptoms and Treatment

Editor: Scarlett Warren

AMERICAN
MEDICAL PUBLISHERS
www.americanmedicalpublishers.com

AMERICAN
MEDICAL PUBLISHERS
www.americanmedicalpublishers.com

Cataloging-in-Publication Data

Ischemic heart disease : causes, symptoms and treatment / edited by Scarlett Warren.
p. cm.
Includes bibliographical references and index.
ISBN 978-1-63927-033-0
1. Coronary heart disease. 2. Coronary heart disease--Etiology.
3. Coronary heart disease--Treatment. 4. Heart--Diseases. I. Warren, Scarlett.
RC685.C6 I83 2022
616.123--dc23

American Medical Publishers,
41 Flatbush Avenue,
1st Floor, New York,
NY 11217, USA

ISBN 978-1-63927-033-0 (Hardback)

Contents

Preface

Every book is a source of knowledge and this one is no exception. The idea that led to the conceptualization of this book was the fact that the world is advancing rapidly; which makes it crucial to document the progress in every field. I am aware that a lot of data is already available, yet, there is a lot more to learn. Hence, I accepted the responsibility of editing this book and contributing my knowledge to the community.

Ischemic heart disease (IHD) also known as coronary artery disease is a condition of the heart in which there is a reduction in the blood flow to the heart muscle. This occurs due to an accumulation of plaque in the arteries of the heart. Sustained obstruction of the blood flow to the heart results in ischemia and myocardial infarction. This leads to damage to the heart and eventual death, if not resolved. Ischemic heart disease can occur in individuals of any age group, but is more common in older adults. It is a leading cause of death in the world today. Nearly half of the cases of IHD have a genetic influence. Smoking and obesity are other risk factors. Chest pain is a common symptom of IHD. Symptoms are often not present and the first sign is a heart attack in many cases. Revascularization, particularly hybrid coronary revascularization, angioplasty and coronary artery bypass grafting are certain procedures for treating acute coronary syndrome. Anti-platelet therapy, calcium channel blockers and beta-blockers, along with lifestyle changes may be recommended for the long-term control of the disease. This book contains some path-breaking studies in the diagnosis and treatment of ischemic heart disease. It outlines the causes and symptoms of ischemic heart disease in detail. A number of latest researches have been included to keep the readers up-to-date with the diverse aspects of this medical condition.

While editing this book, I had multiple visions for it. Then I finally narrowed down to make every chapter a sole standing text explaining a particular topic, so that they can be used independently. However, the umbrella subject sinews them into a common theme. This makes the book a unique platform of knowledge.

I would like to give the major credit of this book to the experts from every corner of the world, who took the time to share their expertise with us. Also, I owe the completion of this book to the never-ending support of my family, who supported me throughout the project.

Editor

1

Transfers to metropolitan hospitals and coronary angiography for rural Aboriginal and non-Aboriginal patients with acute ischaemic heart disease in Western Australia

Derrick Lopez[1*], Judith M Katzenellenbogen[1,2], Frank M Sanfilippo[2], John A Woods[1], Michael ST Hobbs[2], Matthew W Knuiman[2], Tom G Briffa[2], Peter L Thompson[3] and Sandra C Thompson[1]

Abstract

Background: Aboriginal people have a disproportionately higher incidence rate of ischaemic heart disease (IHD) than non-Aboriginal people. The findings on Aboriginal disparity in receiving coronary artery procedures are inconclusive. We describe the profile and transfers of IHD patients admitted to rural hospitals as emergency admissions and investigate determinants of transfers and coronary angiography.

Methods: Person-linked hospital and mortality records were used to identify 28-day survivors of IHD events commencing at rural hospitals in Western Australia. Outcome measures were receipt of coronary angiography, transfer to a metropolitan hospital, and coronary angiography if transferred to a metropolitan hospital.

Results: Compared to non-Aboriginal patients, Aboriginal patients with IHD were more likely to be younger, have more co-morbidities, reside remotely, but less likely to have private insurance. After adjusting for demographic characteristics, Aboriginal people with MI were less likely to be transferred to a metropolitan hospital, and if transferred were less likely to receive coronary angiography. These disparities were not significant after adjusting for comorbidities and private insurance. In the full multivariate model age, comorbidities and private insurance were adversely associated with transfer to a metropolitan hospital and coronary angiography.

Conclusion: Disparity in receiving coronary angiography following emergency admission for IHD to rural hospitals is mediated through the lower likelihood of being transferred to metropolitan hospitals where this procedure is performed. The likelihood of a transfer is increased if the patient has private insurance, however, rural Aboriginal people have a lower rate of private insurance than their non-Aboriginal counterparts. Health practitioners and policy makers can continue to claim that they treat Aboriginal and non-Aboriginal people alike based upon clinical indications, as private insurance is acting as a filter to reduce rural residents accessing interventional cardiology. If health practitioners and policy makers are truly committed to reducing health disparities, they must reflect upon the broader systems in which disparity is perpetuated and work towards a systems improvement.

Keywords: Oceanic ancestry group, Ischaemic heart disease, Myocardial infarction, Healthcare Disparities, Rural Hospitals, Health Insurance, Coronary angiography

* Correspondence: derrick.lopez@uwa.edu.au
[1]Western Australian Centre for Rural Health, The University of Western Australia, Crawley, Western Australia, Australia
Full list of author information is available at the end of the article

Background

Cardiovascular disease is a major cause of mortality in Australia [1] and although age-standardised hospitalisation and mortality rates have fallen [2], health inequalities remain amongst Aboriginal people [2-4], rural and remote residents [2,5], and lower socio-economic status (SES) groups [2,6,7]. In particular, ischaemic heart disease (IHD) is a major contributor to the substantial life expectancy gap between Aboriginal and non-Aboriginal populations, accounting for 14% of the total gap in disease burden [8]. At all levels of remoteness, Aboriginal people have a disproportionately higher incidence rate of myocardial infarction (MI) than non-Aboriginal people [5].

The findings on Aboriginal disparity in receiving coronary artery revascularisation procedures (CARP) are inconclusive with one study showing disparity in their fully adjusted model [9], whilst another showing disparity only in the model adjusted for demographics and admission hospital [10] and yet others showing no disparity in their fully adjusted models [11,12]. However, these analyses considered metropolitan and rural patients together. In Western Australia (WA), the largest and most sparsely populated Australian state, analyses should consider rural patients separately as transfer to metropolitan cardiology centres is a pre-requisite for receiving coronary artery diagnostic and intervention procedures unavailable in rural areas. The determinants of patient transfer are complex, including clinical characteristics and non-medical factors such as age, race, bed availability, insurance status, and patient's previous negative experiences [13-16]. Thus, it is possible that failure to transfer may be partly responsible for disparities in CARP, and may support urban health practitioners' and policy makers' claims of no differential in the treatment of Aboriginal patients.

Our aims were to describe the profile and metropolitan transfer of IHD patients admitted to rural hospitals as emergency admissions; and to investigate determinants (including Aboriginal status) of transfers and coronary angiography, with a specific focus on MI since it is diagnosed based on symptoms, cardiac biomarkers and ECG findings and its diagnosis is likely to be consistently coded throughout the state.

Methods

Study cohort

We identified IHD events in rural residents aged 25–84 years who were admitted to rural hospitals in WA in 2005–09 (Figure 1). Only admissions where patients survived for more than 28 days were included to minimise likely survivor selection bias (fatal cases have less opportunity to be transferred or receive CARP). An emergency admission to a rural hospital with principal discharge diagnosis of IHD marked the starting point for each initial episode of care, defined as a series of contiguous hospital admissions, including inter-hospital transfers. An event included all admissions (booked or emergency) associated with the initial episode of care, or any additional episodes starting within a 28-day period from the initial emergency admission. The 28-day period is consistent with the International Classification of Diseases Australian Modification 10th revision (ICD-10-AM) and major international studies and guidelines [17-19]. A subsequent emergency IHD admission to rural hospitals outside this event definition was considered a new event. Hence, a person could have multiple events over the study period.

Data source

A person-linked file of all WA rural residents admitted to WA rural hospitals with principal discharge diagnosis of IHD and their subsequent hospital admissions (both rural and metropolitan) was extracted from the Hospital Morbidity Data Collection (HMDC) and Death datasets of the WA Data Linkage System [20]. At the admission date of each event, we recorded patient demographic variables, IHD category, MI type, 5-year histories of chronic pulmonary disease, diabetes, heart failure (HF) and kidney disease (ICD-10 codes defined by Quan *et al.* [21]), alcohol-related hospital admissions and smoking. Using principal diagnosis, IHD category was classified as MI (ICD-10-AM: I21), unstable angina (ICD-10-AM: I20.0) or other IHD (all other ICD-10-AM codes between I20-I25). MI type was defined as transmural (ICD-10-AM: I21.0-I21.3), subendocardial (ICD-10-AM: I21.4) or other (ICD-10-AM: I21.9). Using the Accessibility Remoteness Index of Australia Plus (ARIA+) [22], remote residence was defined as ARIA+ categories 4 (remote) and 5 (very remote) while regional included the remaining WA areas, excluding metropolitan Perth (capital of WA). Socio-Economic Indexes for Areas (SEIFA) [23] scores based on the Statistical Local Area of residence were used as a measure of SES. Private insurance status was defined as having private insurance recorded in the HMDC at any admission during the event. As Aboriginal status is under-reported in administrative health data [24,25], patients identified as Aboriginal and/or Torres Strait Islander in any admission since 1980 were classified as Aboriginal. Sensitivity analyses were performed for Aboriginal status based on identification in at least 25% of their hospital admissions or identification at the initial admission for their event.

Study outcomes

As provision of CARP is dependent on the patient's clinical need, suitability and consent (data not available in HMDC), coronary angiography rather than CARP was considered the main outcome, reflecting that the patient had been investigated for diagnostic and therapeutic

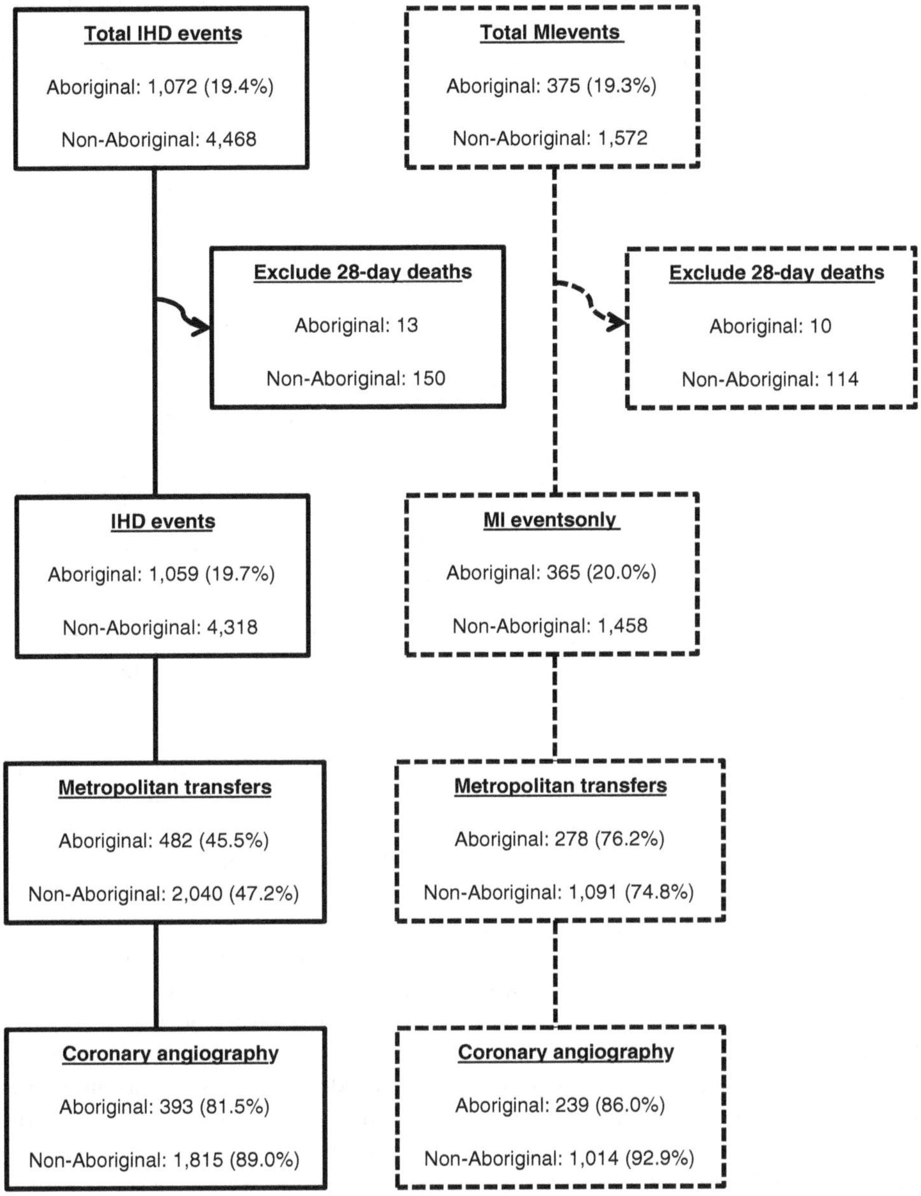

Figure 1 Flow diagram of IHD and MI events from 2005-09 in rural WA by Aboriginal status. IHD = ischaemic heart disease; MI = myocardial infarction.

purposes. Thus, for each event, three 28-day outcomes were identified: (i) receipt of coronary angiography (ICD-10-AM Block 668); (ii) transfer to a metropolitan hospital, defined as any admission to metropolitan hospitals during that event; and (iii) receipt of coronary angiography if transferred to a metropolitan hospital. Angiography was also assumed to have been performed if the patient had a CARP (ICD-10-AM Blocks 669–679) recorded within 28 days of the event admission date where angiography was not separately recorded in the procedure fields. For our third outcome, only rural events associated with a metropolitan transfer were included in the denominator because at the time of the study coronary angiography was performed only in seven metropolitan hospitals in WA and thus receipt of this procedure was contingent on transfer to these metropolitan hospitals. A sensitivity analysis was performed for 90-day events (deaths, transfer to a metropolitan hospital and receipt of coronary angiography within 90 days instead of 28 days) to cover unexpected delays in subsequent care.

Statistical analyses

Analyses were performed using Stata [26]. Baseline characteristics of Aboriginal and non-Aboriginal events were summarized separately with *t*-tests and chi-squared tests used to test for significance in continuous and categorical variables respectively. To model event-based metropolitan transfers and receipt of coronary angiography, the *xtgee* command was used with a Poisson distribution for the dependent variable together with a log link function. This method accounts for repeated measures as some patients had multiple events during 2005–09. With binary outcomes, the exponentiated coefficients from Poisson regression represent risk ratios (RR) instead of incidence-rate ratios [27]. In addition to the unadjusted model that included Aboriginal status only, five models with sequential addition of variables were considered: Model 1 (age, sex); Model 2 (Model 1 + residential area, SES, IHD category/MI type); Model 3 (Model 2 + comorbidities); Model 4 (Model 3 + private insurance); and Model 5 (Model 3 with restriction to patients without private insurance).

Ethics

Ethics approval was obtained from Human Research Ethics Committees of The University of Western Australia, WA Department of Health, WA Country Health Services and WA Aboriginal Health.

Results

Event characteristics

Of the 5,540 acute IHD events identified in rural WA hospitals from 2005–09 (Figure 1), 5,377 (97.1%) survived to 28 days (19.7% Aboriginal). Similar crude proportions of Aboriginal and non-Aboriginal patients with acute IHD were transferred to metropolitan hospitals, although a lower proportion of Aboriginal patients received coronary angiography if transferred (81.5% v 89.0%, $p<0.001$). For MI events, the proportion of Aboriginal people transferred to metropolitan hospitals was not significantly different (76.2% v 74.8%, $p=0.598$) although a lower proportion received coronary angiography if transferred (86.0% v 92.9%, $p<0.001$). Overall, similar proportions of Aboriginal and non-Aboriginal MI patients received coronary angiography (65.5% v 69.5%, $p=0.134$).

Compared to non-Aboriginal patients, Aboriginal patients admitted for IHD or MI events were more likely ($p<0.001$ mostly) to be younger, female, have more risk factors and comorbidities, and live in remote areas, but less likely to have private insurance (Table 1).

Aboriginal disparity in receipt of coronary angiography

Aboriginal people with IHD were less likely to receive coronary angiography after adjusting for demographic factors, IHD category and comorbidities (Model 3: RR_{IHD} 0.87, 95% CI 0.80-0.95) but there was no significant disparity after adjusting for private insurance (Model 4) or restricting to patients without private insurance (Model 5) (Table 2). Aboriginal people with MI were also less likely to receive coronary angiography after adjusting for demographic factors and MI type (Model 2: RR_{MI} 0.81, 95% CI 0.75-0.89) but this disparity was insignificant after adjusting for comorbidities (Model 3) and private insurance (Model 4).

Aboriginal disparity in transfer to metropolitan hospital

Aboriginal people with IHD were less likely to be transferred to metropolitan hospitals after adjusting for demographic factors, IHD category and comorbidities (Model 3: RR_{IHD} 0.91, 95% CI 0.84-0.98) although this disparity was not significant after adjusting for private insurance (Model 4) or restricting to patients without private insurance (Model 5) (Table 2). Aboriginal people with MI were also less likely to be transferred to metropolitan hospitals after adjusting for demographic factors and MI type (Model 2: RR_{MI} 0.89, 95% CI 0.83-0.95); again there was no significant disparity after adjusting for comorbidities and accounting for private insurance.

Aboriginal disparity in receipt of coronary angiography if transferred to metropolitan hospital

After adjusting for demographic factors and IHD category/MI type, Aboriginal people with IHD or MI were less likely to receive coronary angiography when transferred to a metropolitan hospital (Model 2: RR_{IHD} 0.89, 95% CI 0.85-0.94; RR_{MI} 0.91, 95% CI 0.86-0.97). Again, this disparity was not significant after adjusting for comorbidities or for private insurance (Table 2).

Individual characteristics associated with outcomes

In the full multivariate model (presented for MI events only), factors adversely associated with receiving coronary angiography and transfer to metropolitan hospital included older age groups, chronic pulmonary disease, HF and private insurance (Table 3). However, once transferred to a metropolitan hospital, only the oldest age group (75–84 years) and those with HF or kidney disease were less likely to receive coronary angiography. A similar multivariate model but restricted to patients without private insurance resulted in similar RR (Additional file 1).

Sensitivity analyses

Table 4 shows that alternative adjusted RRs for 28-day events using the two other definitions of Aboriginal status were similar to those for Model 4 in Table 2. Adjusted RRs for Aboriginal status based on 28- and 90-day events were also similar.

Discussion

Our study expands on other Australian studies investigating Aboriginal disparities in receipt of coronary angiography by restricting the analysis to rural patients and separating the effects of transfer to metropolitan hospitals

Table 1 Demographic and clinical profile of IHD and MI events originating from rural hospitals in WA

	All IHD (n = 5,377 events)			MI only (n = 1,823 events)		
	Aboriginal	Non-Aboriginal		Aboriginal	Non-Aboriginal	
	n = 1,059 events (794 patients)	n = 4,318 events (3,587 patients)	p value	n = 365 events (342 patients)	n = 1,458 events (1,386 patients)	p value
Age groups			<0.001			<0.001
25-34 years	53 (5.0)	31 (0.7)		25 (6.8)	10 (0.7)	
35-44 years	222 (21.0)	312 (7.2)		83 (22.7)	111 (7.6)	
45-54 years	353 (33.3)	760 (17.6)		116 (31.8)	295 (20.2)	
55-64 years	247 (23.3)	1,073 (24.8)		87 (23.8)	359 (24.6)	
65-74 years	117 (11.0)	1,051 (24.3)		36 (9.9)	333 (22.8)	
75-84 years	67 (6.3)	1,091 (25.3)		18 (4.9)	350 (24.0)	
Sex: female (%)	465 (43.9)	1,419 (32.9)	<0.001	120 (34.2)	368 (25.2)	0.001
Residential area (%)			<0.001			<0.001
Regional	424 (40.0)	3,431 (79.5)		125 (34.2)	1,128 (77.4)	
Remote	635 (60.0)	887 (20.5)		240 (65.8)	330 (22.6)	
SES (%)			<0.001			<0.001
1st quartile[(a)]	576 (54.4)	1,218 (28.2)		209 (57.3)	401 (27.5)	
2nd quartile	209 (19.7)	1,205 (27.9)		63 (17.3)	425 (29.1)	
3rd quartile	166 (15.7)	1,388 (32.1)		50 (13.7)	465 (31.9)	
4th quartile[(b)]	108 (10.2)	507 (11.7)		43 (11.8)	167 (11.5)	
Risk factors (%)						
Alcohol	311 (29.4)	234 (5.4)	<0.001	96 (26.3)	59 (4.0)	<0.001
Smoking	756 (71.4)	2,388 (55.3)	<0.001	263 (72.1)	779.(53.4)	<0.001
Comorbidities (%)						
Chronic pulmonary disease	204 (19.3)	483 (11.2)	<0.001	56 (15.3)	128 (8.8)	<0.001
Diabetes	608 (57.4)	1,113 (25.8)	<0.001	205 (56.2)	340 (23.3)	<0.001
HF	238 (22.5)	666 (15.4)	<0.001	79 (21.6)	230 (15.8)	0.008
Kidney disease	175 (16.5)	316 (7.3)	<0.001	67 (18.4)	110 (7.5)	<0.001
First ever IHD/MI event in 2005–09 (%)	591 (55.8)	3,035 (70.3)	<0.001	263 (72.1)	1,241 (85.1)	<0.001
Private insurance (%)	52 (4.9)	1,181 (27.4)	<0.001	21 (5.8)	470 (32.2)	<0.001
IHD category (%)			0.497			
MI	365 (33.8)	1,458 (33.8)				
Unstable angina	340 (32.1)	1,468 (34.0)				
Other IHD	354 (33.4)	1,392 (32.2)				
MI type (%)[(c)]						
Transmural				167 (45.8)	641 (44.0)	0.078
Subendocardial				144 (39.5)	527 (36.1)	
Other				54 (14.8)	290 (19.9)	

Statistical significance determined using t-test and chi-squared test for continuous and categorical variables respectively.
HF = heart failure; IHD = ischaemic heart disease; MI = myocardial infarction; SES = socio-economic status.
[(a)]most disadvantaged; [(b)]least disadvantaged; [(c)]MI type was based on ICD-10-AM coding terminology.

from receipt of coronary angiography *per se*. After adjusting for age and sex, Aboriginal people presenting to rural hospitals with acute IHD were less likely to be transferred to metropolitan hospitals and if transferred were also less likely to receive coronary angiography. These disparities were mainly explained by the higher prevalence of comorbidities and to a lesser extent by the lower rate of private insurance among Aboriginal people.

Rural WA experienced 5,540 acute IHD events (average 3 events/day) in 2005–09 with Aboriginal people over-represented and their profile being consistent with previous Australian studies [9,10,12]. Our analyses investigated

Table 2 Ratio of Aboriginal to non-Aboriginal risks of coronary angiography, transfer, and coronary angiography if transferred

	IHD		MI	
Aboriginal status = yes	**RR (95% CI)**	**p value**	**RR (95% CI)**	**p value**
(i) Receipt of coronary angiography				
Unadjusted	0.88 (0.80-0.97)	0.010	0.94 (0.87-1.02)	0.162
Model 1	0.77 (0.69-0.85)	<0.001	0.79 (0.73-0.86)	<0.001
Model 2	0.76 (0.70-0.83)	<0.001	0.81 (0.75-0.89)	<0.001
Model 3	0.87 (0.80-0.95)	0.002	0.93 (0.86-1.01)	0.096
Model 4	0.95 (0.88-1.04)	0.283	0.96 (0.88-1.05)	0.366
Model 5	0.93 (0.84-1.03)	0.166	0.97 (0.87-1.07)	0.510
(ii) Transfer to metropolitan hospital				
Unadjusted	0.96 (0.89-1.04)	0.366	1.02 (0.95-1.09)	0.597
Model 1	0.86 (0.79-0.94)	0.001	0.88 (0.83-0.94)	<0.001
Model 2	0.84 (0.78-0.91)	<0.001	0.89 (0.83-0.95)	0.001
Model 3	0.91 (0.84-0.98)	0.012	0.96 (0.90-1.03)	0.256
Model 4	0.99 (0.92-1.07)	0.758	0.99 (0.93-1.06)	0.804
Model 5	0.97 (0.89-1.06)	0.543	1.00 (0.92-1.08)	0.939
(iii) Receipt of coronary angiography if transferred to metropolitan hospital				
Unadjusted	0.92 (0.87-0.96)	<0.001	0.92 (0.88-0.97)	0.003
Model 1	0.88 (0.84-0.93)	<0.001	0.89 (0.84-0.95)	<0.001
Model 2	0.89 (0.85-0.94)	<0.001	0.91 (0.86-0.97)	0.003
Model 3	0.97 (0.92-1.02)	0.188	0.97 (0.92-1.03)	0.304
Model 4	0.98 (0.93-1.03)	0.346	0.97 (0.92-1.03)	0.382
Model 5	0.97 (0.91-1.03)	0.300	0.98 (0.91-1.05)	0.546

Model 1: age group and sex.
Model 2: model 1 + residential area, SES, IHD category (for IHD) or MI type (for MI).
Model 3: model 2 + 5-year histories of chronic pulmonary disease, diabetes, HF, kidney disease.
Model 4: model 3 + private insurance status.
Model 5: model 3 with restriction to patients without private insurance.
RR = risk ratio with reference group being non-Aboriginal patients; 95% CI = 95% confidence interval; HF = heart failure; IHD = ischaemic heart disease; MI = myocardial infarction; SES = socio-economic status.

patients with a principal discharge diagnosis of IHD (which encompasses acute coronary syndrome (ACS) patients) as well as those with a principal discharge diagnosis of MI to increase our specificity. Our results were similar for IHD and MI events and our discussion is focused on MI events.

The proportion of patients who received coronary angiography in our study was higher than that recently reported by Randall *et al.* [10] for both Aboriginal (65.5% v 48.5%) and non-Aboriginal people (69.5% v 54.3%). These differences likely stem from our case selection since we used MI as the principal diagnosis only whereas Randall used MI in principal diagnosis or in second and third diagnoses along with IHD as the principal diagnosis. We found no Aboriginal disparity in receiving coronary angiography when unadjusted but observed significant disparities after adjusting for age and sex which is a reflection of the substantial different age and sex profiles of Aboriginal and non-Aboriginal MI patients [3]. The results of our full model are consistent with Randall's study [10] where an Aboriginal disparity was found in receiving coronary angiography after adjusting for age, sex, admission year, AMI type and admitting hospital (adjusted hazard ratio 0.81, 95% CI 0.74-0.88), which was explained by the higher burden of comorbidities and lower rate of private insurance among Aboriginal people. Similarly, Ranasinghe *et al.* [12] and Roe *et al.* [28] did not find any Aboriginal disparity in their multivariate models, although the latter study was probably under-powered due to small numbers of Aboriginal people. On the other hand, Coory *et al.* [9] found disparities for coronary revascularisation (for which coronary angiography is a pre-requisite) amongst Aboriginal people after adjusting for age, sex, SES, remoteness, hospital characteristics and comorbidities (RR 0.78, 95% CI 0.64-0.94). Whereas Coory's study was a person-based analysis looking at first-ever admission for MI in the 5-year period, ours was an events-based analysis; the former being useful for focussing on outcomes while

Table 3 Full model RR in MI patients for coronary angiography, transfer, and coronary angiography if transferred

	Coronary angiography		Transfer to metropolitan hospital		Coronary angiography if transferred to metropolitan hospital	
	RR (95% CI)	p value	RR (95% CI)	p value	RR (95% CI)	p value
Aboriginal status						
Non-Aboriginal	1.00		1.00		1.00	
Aboriginal	0.96 (0.88-1.05)	0.366	0.99 (0.93-1.06)	0.804	0.97 (0.92-1.03)	0.382
Age groups						
25-34 years	1.11 (0.93-1.31)	0.244	1.04 (0.91-1.20)	0.559	1.07 (0.99-1.17)	0.107
35-44 years	1.04 (0.97-1.12)	0.298	1.05 (0.98-1.12)	0.141	1.00 (0.95-1.05)	0.900
45-54 years	1.00		1.00		1.00	
55-64 years	0.98 (0.92-1.05)	0.541	1.00 (0.95-1.05)	0.959	0.98 (0.94-1.02)	0.331
65-74 years	0.86 (0.79-0.94)	0.001	0.87 (0.80-0.93)	<0.001	1.00 (0.95-1.04)	0.870
75-84 years	0.52 (0.45-0.60)	<0.001	0.59 (0.52-0.66)	<0.001	0.88 (0.82-0.96)	0.002
Sex						
Male	1.00		1.00		1.00	
Female	0.98 (0.91-1.06)	0.648	0.97 (0.91-1.03)	0.290	1.01 (0.97-1.05)	0.786
Residential area						
Regional	1.00		1.00		1.00	
Remote	1.03 (0.96-1.09)	0.488	1.06 (1.00-1.12)	0.035	0.97 (0.93-1.01)	0.147
SES quartiles						
1st quartile[(a)]	1.00		1.00		1.00	
2nd quartile	1.06 (0.99-1.15)	0.115	1.05 (0.98-1.12)	0.153	1.01 (0.97-1.05)	0.691
3rd quartile	1.08 (1.00-1.17)	0.049	1.05 (0.99-1.13)	0.126	1.02 (0.98-1.07)	0.313
4th quartile[(b)]	1.08 (0.98-1.18)	0.107	1.11 (1.04-1.19)	0.003	0.97 (0.91-1.03)	0.278
MI type[(c)]						
Transmural	1.00		1.00		1.00	
Subendocardial/other	0.96 (0.91-1.01)	0.131	0.96 (0.92-1.01)	0.128	0.99 (0.96-1.02)	0.656
Chronic pulmonary disease						
No	1.00		1.00		1.00	
Yes	0.79 (0.67-0.93)	0.005	0.85 (0.74-0.97)	0.019	0.94 (0.85-1.04)	0.183
Diabetes						
No	1.00		1.00		1.00	
Yes	0.97 (0.90-1.04)	0.404	0.99 (0.93-1.05)	0.758	0.98 (0.94-1.02)	0.304
HF						
No	1.00		1.00		1.00	
Yes	0.67 (0.57-0.78)	<0.001	0.74 (0.66-0.84)	<0.001	0.89 (0.81-0.98)	0.014
Kidney disease						
No	1.00		1.00		1.00	
Yes	0.63 (0.51-0.79)	<0.001	0.89 (0.76-1.03)	0.106	0.71 (0.60-0.84)	<0.001
Private insurance						
No	0.84 (0.79-0.88)	<0.001	0.85 (0.81-0.89)	<0.001	0.98 (0.95-1.01)	0.124
Yes	1.00		1.00		1.00	

RR = Risk ratio; 95% CI = 95% confidence interval;
HF = heart failure; MI = myocardial infarction; SES = socio-economic status.
[(a)]most disadvantaged; [(b)]least disadvantaged; [(c)]MI type was based on ICD-10-AM coding terminology.

Table 4 Sensitivity analysis using (i) three definitions for Aboriginal identification, and (ii) 28-day vs 90-day events

	IHD		MI	
Method of identifying Aboriginal status	**RR (95% CI)**	**p value**	**RR (95% CI)**	**p value**
(i) Coronary angiography				
≥25% of admissions: 28-day event	0.94 (0.86-1.03)	0.186	0.94 (0.86-1.03)	0.195
First admission for event: 28-day event	0.97 (0.88-1.06)	0.473	0.96 (0.88-1.06)	0.431
Any admission: 90-day event	0.94 (0.86-1.02)	0.119	0.96 (0.89-1.04)	0.371
(ii) Transfer to metropolitan hospital				
≥25% of admissions: 28-day event	0.96 (0.88-1.04)	0.305	0.98 (0.91-1.05)	0.579
First admission for event: 28-day event	0.97 (0.90-1.06)	0.535	0.99 (0.92-1.07)	0.888
Any admission: 90-day event	1.00 (0.93-1.07)	0.942	1.00 (0.94-1.07)	0.958
(iii) Receipt of coronary angiography if transferred to metropolitan hospital				
≥25% of admissions: 28-day event	0.98 (0.93-1.04)	0.569	0.97 (0.91-1.03)	0.275
First admission for event: 28-day event	1.02 (0.94-1.05)	0.900	0.97 (0.91-1.04)	0.423
Any admission: 90-day event	0.95 (0.90-1.03)	0.061	0.97 (0.92-1.03)	0.338

Results are compared to Model 4 from Table 2 which has been adjusted for age groups, sex, residential area, SES, IHD category (for IHD) or MI type (for MI), 5-year history of chronic pulmonary disease, diabetes, HF, kidney disease and private insurance.
RR = Risk ratio; 95% CI = 95% confidence interval; IHD = ischaemic heart disease; MI = myocardial infarction; SES = socio-economic status; HF = heart failure.

the latter is more useful for health services/management decisions and planning. Restricting our analyses to first-ever MI in the 5-year period produced similar results (Model 6 in Additional file 2). The differences between our and Coory's study may reflect state differences (WA v Queensland) or the time period examined (2005–2009 v 1998–2002) with possible improvement in Aboriginal care more recently.

Our study adds to those of Randall [10], Ranasinghe [12] and Coory [9] by separating from coronary angiography the effects of transfer to a metropolitan hospital (where coronary artery procedures are performed) as the disparity in receiving coronary angiography among rural WA patients could reflect inequity in their transfer to metropolitan hospitals [29]. Therefore, we restricted the analysis to rural patients whereas earlier studies controlled for remoteness of hospitalisation. Aboriginal people of the same demographic profile and MI type were less likely to be transferred to a metropolitan hospital, and when transferred were less likely to receive coronary angiography. These disparities were accounted for by comorbidities (like HF and kidney disease which are associated with adverse outcomes) and private insurance. Although we did not adjust for all comorbidities and risk factors (alcohol, smoking), inclusion of the Charlson comorbidity score and these additional risk factor variables did not change the RR for Aboriginal people (Model 7 in Additional file 2). Our results support those of the Australian and New Zealand SNAPSHOT ACS study [30] in that the burden of comorbidities accentuates the challenges faced in applying evidence-based guidelines among patients in this context.

Patients without private insurance were 16% less likely to receive coronary angiography than those with private insurance. Notably, among demographically and clinically similar patients without private insurance, there was no significant difference between Aboriginal and non-Aboriginal patients in the likelihood of receiving coronary angiography. However, Aboriginal people were substantially less likely to have private insurance than non-Aboriginal people (5.8% versus 32.2%). The effect of private insurance may be two-fold. Firstly, it provides the option of metropolitan transfer to the private hospital system if public beds are not available. Patients in the private system are more likely to receive coronary artery procedures than those in the public system [31,32]. This accords with the anecdotal reports of rural doctors regarding the difficulties they encounter in transferring non ST-elevation MI patients to public metropolitan hospitals, with some of these patients being transferred to the private system if they have private insurance. Secondly, given that we used an ecological measure for SES, private insurance may in fact be a proxy for individual-level SES or educational attainment. Thus, privately insured patients are more affluent, educated, articulate and possibly more likely to demand a transfer to a metropolitan hospital for appropriate care than less affluent patients [33,34]. Private insurance was not a factor in receiving coronary angiography once the patient had been transferred, suggesting that the private insurance-associated disparity in receiving coronary angiography is mediated through patient transfer to metropolitan hospitals.

One of the strengths of this study was the use of person-linked hospital and mortality data with state-wide coverage which allowed us to follow patients throughout the 28-day event. Without such access to person-linked hospital data, we would not be able to determine if the patient had received coronary angiography as this procedure is recorded as a separate admission. Our use of 28-day events was based on previous studies and ICD-10 coding standards [17-19], but repeating the analysis for 90-day events produced similar results, showing that the RRs are relatively robust with respect to the definition of an event.

The limitations of our study are those inherent with reliance on routinely collected administrative data. For example, the absence of individual-level SES data (especially in rural areas where large, heterogeneous areas can be allocated the same SES), more specific clinical information on severity of MI (although HMDC records MI as transmural and subendocardial, providing some indication of severity) and patient decisions to refuse further treatment limits our understanding of these disparities. Aboriginal people may refuse transfer to a metropolitan hospital based on negative experiences of family and friends. In fact, many Aboriginal people, particularly those from remote areas, find tertiary hospitals unwelcoming and are reluctant to attend for diagnosis [15,16]. As we did not have access to either the patient's residential address or hospital name (confidentiality considerations), we could not adjust for the distance of patients' residence from the hospital. Restricted to WA data only, it was possible to overlook patients who were transferred to other states for further treatment, in particular in far North WA where transfer to Royal Darwin Hospital is possible. Although Aboriginal status is under-reported in administrative data, our sensitivity analyses with three methods of Aboriginal identification produced similar results suggesting that our findings are robust with respect to Aboriginal identification.

Conclusion

Our findings question the way in which Australia's universal health insurance scheme is operating to support access of rural residents, especially Aboriginal people, to life-saving treatments. This disparity is particularly relevant in those with MI because the current National Heart Foundation of Australia/Cardiac Society of Australia and New Zealand guidelines [35] recommend coronary angiography in all patients with MI unless there are specific contraindications. Rural residents would benefit from consistent state-wide guidelines, protocols and processes for the management of ACS and system-wide coordination and integration of patient transfer (including central referral coordinating unit and clearly defined roles and responsibilities of individual health professionals) [36]. Our results suggest that urban health practitioners and policy makers can continue to claim that they treat Aboriginal and non-Aboriginal people alike based upon clinical indications, as private insurance is acting as an effective filter to reduce rural residents (where a greater proportion of Aboriginal people live) accessing interventional cardiology. If health practitioners and policy makers are truly committed to reducing health disparities, they must reflect upon the broader systems in which disparity is perpetuated and work towards a systems improvement [37].

Abbreviations

ACS: Acute coronary syndrome; ARIA+: Accessibility Remoteness Index of Australia Plus; CARP: Coronary artery revascularisation procedures; HF: Heart failure; HMDC: Hospital Morbidity Data Collection; ICD-10-AM: International Classification of Diseases Australian Modification 10th revision; IHD: Ischaemic heart disease; MI: Myocardial infarction; RR: Risk ratios; SEIFA: Socio-Economic Indexes for Areas; SES: Socio-economic status; WA: Western Australia.

Competing interests

The authors declare that they have no competing interests.

Authors' contributions

DL, JMK, FMS, SCT, TGB, MSTH and PLT were involved in the concept and design of this study. DL extracted the linked data and performed the statistical analyses, with statistical advice from MWK. DL, JMK, FMS, MWK, JAW and TGB interpreted the results. DL constructed the figure and tables, and, initiated and coordinated the write-up. All authors read and approved the final manuscript.

Acknowledgements

This work was supported by the NHMRC (Grant Number 1031057). JMK is an NHMRC Early Career Fellow (Number 037429). The Western Australian Centre for Rural Health receives funding from the Department of Health and Ageing. Special thanks to the WA Data Linkage Branch, Department of Health Inpatient Data Collections and Registrar General for provision of data.

Author details

[1]Western Australian Centre for Rural Health, The University of Western Australia, Crawley, Western Australia, Australia. [2]School of Population Health, The University of Western Australia, Crawley, Western Australia, Australia. [3]School of Medicine and Pharmacology, Sir Charles Gairdner Hospital Unit, The University of Western Australia, Nedlands, Western Australia, Australia.

References

1. Australian Institute of Health and Welfare: *Australia's health 2012. Australia's health series no.13.* Canberra: Australian Institute of Health and Welfare; 2012.
2. Australian Institute of Health and Welfare: *Cardiovascular disease: Australian facts 2011.* Canberra: Australian Institute of Health and Welfare; 2011.
3. Katzenellenbogen JM, Sanfilippo FM, Hobbs MS, Briffa TG, Ridout SC, Knuiman MW, Dimer L, Taylor KP, Thompson PL, Thompson SC: **Incidence of and case fatality following acute myocardial infarction in Aboriginal and non-Aboriginal Western Australians (2000–2004): a linked data study.** *Heart Lung Circ* 2010, **19**(12):717–725.
4. Katzenellenbogen JM, Sanfilippo FM, Hobbs MS, Briffa TG, Ridout SC, Knuiman MW, Dimer L, Taylor KP, Thompson PL, Thompson SC: **Aboriginal to non-Aboriginal differentials in 2-year outcomes following non-fatal**

first-ever acute MI persist after adjustment for comorbidity. *Eur J Prev Cardiol* 2012, **19**(5):983–990.
5. Katzenellenbogen JM, Sanfilippo FM, Hobbs MST, Briffa TG, Knuiman MW, Dimer L, Thompson PL, Thompson SC: **Complex impact of remoteness on the incidence of myocardial infarction in Aboriginal and non-Aboriginal people in Western Australia.** *Aust J Rural Health* 2012, **20**(6):305–311.
6. Cunningham J: **Socioeconomic disparities in self-reported cardiovascular disease for Indigenous and non-Indigenous Australian adults: analysis of national survey data.** *Popul Health Metr* 2010, **8**:31.
7. Moon L, Waters A: *Socioeconomic inequalities in cardiovascular disease in Australia: current picture and trends since the 1990s. Bulletin No. 37.* Canberra: AIHW; 2006.
8. Vos T, Barker B, Begg S, Stanley L, Lopez AD: **Burden of disease and injury in Aboriginal and Torres Strait Islander Peoples: the Indigenous health gap.** *Int J Epidemiol* 2009, **38**(2):470–477.
9. Coory MD, Walsh WF: **Rates of percutaneous coronary interventions and bypass surgery after acute myocardial infarction in Indigenous patients.** *Med J Aust* 2005, **182**(10):507–512.
10. Randall DA, Jorm LR, Lujic S, O'Loughlin AJ, Eades SJ, Leyland AH: **Disparities in revascularization rates after acute myocardial infarction between aboriginal and non-aboriginal people in Australia.** *Circulation* 2013, **127**(7):811–819.
11. Cunningham J: **Diagnostic and therapeutic procedures among Australian hospital patients identified as indigenous.** *Med J Aust* 2002, **176**(2):58–62.
12. Ranasinghe I, Chew D, Aroney C, Coverdale S, Allen R, Walters D, Brieger D: **Differences in treatment and management of indigenous and non-indigenous patients presenting with chest pain: results of the Heart Protection Partnership (HPP) study.** *Heart Lung Circ* 2009, **18**(1):32–37.
13. Blokker BM, Janssen JH, Van Beeck E: **Referral patterns of patients presenting with chest pain at two rural emergency departments in Western Australia.** *Rural Remote Health* 2010, **10**(3):1558.
14. Gurwitz JH, Goldberg RJ, Malmgren JA, Barron HV, Tiefenbrunn AJ, Frederick PD, Gore JM: **Hospital transfer of patients with acute myocardial infarction: the effects of age, race, and insurance type.** *Am J Med* 2002, **112**(7):528–534.
15. Shahid S, Finn LD, Thompson SC: **Barriers to participation of Aboriginal people in cancer care: communication in the hospital setting.** *Med J Aust* 2009, **190**(10):574–579.
16. Shahid S, Finn L, Bessarab D, Thompson SC: **'Nowhere to room … nobody told them': logistical and cultural impediments to Aboriginal peoples' participation in cancer treatment.** *Aust Health Rev* 2011, **35**(2):235–241.
17. Tunstall-Pedoe H, Vanuzzo D, Hobbs M, Mahonen M, Cepaitis Z, Kuulasmaa K, Keil U, Project WM: **Estimation of contribution of changes in coronary care to improving survival, event rates, and coronary heart disease mortality across the WHO MONICA Project populations.** *Lancet* 2000, **355**(9205):688–700.
18. Rosamond WD, Chambless LE, Heiss G, Mosley TH, Coresh J, Whitsel E, Wagenknecht L, Ni H, Folsom AR: **Twenty-two-year trends in incidence of myocardial infarction, coronary heart disease mortality, and case fatality in 4 US communities, 1987–2008.** *Circulation* 2012, **125**(15):1848–1857.
19. Thygesen K, Alpert JS, Jaffe AS, Simoons ML, Chaitman BR, White HD: **Third universal definition of myocardial infarction.** *Circulation* 2012, **126**(16):2020–2035.
20. Holman CD, Bass AJ, Rouse IL, Hobbs MS: **Population-based linkage of health records in Western Australia: development of a health services research linked database.** *Aust N Z J Public Health* 1999, **23**(5):453–459.
21. Quan H, Sundararajan V, Halfon P, Fong A, Burnand B, Luthi JC, Saunders LD, Beck CA, Feasby TE, Ghali WA: **Coding algorithms for defining comorbidities in ICD-9-CM and ICD-10 administrative data.** *Med Care* 2005, **43**(11):1130–1139.
22. Australian Bureau of Statistics: *Australian Standard Geographical Classification (ASGC).* Canberra: Australian Bureau of Statistics; 2001.
23. Adhikari P: *Socio-Economic Indexes for Areas: Introduction, use and future directions.* Canberra: Australian Bureau of Statistics; 2006.
24. Briffa TG, Sanfilippo FM, Hobbs MS, Ridout SC, Katzenellenbogen JM, Thompson PL, Thompson SC: **Under-ascertainment of Aboriginality in records of cardiovascular disease in hospital morbidity and mortality data in Western Australia: a record linkage study.** *BMC Med Res Methodol* 2010, **10**:111.
25. Australian Institute of Health and Welfare: *Indigenous identification in hospital separations data-quality report. Health Services Series No. 35.* Canberra: Australian Institute of Health and Welfare; 2010.
26. Stata statistical software: *Release 12.1.* College Station, TX: StataCorp LP; 2013.
27. Zou G: **A modified poisson regression approach to prospective studies with binary data.** *Am J Epidemiol* 2004, **159**(7):702–706.
28. Roe YL, Zeitz CJ, Mittinty MN, McDermott RA, Chew DP: **Impact of age, gender and indigenous status on access to diagnostic coronary angiography for patients presenting with non-ST segment elevation acute coronary syndromes in Australia.** *Intern Med J* 2013, **43**(3):317–322.
29. Blustein J, Arons RR, Shea S: **Sequential events contributing to variations in cardiac revascularization rates.** *Med Care* 1995, **33**(8):864–880.
30. Chew DP, French J, Briffa TG, Hammett CJ, Ellis CJ, Ranasinghe I, Aliprandi-Costa BJ, Astley CM, Turnbull FM, Lefkovits J, Redfern J, Carr B, Gamble GD, Lintern KJ, Howell TE, Parker H, Tavella R, Bloomer SG, Hyun KK, Brieger DB: **Acute coronary syndrome care across Australia and New Zealand: the SNAPSHOT ACS study.** *Med J Aust* 2013, **199**(3):185–191.
31. Robertson IK, Richardson JR: **Coronary angiography and coronary artery revascularisation rates in public and private hospital patients after acute myocardial infarction.** *Med J Aust* 2000, **173**(6):291–295.
32. Trafalski S, Briffa T, Hung J, Moorin RE, Sanfilippo F, Preen DB, Einarsdottir K: **Effect of private insurance incentive policy reforms on trends in coronary revascularisation procedures in the private and public health sectors in Western Australia: a cohort study.** *BMC Health Serv Res* 2013, **13**(1):280.
33. Coory M, Scott IA, Baade P: **Differential effect of socioeconomic status on rates of invasive coronary procedures across the public and private sectors in Queensland, Australia.** *J Epidemiol Community Health* 2002, **56**(3):233–234.
34. Wiles R, Higgins J: **Doctor-patient relationships in the private sector: patients' perceptions.** *Sociol Health Ill* 1996, **18**(3):341–356.
35. Chew DP, Aroney CN, Aylward PE, Kelly AM, White HD, Tideman PA, Waddell J, Azadi L, Wilson AJ, Ruta LA: **2011 Addendum to the National Heart Foundation of Australia/Cardiac Society of Australia and New Zealand Guidelines for the management of acute coronary syndromes (ACS) 2006.** *Heart Lung Circ* 2011, **20**(8):487–502.
36. Department of Health Western Australia: *The Model of Care for Acute Coronary Syndromes in Western Australia.* Perth: Department of Health Western Australia; 2009.
37. Durey A, Thompson SC, Wood M: **Time to bring down the twin towers in poor Aboriginal hospital care: addressing institutional racism and misunderstandings in communication.** *Intern Med J* 2012, **42**(1):17–22.

2

The burden of major adverse cardiac events in patients with coronary artery disease

I-Ting Tsai[1,8], Chao-Ping Wang[2,7], Yung-Chuan Lu[3,7], Wei-Chin Hung[2], Cheng-Ching Wu[2,9], Li-Fen Lu[5], Fu-Mei Chung[2], Chia-Chang Hsu[4], Yau-Jiunn Lee[6] and Teng-Hung Yu[2*]

Abstract

Background: Patients with a history of cardiovascular disease are at high risk of developing secondary major adverse cardiac events (MACE). This study aimed to identify independent predictors of MACE after hospital admission which could be used to identify of high-risk patients who may benefit from preventive strategies.

Methods: This study included 1,520 consecutive patients with coronary artery disease (CAD) (654 with acute coronary syndrome (ACS) and 866 with elective percutaneous coronary intervention (PCI) patients) who received PCI and/or stenting. MACE was defined as all-cause mortality or rehospitalization for a cardiovascular- related illness. Cardiovascular-related illnesses included heart failure, reinfarction (nonfatal), recurrence of angina pectoris and repeat PCI or coronary artery bypass graft.

Results: During a mean follow-up period of 32 months, 558 of the 1,520 patients developed at least one MACE. Cox regression analysis showed that the baseline clinical and biochemical variables which associated with MACE were age, being illiterate, a widow or widower, and/or economically dependent, having triple vessel disease, stent implantation, anemia, and/or diabetes mellitus, waist to hip ratio (WHR), diastolic blood pressure, fasting glucose, total cholesterol, high-density lipoprotein cholesterol (HDL-C), creatinine, estimated glomerular filtration rate (eGFR), red blood cell count, hemoglobin, hematocrit, and mean corpuscular-hemoglobin concentration (MCHC) in ACS patients, and age, malnourished, and/or economically dependent, taking hypoglycemic medication, having triple vessel disease, stent implantation, anemia, diabetes mellitus, and/or hypertension, WHR, fasting glucose, HDL-C, uric acid, creatinine, eGFR, high-sensitivity C-reactive protein, mean corpuscular volume, and MCHC in elective PCI patients. Using multivariate Cox regression analysis, we found the MACE's independent factors are triple vessel disease, stent implantation, hypertension, and eGFR in ACS patients, and having triple vessel disease, stent implantation, hypertension, and uric acid in elective PCI patients.

Conclusions: Having triple vessel disease, stent implantation, hypertension, and eGFR or uric acid independently predicted MACE in patients with CAD after long-term follow-up. Fortunately, these factors are modifiable and should be identified and monitored early.

Keywords: Major adverse cardiovascular events, Predictive factors, Coronary artery disease

* Correspondence: gene6623@yahoo.com.tw; tenghungy@yahoo.com.tw
[2]Division of Cardiology, E-Da Hospital, I-Shou University, No. 1, Yi-Da Rd, Jiau-Shu Village, Yan-Chao District, Kaohsiung 82445, Taiwan
Full list of author information is available at the end of the article

Background

Coronary artery disease (CAD) is a major health problem worldwide including Taiwan, and it is expected to be the leading cause of death by 2020 [1–3]. With advances in both coronary artery bypass graft (CABG) surgery and percutaneous coronary intervention (PCI), mortality from CAD has significantly decreased [4]. Moreover, PCI or PCI with stenting and CABG were associated with a long-term safety profile and improving patient outcomes [5, 6]. However, the poor prognosis and high cost of medical care for patients with CAD impose a considerable burden on both their families and society. Therefore, identifying risk factors that affect the prognosis of patients undergoing revascularization is necessary.

Major adverse cardiac events (MACE) are important causes of morbidity and mortality in CAD patients undergoing PCI. The detection and treatment of the risk factors for MACE are critical to improve health and longevity. As expected, the traditional risk factors (e.g. age, sex, total cholesterol, low-density lipoprotein (LDL) cholesterol, high-density lipoprotein (HDL) cholesterol, systolic blood pressure, and smoking) [7] for CAD are associated with disease progression. Using Intravascular ultrasound monitoring of changes in atheroma burden in 3,473 patients, Chhatriwalla et al. demonstrated that the patients with a very low LDL level (≤70 mg/dL) and normal systolic blood pressure (SBP) (≤120 mmHg) had the slowest CAD progression [8]. In addition, in patients with LDL levels ≤70 mg/dL, progression of native coronary atherosclerotic disease was associated with the presence of residual risk factors including high baseline glucose levels, increased level of triglycerides, and small decrease in apolipoprotein B [9]. Previous study also reported that baseline diabetes was the strongest significant cardiovascular disease-related factor for disease progression [10]. Therefore, the purpose of this study was to evaluate whether baseline risk factors such as demographic and clinical characteristics, lipid levels, inflammation, triple vessel disease, stent implantation, anemia, diabetes mellitus (DM), hypertension, and chronic kidney disease (CKD) were associated with the development of MACE in patients with CAD receiving PCI. The results could be important in increasing physicians' awareness on the importance of regular baseline risk factors screening when caring for patients with CAD.

Methods

Study Subjects

In this prospective study, from June 2007 to June 2015, we studied 1,644 patients with CAD who made consecutive visits to the Taiwan I-Shout University E-Da Hospital's Emergency Room and Cardiovascular Clinic (Fig. 1). All

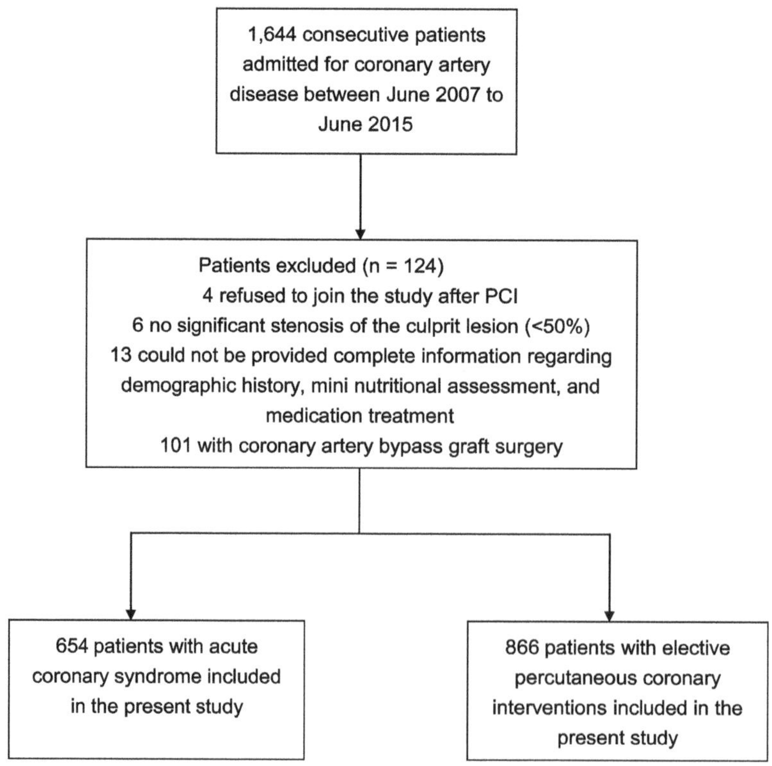

Fig. 1 Study flowchart

the demographic data, clinical information, and current medications of the patients were examined and recorded by two healthcare professionals with expertise in CAD care, via a web-based case report form in the clinical data management system of the E-Da Hospital, with special attention being paid to cardiovascular risk factors and co-morbidities. The clinical data system at the E-Da Hospital documented all the clinical consecutive variables and values when patient admitted to the Cardiovascular Clinic or Ward due to CAD or other heart diseases. Age, sex, smoking habits, hyperlipidemia, arterial hypertension, DM, CAD, history of stroke and acute myocardial infarction were evaluated. Medical history survey, physical examinations, blood test, and urinalysis were conducted. Patients presenting with stage 5 CKD, concomitant inflammatory diseases such as infection or sepsis, and other medical history of malignancy, liver disease or collagen disease, those using steroids, and those who had undergone any type of surgery in the month prior to admission or refused to participate in the study were excluded. Data were evaluated on the day of patients discharge after interobserver agreement gained. In cases of discrepancy, reevaluation by both investigators and a consensus was performed. To detect undiagnosed diabetes, fasting blood glucose concentration was determined at admission. During the hospital stay, repeat blood pressure measurements were conducted to discover undiagnosed hypertension. Written informed consent was given by each CAD patient before enrollment. If patients were unable to give consent because of disease severity, informed consent was obtained from a relative or legal representative. The study protocol and informed consent procedure were approved by the Ethics Committee of I-Shou University E-Da Hospital.

Laboratory Measurements

Plasma biochemical parameters were measured after an overnight fast. Levels of plasma triglycerides, total cholesterol, LDL-cholesterol, HDL-cholesterol, uric acid, creatinine, and glucose were determined by standard commercial methods using a parallel-multichannel analyzer (Hitachi 7170A, Tokyo, Japan), as described previously [11]. Levels of plasma C-reactive protein (CRP) were measured using a high-sensitivity method (IMMAGE; Beckman Coulter, Immunochemistry Systems, Brea, CA) with a detection limit of 0.2 mg/L. The intra-assay coefficient of variation was 4.2% to 8.7% for high-sensitivity CRP (hs-CRP). Samples were measured in duplicate in a single experiment. Estimated glomerular filtration rate (eGFR) was calculated using the CKD-EPI two-level race equation [12]. Anthropometric parameters including body mass index (BMI) and waist to hip ratio (WHR) were measured. Waist and hip circumferences were measured to the nearest 0.1 cm at the narrowest point between the lowest rib and the uppermost lateral border of the right iliac crest. Hips were measured at their widest point. Seated blood pressure was measured by a trained nurse with a digital automatic blood pressure monitor (model HEM-907; Omron, Omron, Japan) after the subjects had rested for 5 minutes.

Study End-points

The patients were followed-up after admission using a standardized protocol that included outpatient visits, telephone contact and the recording of recurrent cardiac events. The endpoints were the composite occurrence of MACE, including all-cause mortality or re-hospitalization for a cardiovascular-related illness. Cardiovascular-related illnesses included heart failure, reinfarction (nonfatal), recurrence of angina pectoris and repeat PCI or CABG [13]. The heart failure endpoint was investigated on the basis of clinical parameters suggestive of pulmonary congestion and/or signs of low cardiac output. Angina was definitions of dull diffuse substernal chest discomfort precipitated by exertion or emotion and relieved by rest or nitroglycerin. Non-fatal reinfarction was defined as angina or anginal equivalent accompanied by a new ST-segment elevation in leads consistent with those of the territory of the artery affected in the index event. Revascularization was characterized by the need for percutaneous or surgical intervention motivated by instability of the clinical picture (elective revascularization were not considered endpoints).

Follow-up

The patients were clinically reevaluated at 3, 6, and 12 months after hospital discharge and then annually until June 2015. All participants had entered a disease management program at our Cardiovascular Clinic. All of the patients received a follow-up questionnaire from a trained nurse during June 2015 to re-evaluate the occurrence of MACE during the whole follow-up period. For the patients did not respond to the questionnaire, personal telephone contact was made. In addition, all hospital discharge reports relating to any other re-admission during the follow-up period were also been reviewed. The performance of PCI and CABG was validated by reviewing the original procedure protocols. Outcomes were assessed by two research physicians with expertise in Cardiology; they have 11 years clinical experience in catheriterization procedure and were active member of the Taiwan Society of Cardiology. Two research physicians were blinded to the patients' all baseline clinical data. In case of disagreement, consensus was sought. Finally, a cardiovascular interventionist, whose judgment was considered decisive, reviewed all events. In addition, the type of objective information included medical records, radiography, reports of cardiac catheterization, EKG, and cardiac echo, and pathology that were provided the adjudicators to make their assessments according to the endpoint definitions.

Definitions

In our study, the diagnosis of CAD was confirmed by coronary angiography. Significant coronary stenosis was defined as a vessel luminal diameter decrease of greater than or equal to 70% in either one of 15 coronary segments. If PCI was considered, balloon angioplasty or stenting was performed according the vessel condition. However, for left main and severe triple vessel disease, CABG was suggested to the patients. Hypertension was defined as systolic blood pressure of ≥140 mmHg, diastolic blood pressure of ≥90 mmHg or both, or the use of anti-hypertensive drugs. Hyperlipidemia was defined as a triglyceride level ≥150 mg/dL, and/or a HDL-cholesterol level of <35 mg/dL for men and <39 mg/dL for women, and/or a total cholesterol level of ≥200 mg/dL, and/or a LDL-cholesterol level of ≥130 mg/dL, or those undergoing treatment for lipid disorders according to the ATP III criteria [14]. DM was defined as a glucose level >126 mg/dl [15], or having received treatment for DM. Malnutrition indicator score was defined as normal nutritional status 24 to 30 points, at risk of malnutrition 17 to 23.5 points, and malnourished less than 17 points using the Mini Nutritional Assessment. Patients' smoking status was classified as never having smoked, former smoker (ceased smoking for at least 1 year), or current smoker. In this study, former and current smokers were analyzed as a group and compared with those who had never smoked.

Statistical Analysis

Continuous variables were presented as mean ± SD, and categorical variables as a percentage of the total. All statistical analyses were performed using SAS software version 10.0 (SAS Institute, Cary, NC). Baseline characteristics of the patients with MACE and without MACE were compared using the Student's t test or χ^2 test. Cox regression univariate analysis was performed. The outcome was defined as the time elapsed until the development of the MACE, and all the patients were followed until they developed a MACE. Hazard ratios (HRs) with 95% confidence intervals were estimated by Cox proportional hazards model. The variables with a p value less than 0.25 in the univariate Cox regression analysis were entered into the multivariate model. The proportional hazards assumption was further verified by Schoenfeld residuals analysis and assessment of the survival function versus the survival time graph. Model discrimination was assessed by area under the receiver operating characteristic (ROC) curve (AUC) analysis, which is a measure of overall predictive discrimination. The AUC is an overall summary of diagnostic accuracy. AUC equals 0.5 when the ROC curve corresponds to random chance and 1.0 for perfect accuracy. On rare occasions, the estimated AUC is <0.5, indicating that the test does worse than chance [16]. All of the statistical analyses were two-sided, and a p value less than 0.05 was considered to be significant.

Results

Among 1,644 consecutive CAD patients, 124 were excluded due to the following reasons: four patients refused to join the study after PCI, six patients had no significant stenosis of the culprit lesion (<50%), one hundred and one with coronary artery bypass graft surgery, and 13 patients could not be provided complete information regarding demographic history, mini nutritional assessment, and medication treatment. The final study population included 1,520 patients (654 with ACS and 866 with elective PCI patients; Fig. 1). Of the 1,520 patients, 1,107 (72.8%) men and 413 (27.2%) women, mean age of patients is 69 ± 12 years (range, 30 to 99 years). 582 (38.3%) had DM, 949 (62.4%) had hyperlipidemia, and 1,092 (71.8%) had hypertension (Tables 1 and 2).

Baseline Characteristics

All patients received clinical follow-up with a median duration of 23 months (interquartile range: 5–55 months). During the follow-up period, the incidence of MACE was 36.7% (558 of 1,520 patients). The baseline clinical characteristics and data for all of the patients are presented in Table 1. The patients who developed a MACE had higher rates of illiteracy, at risk of malnutrition, malnourished, being economically dependent, taking statins and hypoglycemic medications, and/or having triple vessel disease, stent implantation, anemia, DM, hypertension, and cause of admission for ACS than the patients without a MACE. In addition, the patients who developed a MACE were older and had a higher waist circumference, WHR, HbA1C, fasting glucose, creatinine, uric acid, hs-CRP, white blood cell count, lower diastolic blood pressure, HDL-cholesterol, eGFR, red blood cell count, hemoglobin, hematocrit, mean corpuscular-hemoglobin concentration (MCHC), and malnutrition indicator score than the patients without a MACE (Table 2). Additionally, there was no statistically significant difference in rate of MACE among 4 operators (37.7% vs. 34.1% vs. vs. 39.7% vs. 42.7%, $p = 0.105$).

Association of the Baseline Clinical and Biochemical Risk Factors for the Development of MACE

After univariate Cox regression analysis, the baseline clinical and biochemical variables associated with MACE were age, being illiterate, a widow or widower, economically dependent, having triple vessel disease, stent implantation, anemia, and DM, WHR, diastolic blood pressure, fasting

Table 1 Baseline characteristics and clinical data of the study participants with and without major adverse cardiovascular events

Variable	Total *n* (%)	With MACE *n* (%)	Without MACE *n* (%)	*P* value
No	1520	558 (36.7)	962 (63.3)	
Gender				
Women	413 (27.2)	140 (25.1)	273 (28.4)	0.165
Men	1107 (72.8)	418 (74.9)	689 (71.6)	0.165
Education				
Illiterate	256 (16.8)	120 (21.5)	136 (14.1)	0.002
Elementary school	586 (38.6)	228 (40.9)	358 (37.2)	0.240
Junior high school	225 (14.8)	77 (13.8)	148 (15.4)	0.497
High school	336 (22.1)	96 (17.2)	240 (24.9)	0.003
College	119 (7.8)	38 (6.8)	81 (8.4)	0.315
Marital status				
Single	54 (3.6)	18 (3.2)	36 (3.7)	0.695
Married	1222 (80.4)	442 (79.2)	780 (81.1)	0.405
Divorced	54 (3.6)	18 (3.2)	36 (3.7)	0.695
Widow or widower	187 (12.3)	80 (14.3)	107 (11.1)	0.121
Mini nutritional assessment				
Normal nutritional status	1082 (71.2)	326 (58.4)	756 (78.6)	0.001
At risk of malnutrition	376 (24.7)	184 (33.0)	192 (20.0)	0.025
Malnourished	61 (4.0)	48 (8.6)	13 (1.4)	0.009
Economic situation, dependent	766 (50.4)	336 (60.2)	430 (44.7)	<0.0001
Smoking	722 (47.5)	267 (47.9)	455 (47.3)	0.809
Drinking	463 (30.5)	164 (29.4)	299 (31.1)	0.503
Regular exercise	617 (40.6)	219 (39.3)	398 (41.4)	0.488
Antihypertensive medication	824 (54.2)	312 (55.9)	512 (53.2)	0.310
Statin	487 (32.0)	201 (36.0)	286 (29.7)	0.011
Hypoglycemic medication	223 (14.7)	108 (19.4)	115 (12.0)	<0.0001
Triple vessel disease	435 (28.6)	228 (40.9)	207 (21.5)	<0.0001
Stents placed	444 (29.2)	198 (35.5)	246 (25.6)	<0.0001
Anemia	356 (23.4)	155 (27.8)	201 (20.9)	0.003
Diabetes mellitus	582 (38.3)	260 (46.6)	322 (33.5)	<0.0001
Hypertension	1092 (71.8)	435 (78.0)	657 (68.3)	<0.0001
Hyperlipidemia	949 (62.4)	364 (65.2)	585 (60.8)	0.088
Cause of admission				
Acute coronary syndrome	654 (43.0)	311 (55.7)	343 (35.7)	<0.0001
Elective PCI	866 (57.0)	247 (44.3)	619 (64.4)	<0.0001

MACE major adverse cardiovascular events; *PCI* percutaneous coronary intervention

glucose, total cholesterol, HDL-cholesterol, creatinine, eGFR, red blood cell count, hemoglobin, hematocrit, and MCHC in ACS patients, and age, malnourished, economically dependent, taking hypoglycemic medication, having triple vessel disease, stent implantation, anemia, DM, and hypertension, WHR, fasting glucose, HDL-C, uric acid, creatinine, eGFR, high-sensitivity C-reactive protein, mean corpuscular volume, and MCHC in elective PCI patients. Using multivariate Cox regression analysis, we found the independent factors associated with the development of MACE were triple vessel disease [HR 3.66 (1.38–9.97)], stent implantation [HR 3.61 (1.47–9.05)], hypertension [HR1.73 (1.06–2.21)], and eGFR [HR 0.99 (0.98–1.00)] in ACS patients, and having triple vessel disease [HR 3.12 (1.43–6.82)], stent implantation [HR 4.10 (2.09–8.13)], hypertension [HR

Table 2 Baseline characteristics and biochemical data of the study participants with and without major adverse cardiovascular events

Variable	Total	With MACE	Without MACE	*P*-value
No	1520	558	962	
Age (years)	68.9 ± 12.0	71.9 ± 11.7	67.2 ± 11.9	<0.0001
Body mass index (kg/m^2)	25.7 ± 10.6	25.2 ± 4.4	26.0 ± 12.9	0.186
Waist circumference (cm)	91.0 ± 10.4	91.9 ± 10.5	90.4 ± 10.2	0.021
Waist to hip ratio	0.94 ± 0.11	0.95 ± 0.14	0.93 ± 0.08	<0.0001
Systolic BP (mmHg)	133 ± 22	133 ± 24	132 ± 21	0.298
Diastolic BP (mmHg)	77 ± 14	75 ± 14	77 ± 13	0.008
HbA1C (%)	7.0 ± 1.8	7.1 ± 1.9	6.9 ± 1.7	0.012
Fasting glucose (mg/dl)	144.9 ± 77.0	159.5 ± 88.7	136.4 ± 68.0	<0.0001
Total cholesterol (mg/dl)	177.1 ± 45.5	174.9 ± 45.3	178.4 ± 45.5	0.156
Triglycerides (mg/dl)	143.8 ± 105.2	138.1 ± 93.3	147.0 ± 111.2	0.116
HDL-cholesterol (mg/dl)	40.2 ± 12.0	38.6 ± 11.9	41.0 ± 12.0	0.0002
LDL-cholesterol (mg/dl)	103.7 ± 35.4	104.4 ± 37.1	103.2 ± 34.3	0.518
Creatinine (mg/dl)	1.74 ± 1.83	2.0 ± 2.3	1.6 ± 1.5	<0.0001
Uric acid (mg/dl)	6.8 ± 2.7	7.0 ± 2.1	6.6 ± 3.0	0.017
eGFR (ml/min/1.73 m^2)	57.2 ± 23.1	51.4 ± 23.0	60.5 ± 22.6	<0.0001
Hs-CRP (mg/L)	12.2 ± 32.4	14.0 ± 36.8	11.0 ± 29.1	0.001
White blood cell (10^9/l)	8.469 ± 3.877	8.795 ± 3.699	8.279 ± 3.967	0.012
Red blood cell (10 ^{6}/μl)	4.54 ± 1.21	4.46 ± 0.94	4.58 ± 1.34	0.030
Hemoglobin (g/dl)	13.2 ± 2.3	13.1 ± 2.6	13.3 ± 2.1	0.033
Hematocrit (%)	39.5 ± 6.1	39.1 ± 6.3	39.8 ± 5.9	0.039
Mean corpuscular volume (fL)	88.4 ± 7.7	88.6 ± 7.9	88.2 ± 7.6	0.320
MCH (pg/cell)	29.8 ± 7.4	29.6 ± 3.0	30.0 ± 9.1	0.323
MCHC (g/dL)	33.4 ± 1.3	33.3 ± 1.4	33.5 ± 1.2	<0.0001
Malnutrition indicator score	24.7 ± 3.5	23.9 ± 3.6	25.1 ± 3.3	0.010

Data are means ± SD. *MACE* major adverse cardiovascular events, *HDL-C* high-density lipoprotein cholesterol *LDL-C* low-density lipoprotein cholesterol, *Hs-Crp* high-sensitivity C-reactive protein, *MCH* mean corpuscular hemoglobin, *MCHC* mean corpuscular-hemoglobin concentration, *eGFR* = estimated glomerular filtration rate calculated by the chronic kidney disease-EPI two-level race equation [12]

1.07 (1.02–2.37)], and uric acid [HR 1.14 (1.01–1.28)] in elective PCI patients (Tables 3 and 4).

AUC analysis

We then evaluated the ability of triple vessel disease, stent implantation, hypertension, and eGFR or uric acid to predict the risk of MACE. In ACS patients, the AUC for triple vessel disease was 0.574 ($p < 0.0001$). When stent implantation, hypertension, and eGFR were added to this multivariate model, the AUC increased to 0.606 ($p = 0.0004$) for triple vessel disease and stent implantation, 0.615 for triple vessel disease, stent implantation, and hypertension, 0.655 ($p = 0.004$) for triple vessel disease, stent implantation, hypertension, and eGFR (Fig. 2a). In elective PCI patients, the AUC for triple vessel disease was 0.610 ($p < 0.0001$). When stent implantation, hypertension, and uric acid were added to this multivariate model, the AUC increased to 0.627 ($p = 0.045$) for triple vessel disease and stent implantation, 0.644 for triple vessel disease, stent implantation, and hypertension, 0.678 ($p = 0.001$) for triple vessel disease, stent implantation, hypertension, and uric acid (Fig. 2b).

Basic characteristics and biochemical data of the study participants with and without stent implantation

In the present study, we found that stent implantation was associated with the development of MACE. Hence, we further subgrouped our study subjects according to their stent implantation status to examine what reason the stent implantation was associated with MACE. Table 5 lists the basic characteristics and biochemical data of the study participants with and without stent implantation. Patients with stent implantation were younger and had higher frequencies of male gender, triple vessel disease, and hyperlipidemia; higher BMI, HbA1C, total cholesterol, LDL-cholesterol, hs-CRP, and white

Table 3 Cox proportional hazard model of baseline clinical risk factors for the development of major adverse cardiovascular events stratified by acute coronary syndrome and elective PCI subjects

	Acute coronary syndrome				Elective PCI			
Baseline data	Univariate analysis HR (95% CI)	*P* value	Multivariate model HR (95% CI)	*P* value	Univariate analysis HR (95% CI)	*P* value	Multivariate model HR (95% CI)	*P* value
Age	1.02 (1.02–1.03)	<0.0001			1.03 (1.01–1.04)	<0.0001		
Gender	1.10 (0.85–1.45)	0.486			1.15 (0.88–1.54)	0.317		
Education (illiterate)	1.63 (1.19–2.18)	0.002			1.25 (0.85–1.79)	0.257		
Marital status (widow or widower)	1.44 (1.02–1.98)	0.040			0.90 (0.55–1.40)	0.662		
Malnourished	2.87 (0.86–7.21)	0.082			4.00 (1.20–9.91)	0.027		
Economic situation (dependent)	1.52 (1.18–1.97)	0.001			1.81 (1.34–2.45)	0.0001		
Smoking	1.11 (0.89–1.39)	0.369			0.98 (0.76–1.26)	0.857		
Drinking	0.90 (0.68–1.17)	0.414			0.97 (0.71–1.31)	0.849		
Regular exercise	0.85 (0.65–1.11)	0.236			0.79 (0.57–1.07)	0.127		
Antihypertensive medication	0.98 (0.78–1.24)	0.885			0.95 (0.73–1.22)	0.661		
Statins	0.87 (0.69–1.09)	0.222			0.98 (0.74–1.29)	0.909		
Hypoglycemic medication	1.17 (0.89–1.53)	0.262			1.43 (1.01–1.98)	0.042		
Triple vessel disease	1.67 (1.33–2.10)	<0.0001	3.66 (1.38–9.97)	0.009	2.27 (1.75–2.93)	<0.0001	3.12 (1.43–6.82)	0.005
Stent implantation	1.50 (1.18–1.90)	0.001	3.61 (1.47–9.05)	0.005	1.47 (1.12–1.91)	0.005	4.10 (2.09–8.13)	0.0001
Anemia	1.42 (1.10–1.81)	0.007			1.47 (1.09–1.95)	0.011		
Diabetes mellitus	1.78 (1.42–2.23)	<0.0001			1.35 (1.04–1.74)	0.024		
Hypertension	1.27 (0.97–1.67)	0.079	1.73 (1.06–2.21)	0.020	1.50 (1.11–2.07)	0.008	1.07 (1.02–2.37)	0.014
Hyperlipidemia	0.99 (0.78-1.28)	0.960			1.03 (0.79-1.34)	0.839		

HR Hazard ratio, *PCI* percutaneous coronary intervention

blood cell count; and lower frequencies of being a widow or widower than those without stent implantation patients.

Discussion

The goal of this study was to determine the predictors of MACE in Chinese patients with CAD who underwent PCI and/or stenting. Of the 1,520 consecutive patients evaluated, the incidence of MACE was 36.7% after a median duration of 23 months (interquartile range: 5–55 months) of follow-up. Triple vessel disease, stent implantation, hypertension, and eGFR or uric acid all contributed to the risk of a MACE between ACS and elective PCI patients. To the best of our knowledge, this study is the first observational clinical study to identify the independent risk factors for adverse cardiac events in a Chinese cohort of patients, who have distinct differences in presentation from those in western countries [17].

In addition to the most common predictors of MACE in CAD patients such as age [18], female gender [19], hypertension, number of stents placed [19–21], chronic heart failure [20], eGFR [22, 23], anemia [24], HDL-cholesterol [25], and hs-CRP [26], the development of MACE in our population was further determined by triple vessel disease, stent implantation, hypertension, and eGFR or uric acid. Furthermore, we found that triple vessel disease, stent implantation, hypertension, and eGFR predicted the development of MACE in multivariate analysis, with an AUC of 0.655 in ACS patients, and triple vessel disease, stent implantation, hypertension, and uric acid predicted the development of MACE in multivariate analysis, with an AUC of 0.678 in elective PCI patients. In addition, consistent with several previous reports [19, 20] but in contrast to others [26–28], in the present study, DM did not predict the development of a MACE in our patients. Previous studies investigating the impact of DM on clinical outcomes yielded inconsistent results, which likely reflect differences in clinical diagnosis [29–31].

In the current study the levels of eGFR at baseline were inversely associated with the development of MACE in ACS patients, so a low eGFR may have higher risk of MACE, which is consistent with other studies where a lower eGFR was associated with the risk of death, cardiovascular events, and hospitalization [32, 33]. The mechanisms that underlie the association between renal dysfunction and CAD have not been elucidated fully. Previous studies have shown that renal dysfunction is associated with low-grade inflammation

Table 4 Cox proportional hazard model of baseline biochemical risk factors for the development of major adverse cardiovascular events stratified by acute coronary syndrome and elective PCI subjects

	Acute coronary syndrome				Elective PCI			
Baseline data	Univariate analysis HR (95% CI)	*P* value	Multivariate model HR (95% CI)	*P*-value	Univariate analysis HR (95% CI)	*P* value	Multivariate model HR (95% CI)	*P* value
Body mass index	0.98 (0.95–1.01)	0.135			0.99 (0.97–1.03)	0.942		
Waist circumference	1.01 (0.99–1.02)	0.131			1.01 (0.99–1.02)	0.172		
Waist to hip ratio	3.45 (1.30–7.40)	0.016			3.56 (1.29–7.03)	0.019		
Systolic BP	0.99 (0.99–1.00)	0.701			1.01 (0.99–1.01)	0.146		
Diastolic BP	0.24 (0.07–0.90)	0.034			0.15 (0.02–0.97)	0.046		
HbA1C	1.06 (0.99–1.11)	0.063			1.06 (0.99–1.16)	0.192		
Fasting glucose	3.98 (2.24–6.98)	<0.0001			3.82 (1.85–7.66)	0.0004		
Total cholesterol	0.43 (0.24–0.91)	0.030			1.04 (0.30–3.61)	0.946		
Triglyceride	0.99 (0.99–1.00)	0.121			0.99 (0.99–1.00)	0.154		
HDL-cholesterol	0.29 (0.11–0.77)	0.014			0.30 (0.11–0.83)	0.021		
LDL-cholesterol	1.00 (0.99–1.00)	0.447			1.00 (0.99–1.01)	0.221		
Uric acid	1.00 (0.96–1.03)	0.981			1.17 (1.09–1.26)	<0.0001	1.14 (1.01–1.28)	0.041
Creatinine	1.10 (1.03–1.16)	0.005			1.09 (1.05–1.13)	0.0004		
eGFR	0.46 (0.32–0.66)	0.0001	0.20 (0.05–0.86)	0.031	0.32 (0.23–0.48)	<0.0001		
Hs-CRP	1.00 (0.99–1.01)	0.713			1.01 (1.00–1.01)	0.013		
White blood cell	1.02 (0.99–1.05)	0.148			1.01 (0.97–1.05)	0.653		
Red blood cell	0.84 (0.73–0.97)	0.017			0.88 (0.73–1.04)	0.158		
Hemoglobin	0.93 (0.89–0.98)	0.004			0.95 (0.89–1.02)	0.143		
Hematocrit	0.98 (0.96–0.99)	0.003			0.98 (0.95–1.00)	0.073		
MCV	1.00 (0.98–1.01)	0.656			1.02 (1.00–1.04)	0.047		
MCH	0.97 (0.94–1.01)	0.099			1.00 (0.97–1.01)	0.687		
MCHC	0.91 (0.84–0.99)	0.029			0.89 (0.81–0.98)	0.016		

PCI, percutaneous coronary intervention; HR, hazard ratio; HDL-C, high-density lipoprotein cholesterol; LDL-C, low-density lipoprotein cholesterol; MCV, mean corpuscular volume; MCH, mean corpuscular hemoglobin; MCHC, mean corpuscular-hemoglobin concentration. eGFR = estimated glomerular filtration rate calculated by the chronic kidney disease-EPI two-level race equation [12]

and activation of the sympathetic nervous system or the rennin-angiotensinaldosterone system [34–36]. Foley et al. demonstrated that calcium-phosphate production and oxidative stress were shown to promote renal dysfunction [37]. Muntner et al. showed that apolipoprotein A1 levels are decreased and levels of homocysteine, lipoprotein (a), fibrinogen, and CRP are increased among patients with CKD [38]. These factors above could also contribute to the pathogenesis of atherosclerosis. Herzog and colleagues also described pressure overload, volume overload, and CKD associated non-hemodynamic factors that have enhanced CKD to alter the myocardium [39]. Renal insufficiency is an independent risk factor for cardiovascular outcomes and in-hospital and late mortality [40, 41]. Increased uremic toxins such as total indoxyl sulfate and *p*-cresylsulphate may be involved in the pathogenesis of coronary atherosclerosis, prolonged QTc interval, left ventricular systolic dysfunction, and elevated risk of MACE in CAD patients with low estimated glomerular filtration rate, and it is considered a coronary heart disease risk equivalent [42–46]. In addition, we found that uric acid was an independent risk factor for developing a MACE in elective PCI patients. Previous clinical investigations have demonstrated that hyperuricemia is an independent predictor of mortality in patients with cardiovascular disease [47–49]. Uric acid is the final oxidation product of purine catabolism in humans. It is formed from the breakdown of adenosine and guanine. When the purine breakdown products xanthine and hypoxanthine are converted to uric acid through the enzymatic action of xanthine oxidase, molecular oxygen is reduced and the free radical superoxide is generated. Oxygen-free radicals are postulated to play a key role in vascular injury in cardiovascular and kidney disease. George et al. suggested that uric acid was harm to endothelial function leading to cause of cardiovascular disease because uric acid levels may act as a marker of xanthine oxidase activity [50]. Previous studies have also shown that uric acid has directly contributed proliferative,

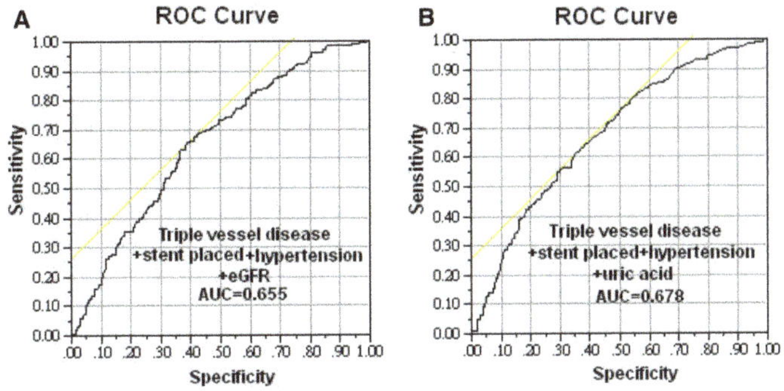

Parameter	AUC	Odds ratio (95%CI)	p-value
Triple vessel disease	0.574	1.98(1.42-2.76)	<0.0001
Triple vessel disease +stent implantation	0.606	1.89(1.33-2.70)	0.0004
Triple vessel disease +stent implantation +hypertension	0.615	1.32(0.92-1.89)	0.135
Triple vessel disease +stent implantation +hypertension +eGFR	0.655	1.63(1.17-2.29)	0.004

Parameter	AUC	Odds ratio (95%CI)	p-value
Triple vessel disease	0.610	2.94(2.13-4.07)	<0.0001
Triple vessel disease +stent implantation	0.627	1.21(1.07-1.68)	0.045
Triple vessel disease +stent implantation +hypertension	0.644	1.76(1.23-2.55)	0.002
Triple vessel disease +stent implantation +hypertension +uric acid	0.678	4.87(1.87-12.65)	0.001

Fig. 2 Comparison of the receiver operating characteristic (ROC) curves with area under the curves (AUC) for the risk of major adverse cardiac events (MACE) of acute coronary syndrome subjects with four factors (triple vessel disease, stent implantation, hypertension, and estimated glomerular filtration rate (eGFR)). The AUC using triple vessel disease was calculated first, then stent implantation was added to this model, and then hypertension and eGFR (**a**). In addition, comparison of the ROC curves with area under the curves (AUC) for the risk of MACE of elective percutaneous coronary interventions subjects with four factors (triple vessel disease, stent implantation, hypertension, and uric acid). The AUC using triple vessel disease was calculated first, then stent implantation was added to this model, and then hypertension and uric acid (**b**)

proinflammatory, and proatherogenic effects on human vascular smooth muscle cells and endothelial cells through upregulate CRP, an active component in the inflammatory process, which can lead to both hypertension and vascular disease [51–53]. Taken together, these findings highlight the clinical and public health importance of chronic renal insufficiency and hyperuricemia.

In this study, we found that hypertension was an independent risk factor for developing a MACE not only in ACS patients but also in elective PCI patients. This is consistent with reports in which a history of hypertension was one of the risk factors for a MACE [21, 54]. Madan et al. enrolled 9,494 patients and found that hypertension was an independent predictor of adverse cardiac events after PCI [20]. In the other hand, chronic hypertension is also one of the important cardiovascular risk factors for development of atherosclerosis [55] and an increased incidence of CAD [56], CKD [57], peripheral vascular disease [58], and cerebrovascular disease [59]. Moreover, hypertension is also known as an important risk factor for myocardial infarction, stroke, heart failure, and cardiovascular death [60, 61]. The relation between hypertension and myocardial infarction could be explained underscoring two key factors: (1) common risk factors, such as sympathetic hyperactivity, insulin resistance, vasoactive substances (i.e., angiotensin II), and genetic risk profiles and (2) hypertension is a risk factor of atherosclerosis, which contributes to progression of myocardial infarction [62]. Genetic risk factors such as gene polymorphisms of the angiotensinogen-converting enzyme and of the renin-angiotensin-aldosterone system, could cause myocardial infarction, hypertension, and cardiovascular complications [63, 64]. Furthermore, in hypertensive patients, a hyperactivity of sympathetic tone which causes sympathetic vasoconstriction on glucose extraction in skeletal muscle, beta-adrenergic receptor-mediated insulin resistance, and vascular rarefaction; may contribute atherosclerosis by worsening insulin resistance. Previous study suggested that sympathetic hyperactivity itself also contributes higher risk of coronary spasm, coronary thrombosis, and sudden death [65].

Besides the classical risk factors, others risk factors may also influence the development of MACE [20]. In the present study, we also found that triple vessel disease and stent implantation were associated with the development of MACE. Studies by Chow et al. and de Waha et al. both reported that the severity of CAD and multivessel CAD not only predicted all-cause mortality but also were high-risk factors for adverse clinical outcomes [66, 67]. The higher morbidity and mortality are seen in ST-segment elevation myocardial infarction patients with multi-vessel CAD. The mechanism is multifactorial, including total ischemic burden, the presence of diffuse atherosclerosis as a harbinger of plaque instability, and

Table 5 Baseline characteristics and biochemical data of the study participants with and without stent implantation

Variable	With stent implantation	Without stent implantation	*P*-value
No	458	1062	
Age (years)	67.2 ± 11.1	69.5 ± 12.3	0.001
Gender (male)	352(76.9)	751(70.7)	0.004
Education (illiterate)	62(13.5)	194(18.3)	0.053
Marital status (widow or widower)	41(9.0)	145(13.7)	0.028
Malnourished	11(2.4)	49(4.6)	0.406
Economic situation (dependent)	215(46.9)	552(52.0)	0.128
Smoking	235(51.3)	490(46.1)	0.077
Triple vessel disease	174(38.0)	254(23.9)	<0.0001
Anemia	103(22.5)	249(23.5)	0.661
Diabetes mellitus	188(41.1)	396(37.3)	0.168
Hypertension	341(74.5)	750(70.6)	0.137
Hyperlipidemia	335(73.1)	613(57.7)	<0.0001
Body mass index (kg/m^2)	26.7 ± 18.5	25.3 ± 4.4	0.017
Systolic BP (mmHg)	133 ± 21	132 ± 22	0.864
Diastolic BP (mmHg)	77 ± 13	76 ± 14	0.242
HbA1C (%)	7.1 ± 1.7	6.9 ± 1.8	0.048
Fasting glucose (mg/dl)	146.0 ± 75.5	144.3 ± 77.6	0.700
Total cholesterol (mg/dl)	180.7 ± 46.6	175.4 ± 44.7	0.039
Triglycerides (mg/dl)	148.6 ± 108.1	141.3 ± 103.0	0.220
HDL-cholesterol (mg/dl)	39.4 ± 12.7	40.5 ± 11.8	0.110
LDL-cholesterol (mg/dl)	106.7 ± 37.8	102.1 ± 34.0	0.023
Creatinine (mg/dl)	1.9 ± 2.4	1.7 ± 1.5	0.090
Uric acid (mg/dl)	6.9 ± 3.7	6.8 ± 2.2	0.622
eGFR (ml/min/1.73 m^2)	57.8 ± 22.7	57.3 ± 23.2	0.686
Hs-CRP (mg/L)	13.6 ± 35.5	9.0 ± 24.2	0.044
White blood cell (10^9/l)	8.652 ± 4.151	8.010 ± 3.128	0.004
Red blood cell (10 ^{6}/μl)	4.54 ± 0.85	4.54 ± 1.33	0.952
Hemoglobin (g/dl)	13.3 ± 2.1	13.2 ± 2.3	0.482
Hematocrit (%)	39.7 ± 5.6	39.5 ± 6.2	0.720

Data are means ± SD or number (%). *HDL-C* high-density lipoprotein cholesterol, *LDL-C* low-density lipoprotein cholesterol; *Hs-CRP* high-sensitivity C-reactive protein. eGFR = estimated glomerular filtration rate calculated by the chronic kidney disease-EPI two-level race equation [12]

impaired contractility of non-infarct zones in the presence of multiple obstructive stenosis [68]. Interestingly, in our study, the stent implantation was found to be a surrogate marker of MACE. When we further subgrouped our study subjects according to their stent implantation status, the results found that patients with stent implantation had higher rates of triple vessel disease and hyperlipidemia; higher BMI, HbA1C, total cholesterol, LDL-cholesterol, hs-CRP, and white blood cell count than those without stent implantation patients. Hyperlipidemia and obesity are recognized as a risk factor for CAD and coronary mortality [69, 70]. Furthermore, several reports have suggested that delayed arterial healing and vessel remodeling due to chronic inflammation have been reported as reasons for the high rates of very late stent thrombosis with drug-eluting stent [71–75]. Previously, studies have indicated that this reduction in restenosis might have been obtained at the expense of a higher incidence of stent thrombosis that links stent implantation and adverse cardiac events such as recurrent myocardial infarction or death [76, 77]. Hence, we think multifactorial occurrence, including triple vessel disease, hyperlipidemia, higher BMI, HbA1C, and inflammation response that promote the association of stent implantation with the MACE in our study [66, 67, 69, 70, 75, 78]. In addition, there was no statistically significant difference in rate of MACE among 4 operators in the present study. This indicated that operators issue did not affect the finding of stent implantation association with MACE.

There are several limitations to this study. First, the results may be skewed by procedural preferences and the patients seen at our institution. Second, we did not assess several complications that are common after PCI such as contrast nephropathy and access-site vascular complications. Third, we did not examine the relationship between operator procedure volume and cardiac complications. Four, this is an observational study in only one centre. Hence, further work is required to confirm these findings in populations of different races and these exploratory results should be confirmed in a larger study and other centre. Finally, although the current model has been validated for the contemporary practice of PCI, further advances in PCI techniques and technology may reduce the discriminatory ability and predictive accuracy of the model. Thus, the model may need to be recalibrated in the future.

Conclusion

The present study indicates that having triple vessel disease, stent implantation, hypertension, and eGFR or uric acid levels independently predicted the development of MACE in patients with CAD after long-term follow-up. We suggest that uric acid, eGFR, and blood pressure should be closely monitored in patients with CAD.

Abbreviations

ACS: acute coronary syndrome; AUC: area under the curves; BMI: body mass index.; CABG: coronary artery bypass graft; CAD: Coronary artery disease; CKD: Chronic kidney disease; eGFR: Estimated glomerular filtration rate; HbA1c: Hemoglobin A1c; HDL: High-density lipoprotein; HF: Heart failure; CRP: C-reactive protein; HR: Hazard ratio; LDL: Low-density lipoprotein; MACE: Major adverse cardiac events; MCHC: Mean corpuscular-hemoglobin concentration; MI: Myocardial infarction; PCI: Percutaneous coronary intervention; RBC: Red blood cell; ROC: Receiver operating characteristic; WBC: White blood cell; WHR: Waist to hip ratio

Acknowledgments

We are grateful to the staff and members of the heart care teams for their assistance with various measurements and other organizational aspects of this study.

Funding

This work was supported by grants from the E-Da Hospital of the Republic of China, Taiwan (contract no. EDAHP-104064).

Authors' contributions

Of the 10 authors, I-TT is the first author who conceived and designed the study and interpreted the data. Y-CL, C-CH, C-PW, W-CH, and Y-JL contributed to drafting of the manuscript or revising it critically for important intellectual content. L-FL and C-CW acquired data, drafted the manuscript and designed the study. Dr. F-MC participated in the design of the study and performed the statistical analysis. Dr. T-HY is the corresponding author and contributed to the final approval of the manuscript as submitted. All authors read and approved the final version of the manuscript.

Competing interests

The authors declare that they have no competing interests.

Author details

[1]Department of Emergency, E-Da Hospital, I-Shou University, Kaohsiung 82445, Taiwan. [2]Division of Cardiology, E-Da Hospital, I-Shou University, No. 1, Yi-Da Rd, Jiau-Shu Village, Yan-Chao District, Kaohsiung 82445, Taiwan. [3]Division of Endocrinology and Metabolism, E-Da Hospital, I-Shou University, Kaohsiung 82445, Taiwan. [4]Division of Gastroenterology and Hepatology, Department of Internal Medicine, E-Da Hospital, I-Shou University, Kaohsiung 82445, Taiwan. [5]Division of Cardiac Surgery, Department of Surgery, E-Da Hospital, I-Shou University, Kaohsiung 82445, Taiwan. [6]Lee's Endocrinology Clinic, Pingtung 90000, Taiwan. [7]School of Medicine for International Students, E-Da Hospital, I-Shou University, Kaohsiung 82445, Taiwan. [8]Department of Nursing, I-Shou University, Kaohsiung 82445, Taiwan. [9]Department of Biomedical Engineering, National Cheng Kung University, Tainan 70101, Taiwan.

References

1. Directorate-general of budget, accounting and statistics Executive Yuan, Republic of China Statistical Yearbook of the Republic of China. Health. 2010;114:109–116.
2. Chen CL, Chen L, Yang WC. The influences of Taiwan's generic grouping price policy on drug prices and expenditures: Evidence from analysing the consumption of the three most-used classes of cardiovascular drugs. BMC Public Health. 2008;8:118.
3. Murray CJ, Lopez AD. Alternative projections of mortality and disability by cause 1990–2020: Global burden of disease study. Lancet. 1997;349:1498–504.
4. Deb S, Wijeysundera HC, Ko DT, Tsubota H, Hill S, Fremes SE. Coronary artery bypass graft surgery vs percutaneous interventions in coronary revascularization: a systematic review. JAMA. 2013;310:2086–95.
5. Schömig A, Mehilli J, de Waha A, Seyfarth M, Pache J, Kastrati A. A meta-analysis of 17 randomized trials of a percutaneous coronary intervention-based strategy in patients with stable coronary artery disease. J Am Coll Cardiol. 2008;52:894–904.
6. Daemen J, Boersma E, Flather M, Booth J, Stables R, Rodriguez A, et al. Long- term safety and efficacy of percutaneous coronary intervention with stenting and coronary artery bypass surgery for multivessel coronary artery disease: a meta-analysis with 5-year patient-level data from the ARTS, ERACI-II, MASS-II, and SoS trials. Circulation. 2008;118:1146–54.
7. Yusuf S, Hawken S, Ounpuu S, Dans T, Avezum A, Lanas F, et al. INTERHEART Study Investigators. Effect of potentially modifiable risk factors associated with myocardial infarction in 52 countries (the INTERHEART study): case–control study. Lancet. 2004;364:937–52.
8. Chhatriwalla AK, Nicholls SJ, Wang TH, Wolski K, Sipahi I, Crowe T, et al. Low levels of low-density lipoprotein cholesterol and blood pressure and progression of coronary atherosclerosis. J Am Coll Cardiol. 2009;53:1110–5.
9. Bayturan O, Kapadia S, Nicholls SJ, Tuzcu EM, Shao M, Uno K, et al. Clinical predictors of plaque progression despite very low levels of low-density lipoprotein cholesterol. J Am Coll Cardiol. 2010;55:2736–42.
10. Schoenenberger AW, Jamshidi P, Kobza R, Zuber M, Stuck AE, Pfisterer M, et al. Progression of coronary artery disease during long-term follow-up of the Swiss Interventional Study on Silent Ischemia Type II (SWISSI II). Clin Cardiol. 2010;33:289–95.
11. Hung WC, Yu TH, Hsu CC, Lu LF, Chung FM, Tsai IT, et al. Plasma visfatin levels are associated with major adverse cardiovascular events in patients with acute ST-elevation myocardial infarction. Clin Invest Med. 2015;38: E100–9.
12. Kong X, Ma Y, Chen J, Luo Q, Yu X, Li Y, et al. Chinese eGFR Investigation Collaboration. Evaluation of the Chronic Kidney Disease Epidemiology Collaboration equation for estimating glomerular filtration rate in the Chinese population. Nephrol Dial Transplant. 2013;28:641–51.

13. Califf RM, Bengtson JR. Cardiogenic shock. N Engl J Med. 1994;330:1724–30.
14. Expert Panel on Detection, Evaluation, and Treatment of High Blood Cholesterol in Adults. Executive summary of the third report of the National Cholesterol Education Program (NCEP) Expert Panel on Detection, Evaluation, And Treatment of High Blood Cholesterol In Adults (Adult Treatment Panel III). JAMA. 2001;285:2486–97.
15. American Diabetes Association. Diagnosis and classification of diabetes mellitus. Diabetes Care. 2012;35 Suppl 1:S64–71.
16. Hanley JA, McNeil BJ. The meaning and use of the area under a receiver operating characteristic (ROC) curve. Radiology. 1982;143:29–36.
17. Brieger DB, Chew DP, Redfern J, Ellis C, Briffa TG, Howell TE, et al. Survival after an acute coronary syndrome: 18-month outcomes from the Australian and New Zealand SNAPSHOT ACS study. Med J Aust. 2015;203:368.
18. Bae MH, Lee JH, Yang DH, Park HS, Cho Y, Chae SC. Usefulness of surgical parameters as predictors of postoperative cardiac events in patients undergoing non-cardiac surgery. Circ J. 2014;78:718–23.
19. Xu L, Yu C, Jiang J, Zheng H, Yao S, Pei L, et al. Major adverse cardiac events in elderly patients with coronary artery disease undergoing noncardiac surgery: A multicenter prospective study in China. Arch Gerontol Geriatr. 2015;61:503–9.
20. Madan P, Elayda MA, Lee VV, Wilson JM. Predicting major adverse cardiac events after percutaneous coronary intervention: the Texas Heart Institute risk score. Am Heart J. 2008;155:1068–74.
21. Omstedt Å, Höijer J, Djärv T, Svensson P. Hypertension predicts major adverse cardiac events after discharge from the emergency department with unspecified chest pain. Eur Heart J Acute Cardiovasc Care. 2016, in press.
22. Huang H, Zeng C, Ma Y, Chen Y, Chen C, Liu C, et al. Effects of Long-Term Statin Therapy in Coronary Artery Disease Patients with or without Chronic Kidney Disease. Dis Markers. 2015;2015:252564.
23. Édes IF, Ruzsa Z, Szabó G, Nardai S, Becker D, Benke K, et al. Clinical predictors of mortality following rotational atherectomy and stent implantation in high-risk patients: A single center experience. Catheter Cardiovasc Interv. 2015;86:634–41.
24. Wang X, Qiu M, Li J, Wang H, Qi J, Wang G, et al. Impacts of anemia on 3-year ischemic events in patients undergoing percutaneous coronary intervention: a propensity-matched study. J Thorac Dis. 2015;7:1951–9.
25. Lu Q, Tian G, Zhang Y, Lu M, Lin X, Ma A. Low HDL-C predicts risk and PCI outcomes in the Han Chinese population. Atherosclerosis. 2013;226:193–7.
26. Pan HC, Sheu WH, Lee WJ, Lee WL, Liao YC, Wang KY, et al. Coronary severity score and C-reactive protein predict major adverse cardiovascular events in patients with stable coronary artery disease (from the Taichung CAD study). Clin Chim Acta. 2015;445:93–100.
27. Elezi S, Kastrati A, Pache J, Wehinger A, Hadamitzky M, Dirschinger J, et al. Diabetes mellitus and the clinical and angiographic outcome after coronary stent placement. J Am Coll Cardiol. 1998;32:1866–73.
28. Zhu L, Liu J, Gao C, Zhao W, Que J, Wang X, et al. Comparison of coronary plaque, coronary artery calcification and major adverse cardiac events in Chinese outpatients with and without type 2 diabetes. Springerplus. 2016; 5(1):1678.
29. Park DW, Flaherty JD, Davidson CJ, Yun SC, Lee SW, Kim YH, et al. Prognostic influence of diabetes mellitus on long-term clinical outcomes and stent thrombosis after drug-eluting stent implantation in Asian patients. Am J Cardiol. 2009;103:646–52.
30. Lee MS, Jurewitz D, Zimmer R, Pessegueiro A, Bhatia R, Currier J, et al. Impact of diabetes and acute coronary syndrome on survival in patients treated with drug-eluting stents. Catheter Cardiovasc Interv. 2008;72:909–14.
31. Kedhi E, Généreux P, Palmerini T, McAndrew TC, Parise H, Mehran R, et al. Impact of coronary lesion complexity on drug-eluting stent outcomes in patients with and without diabetes mellitus: analysis from 18 pooled randomized trials. J Am Coll Cardiol. 2014;63:2111–8.
32. Go AS, Chertow GM, Fan D, McCulloch CE, Hsu CY. Chronic kidney disease and the risks of death, cardiovascular events, and hospitalization. N Engl J Med. 2004;351:1296–305.
33. Anavekar NS, McMurray JJ, Velazquez EJ, Solomon SD, Kober L, Rouleau JL, et al. Relation between renal dysfunction and cardiovascular outcomes after myocardial infarction. N Engl J Med. 2004;351:1285–95.
34. Schiffrin EL, Lipman ML, Mann JF. Chronic kidney disease: Effects on the cardiovascular system. Circulation. 2007;116:85–97.
35. Manabe I. Chronic inflammation links cardiovascular, metabolic and renal diseases. Circ J. 2011;75:2739–48.
36. Iwanaga Y, Miyazaki S. Heart failure, chronic kidney disease, and biomarkers: An integrated viewpoint. Circ J. 2010;74:1274–82.
37. Foley RN, Collins AJ, Ishani A, Kalra PA. Calcium-phosphate levels and cardiovascular disease in community-dwelling adults: The atherosclerosis risk in communities (ARIC) study. Am Heart J. 2008;156:556–63.
38. Muntner P, Hamm LL, Kusek JW, Chen J, Whelton PK, He J. The prevalence of nontraditional risk factors for coronary heart disease in patients with chronic kidney disease. Ann Intern Med. 2004;140:9–17.
39. Herzog CA, Asinger RW, Berger AK, Charytan DM, Díez J, Hart RG, et al. Cardiovascular disease in chronic kidney disease. A clinical update from Kidney Disease: Improving Global Outcomes (KDIGO). Kidney Int. 2011; 80:572–86.
40. Kwok CS, Hulme W, Olier I, Holroyd E, Mamas MA. Review of early hospitalisation after percutaneous coronary intervention. Int J Cardiol. 2016. doi:10.1016/j.ijcard.2016.11.050. [Epub ahead of print].
41. Chew DP, Astley C, Molloy D, Vaile J, De Pasquale CG, Aylward P. Morbidity, mortality and economic burden of renal impairment in cardiac intensive care. Intern Med J. 2006;36:185–92.
42. Wang CP, Lu LF, Yu TH, Hung WC, Chiu CA, Chung FM, et al. Associations among chronic kidney disease, high total p-cresylsulfate and major adverse cardiac events. J Nephrol. 2013;26:111–8.
43. Wang CP, Lu LF, Yu TH, Hung WC, Chiu CA, Chung FM, et al. Serum levels of total p-cresylsulphate are associated with angiographic coronary atherosclerosis severity in stable angina patients with early stage of renal failure. Atherosclerosis. 2010;211:579–83.
44. Tang WH, Wang CP, Chung FM, Huang LL, Yu TH, Hung WC, et al. Uremic retention solute indoxyl sulfate level is associated with prolonged QTc interval in early CKD patients. PLoS One. 2015;10:e0119545.
45. Lu LF, Tang WH, Hsu CC, Tsai IT, Hung WC, Yu TH, et al. Associations among chronic kidney disease, high total p-cresylsulfate and left ventricular systolic dysfunction. Clin Chim Acta. 2016;457:63–8.
46. Hsu CC, Lu YC, Chiu CA, Yu TH, Hung WC, Wang CP, et al. Levels of indoxyl sulfate are associated with severity of coronary atherosclerosis. Clin Invest Med. 2013;36:E42–9.
47. Ioachimescu AG, Brennan DM, Hoar BM, Hazen SL, Hoogwerf BJ. Serum uric acid is an independent predictor of all-cause mortality in patients at high risk of cardiovascular disease. Arthritis Rheum. 2008;58:623–30.
48. Fang J, Alderman MH. Serum uric acid and cardiovascular mortality the NHANES I epidemiologic follow-up study, 1971–1992. National Health and Nutrition Examination Survey. JAMA. 2000;283:2404–10.
49. Niskanen LK, Laaksonen DE, Nyyssönen K, Alfthan G, Lakka HM, Lakka TA, et al. Uric acid level as a risk factor for cardiovascular and all-cause mortality in middle-aged men: A prospective cohort study. Arch Intern Med. 2004;164:1546–51.
50. George J, Carr E, Davies J, Belch JJ, Struthers A. High-dose allopurinol improves endothelial function by profoundly reducing vascular oxidative stress and not by lowering uric acid. Circulation. 2006;114:2508–16.
51. Kang DH, Park SK, Lee IK, Johnson RJ. Uric acid induced C-reactive protein (CRP) expression: Implication on cell proliferation and nitric oxide production in human vascular cells. J Am Soc Nephrol. 2005;16:3553–62.
52. Rao GN, Corson MA, Berk BC. Uric acid stimulates vascular smooth muscle cell proliferation by increasing plateletderived growth factor A-chain expression. J Biol Chem. 1991;266:8604–8.
53. Kang DH, Han L, Ouyang X, Kahn AM, Kanellis J, Li P, et al. Uric acid causes vascular smooth muscle cell proliferation by entering cells via a functional urate transporter. Am J Nephrol. 2005;25:425–33.
54. Howell SJ, Sear YM, Yeates D, Goldacre M, Sear JW, Foëx P. Risk factors for cardiovascular death after elective surgery under general anaesthesia. Br J Anaesth. 1998;80:14–9.
55. Dzau VJ. Atherosclerosis and hypertension: mechanisms and interrelationships. J Cardiovasc Pharmacol. 1990;15 Suppl 5:S59–64.
56. Levy D, Wilson PW, Anderson KM, Castelli WP. Stratifying the patient at risk from coronary disease: new insights from the Framingham Heart Study. Am Heart J. 1990;119:712–7.
57. Adamczak M, Zeier M, Dikow R, Ritz E. Kidney and hypertension. Kidney Int Suppl. 2002;80:62–7.
58. Murabito JM, D'Agostino RB, Silbershatz H, Wilson WF. Intermittent claudication. A risk profile from The Framingham Heart Study. Circulation. 1997;96:44–9.
59. Lewington S, Clarke R, Qizilbash N, Peto R. Collins R; Prospective Studies Collaboration. Age-specific relevance of usual blood pressure to vascular mortality: a meta-analysis of individual data for one million adults in 61 prospective studies. Lancet. 2002;360:1903–13.

60. Richards AM, Nicholls MG, Troughton RW, Lainchbury JG, Elliott J, Frampton C, et al. Antecedent hypertension and heart failure after myocardial infarction. J Am Coll Cardiol. 2002;39:1182–8.
61. Miura K, Daviglus ML, Dyer AR, Liu K, Garside DB, Stamler J, et al. Relationship of blood pressure to 25-year mortality due to coronary heart disease, cardiovascular diseases, and all causes in young adult men: the Chicago Heart Association Detection Project in Industry. Arch Intern Med. 2001; 161:1501–8.
62. Rakugi H, Yu H, Kamitani A, Nakamura Y, Ohishi M, Kamide K, et al. Links between hypertension and myocardial infarction. Am Heart J. 1996;132:213–21.
63. Hata A, Namikawa C, Sasaki M, Sato K, Nakamura T, Tamura K, et al. Angiotensinogen as a risk factor for essential hypertension in Japan. J Clin Invest. 1994;93:1285–7.
64. Iwai N, Shimoike H, Ohmichi N, Kinoshita M. Angiotensinogen gene and blood pressure in the Japanese population. Hypertension. 1995;25:688–93.
65. Julius S. Corcoran Lecture. Sympathetic hyperactivity and coronary risk in hypertension. Hypertension. 1993;21:886–93.
66. Chow BJ, Wells GA, Chen L, Yam Y, Galiwango P, Abraham A, et al. Prognostic value of 64-slice cardiac computed tomography severity of coronary artery disease, coronary atherosclerosis, and left ventricular ejection fraction. J Am Coll Cardiol. 2010;55:1017–28.
67. de Waha S, Eitel I, Desch S, Fuernau G, Pöss J, Schuler G, et al. Impact of multivessel coronary artery disease on reperfusion success in patients with ST-elevation myocardial infarction: A substudy of the AIDA STEMI trial. Eur Heart J Acute Cardiovasc Care. 2015, in press.
68. Goldstein JA, Demetriou D, Grines CL, Pica M, Shoukfeh M, O'Neill WW. Multiple complex coronary plaques in patients with acute myocardial infarction. N Engl J Med. 2000;343:915–22.
69. National Cholesterol Education Program. Second Report of the Expert Panel on Detection, Evaluation, and Treatment of High Blood Cholesterol in Adults (Adult Treatment Panel II). Circulation. 1994;89:1333–445.
70. Sharma S, Batsis JA, Coutinho T, Somers VK, Hodge DO, Carter RE, et al. Normal-Weight Central Obesity and Mortality Risk in Older Adults With Coronary Artery Disease. Mayo Clin Proc. 2016;91:343–51.
71. Kotani J, Awata M, Nanto S, Uematsu M, Oshima F, Minamiguchi H, et al. Incomplete neointimal coverage of sirolimus-eluting stents: Angioscopic findings. J Am Coll Cardiol. 2006;47:2108–11.
72. Awata M, Kotani J, Uematsu M, Morozumi T, Watanabe T, Onishi T, et al. Serial angioscopic evidence of incomplete neointimal coverage after sirolimus-eluting stent implantation: Comparison with baremetal stents. Circulation. 2007;116:910–6.
73. Alfonso F, Pérez-Vizcayno MJ, Ruiz M, Suárez A, Cazares M, Hernández R, et al. Coronary aneurysms after drug-eluting stent implantation: Clinical, angiographic, and intravascular ultrasound findings. J Am Coll Cardiol. 2009; 53:2053–60.
74. Guagliumi G, Costa MA, Sirbu V, Musumeci G, Bezerra HG, Suzuki N, et al. Strut coverage and late malapposition with paclitaxel-eluting stents compared with bare metal stents in acute myocardial infarction: Optical coherence tomography substudy of the Harmonizing Outcomes with Revascularization and Stents in Acute Myocardial Infarction (HORIZONS-AMI) Trial. Circulation. 2011;123:274–81.
75. Virmani R, Guagliumi G, Farb A, Musumeci G, Grieco N, Motta T, et al. Localized hypersensitivity and late coronary thrombosis secondary to a sirolimus-eluting stent: Should we be cautious? Circulation. 2004;109:701–5.
76. Cutlip DE, Baim DS, Ho KK, Popma JJ, Lansky AJ, Cohen DJ, et al. Stent thrombosis in the modern era: a pooled analysis of multicenter coronary stent clinical trials. Circulation. 2001;103:1967–71.
77. Ong AT, Hoye A, Aoki J, van Mieghem CA, Rodriguez Granillo GA, Sonnenschein K, et al. Thirty-day incidence and six-month clinical outcome of thrombotic stent occlusion after bare-metal, sirolimus, or paclitaxel stent implantation. J Am Coll Cardiol. 2005;45:947–53.
78. Tsai JP, Tian J, Wang WY, Ng AC. Glycated hemoglobin vs fasting plasma glucose as a predictor of left ventricular dysfunction after ST-elevation myocardial infarction. Can J Cardiol. 2015;31:44–9.

3

Association between appropriateness of coronary revascularization and quality of life in patients with stable ischemic heart disease

Harindra C Wijeysundera[1,2,3,4*], Feng Qiu[3], Paul Fefer[1,5], Maria C Bennell[1], Peter C Austin[2,3] and Dennis T Ko[1,2,3]

Abstract

Background: The relationship between appropriateness score, treatment strategy and quality of life (QOL) among patients with stable ischemic heart disease (SIHD) is not known. In this prospective cohort study, we evaluated changes in generic and cardiac-specific quality of life in patients with documented SIHD, comparing patients with revascularization versus those with medical therapy alone, stratified by their appropriateness scores.

Methods: Consecutive patients with SIHD undergoing elective coronary angiogram from November 1st 2008 to December 1st 2009 completed the Seattle Angina Questionnaire (SAQ) and EQ-5D at the time of procedure and at 1 year. The appropriateness for coronary revascularization was determined at the time of coronary angiography.

Results: Our final cohort consisted of 425 patients, 69.4% of whom underwent revascularization. In the overall cohort, 272 (64.0%) had appropriate indications for revascularization, while 57 (13.4%) had inappropriate indications and 96 (22.6%) had uncertain indications. On average, patients improved in most QOL domains, regardless of treatment strategy and appropriateness score. In patients with appropriate indications, revascularized patients had greater improvements in both generic (0.073; 95% CI 0.003-0.144; p-value 0.04) and disease-specific indices, including angina stability (14.6; 95% CI 0.85-28.3; p-value 0.04), physical limitation (9.3; 95% CI 0.71-17.8; p-value 0.03) and disease perception (12.7; 95% CI4.3-21.1; p-value 0.003) compared to medically treated patients. However, patients with uncertain and inappropriate indications also had improvements in physical limitation and disease perception with revascularization compared to medical therapy.

Conclusions: Patients who had appropriate revascularization derived the greatest improvement in QOL compared with medical therapy.

Keywords: Quality of life, Angina, Appropriateness

Background

Landmark randomized controlled trials have consistently shown no difference in death or myocardial infarction between patients with stable ischemic heart disease (SIHD) who are treated with optimal medications alone compared to those treated with revascularization, with either coronary artery bypass grafting (CABG) or percutaneous coronary intervention (PCI) [1-3]. Despite this, there is wide regional variation in the use of coronary revascularization, suggesting the possible misuse of these invasive therapies [4,5].

The appropriate use criteria for coronary revascularization were designed to assist physicians balance the potential benefits of revascularization against its potential harms [6,7]. Organized jointly by six international cardiovascular societies, an expert panel used a modified Delphi process to categorize clinical scenarios into appropriate, uncertain and inappropriate indications for coronary revascularization [6,7]. The rationale for the appropriate use criteria in identifying candidates for revascularization will be strengthened if one demonstrates a strong relationship between improved outcomes and revascularization decisions based on the appropriateness score. Arguably,

* Correspondence: harindra.wijeysundera@sunnybrook.ca
[1]Schulich Heart Centre, Division of Cardiology, Sunnybrook Health Sciences Centre, University of Toronto, Toronto, Ontario, Canada
[2]Institute of Health Policy, Management and Evaluation, University of Toronto, Toronto, Ontario, Canada
Full list of author information is available at the end of the article

the most important indication for revascularization in SIHD is reducing symptomatic angina and improving quality of life, given the equivalence between optimal medical therapy and revascularization in reducing hard clinical outcomes. To the best of our knowledge, there are no data on the relationship between the appropriateness of revascularization and its impact on quality of life.

Accordingly, our objective in this prospective cohort study was to address this gap in knowledge by evaluating changes in generic and cardiac-specific quality of life over one year in patients with documented SIHD based on non-emergent coronary angiography, comparing patients with revascularization versus those with medical therapy, stratified by their appropriateness scores.

Methods

This study was approved by the Institutional Research Ethics Boards at Sunnybrook Health Sciences Center at the University of Toronto. All enrolled patients provided informed consent to participate in the study.

i. Data source

Our study cohort consisted of consecutive patients with stable chronic coronary artery disease who underwent coronary angiography at the Schulich Heart Center, Sunnybrook Health Sciences Centre in Toronto, Ontario, Canada. Patients were recruited from November 1st 2008 to December 1st 2009. We excluded patients whose indications for angiography were myocardial infarction, acute coronary syndrome, or valvular heart disease. We also excluded patients under the age of 20 years and those with normal coronary arteries, or only mild coronary artery disease, defined as stenosis less than 70% in severity (or less than 50% in the left main artery).

Socio-demographic features, co-morbidities, baseline medications, coronary anatomy, left ventricular (LV) function, as well as pre-procedural stress testing were collected. Patients completed two self-administered quality of life surveys, the Seattle Angina Questionnaire (SAQ) and the EQ-5D just prior to the baseline angiogram, with follow-up at 1 year. The questionnaires were mailed to patients for completion, with telephone reminders provided. Abstracted data were linked using unique patient identifiers to population-based administrative databases housed at the Institute for Clinical Evaluative Sciences (ICES). Death was ascertained through linkage with the Ontario Registered Persons Database (RPDB). Subsequent cardiac procedures were determined through linkage with the Canadian Institute for Health Information Discharge Abstract Database (CIHI-DAD) and Same-Day Surgery database (CIHI-SDS). These contain data on all in-hospital and outpatient procedures, as well as acute hospitalizations.

ii. Measures

a. Seattle Angina Questionnaire (SAQ)

The SAQ is a 19-item descriptive, self-administered questionnaire that focuses on impairments in health unique to coronary disease, across five dimensions: physical limitation, anginal stability, anginal frequency, disease perception and treatment satisfaction [8]. Each dimension is scored and analyzed separately on a continuous scale with a range from 0 to 100, with higher scores indicating better quality of life [8]. A clinically relevant improvement in the SAQ that reflects a change that is perceptible to patients is an improvement of 10 points, while a substantial improvement in clinical status is considered to be an increase of 20 points [8].

b. EQ-5D

The EQ-5D measures the preference for health status using a single index score that has two anchors, with a low score of 0 representing death, and an upper ceiling of 1, representing perfect health [9]. The EQ-5D covers five dimensions of health: mobility, self-care, usual activities, pain/discomfort, and anxiety/depression [9]. Each dimension is measured using a three-level ordinal scale and a unique health state is defined by a combination of values on each of the five dimensions [9]. Each of the 243 potential health states is assigned a score by applying a country-specific tariff. US tariffs were used in this study [9]. To provide clinical context, previous studies have found that Canadian Cardiovascular Class (CCS) 2 is associated with an EQ-5D score of 0.77, while CCS 4 is associated with a score of 0.72 [10].

iii. Treatment category

Patients were assigned to the revascularization category if they underwent a PCI or CABG within 90 days of index angiogram. All other patients were assigned to the medical therapy category.

iv. Appropriateness category

The appropriateness for coronary revascularization was determined based on data collected at the time of the index angiogram. For this study, we used the 2009 appropriate use criteria, and restricted our analyses to the 59 indications related to SIHD [7]. Briefly, each patient was assigned an appropriateness score from 1 to 9, based broadly on coronary anatomy (single versus double versus triple vessel coronary artery disease), the severity of symptoms (based on Canadian Cardiovascular (CCS) class), the intensity of anti-anginal medications and the extent of ischemia on non-invasive stress testing [6,7]. For each patient, the score was calculated automatically using a computer algorithm. Patients were categorized into those with appropriate indications for revascularization (score of 7–9), uncertain indications (score of

4–6) and inappropriate indications (score of 1–3). Patients that could not be assigned appropriateness scores were excluded from the analyses [6,7].

v. Analysis

a. Missing data

In our primary analyses for each quality of life measure, we included all patients with complete data at baseline and 1 year for that particular quality of life indicator. As we anticipated that the same patient may have varying degrees of missingness for each outcome, this would result in potentially different sample sizes for the primary analyses for each outcome. Importantly, to determine if our conclusions were affected by missing data, we created five imputed datasets, using Markov Chain Monte Carlo methods to impute missing data, which were assumed to be missing at random. Regression coefficient estimates were then combined from each imputed dataset to allow for valid statistical inference.

b. Model development

Comparison of baseline characteristics between patients in each treatment group was evaluated using the Wilcoxon Rank Sum test for continuous data, and Chi-square or Fisher exact tests for categorical data.

We created six unadjusted linear regression models, each with the scores from the EQ-5D or one of the five domains of the SAQ, treated as a continuous dependent variable. The unit of analysis for all models was the individual patient. To account for the repeated measures per patient, we used generalized estimating equation (GEE) methods, with each patient having both a baseline and a 1-year score. Variables included in the model were time (baseline versus 1 year), treatment strategy (medical therapy versus revascularization), appropriateness category (appropriate versus inappropriate versus uncertain) and all 2-way and 3-way interactions between time, appropriateness category and treatment strategy. In this manner, we were able to contrast quality of life changes from baseline to 1 year for patients treated with revascularization compared to medical therapy alone, within each appropriateness category. Finally, fully adjusted models comparing within and between group changes over time were developed as above, by forcing in all baseline characteristics into the regression. In these models, we adjusted for factors that may impact the quality of life, independent of the choice of revascularization. These included baseline age, gender, LV function, serum creatinine, presence of diabetes mellitus, hypertension, hyperlipidemia, stroke, peripheral vascular disease, smoking, malignancy, heart failure, in addition to having a prior MI, CABG or PCI.

Sensitivity analyses

Given the higher clinical threshold for considering CABG, as opposed to PCI, as well as the potential for differential benefit between the two treatments, we repeated all the adjusted models, stratified by the type of revascularization modality.

Statistical analyses were performed using SAS version 9.3 (SAS corporation). Results were considered statistically significant with a 2-sided p-value of <0.05.

Results

During the 1 year of patient accrual, 761 consecutive patients were enrolled. Of these, 282 patients had either mild coronary disease or normal coronaries arteries. A further 54 (7.1%) patients could not be assigned an appropriateness score because they had missing data on a previous stress testing. Our final cohort consisted of 425 patients, with 295 (69.4%) patients treated with revascularization within 90 days of their index angiogram. Of these, 78 (26.4%) patients underwent CABG, with a mean delay of 16.7 days (median 10, interquartile range 0–29 days), while 217 (73.6%) underwent PCI, at a mean delay of 2.5 days (median 0, interquartile range 0–0 days).

Within the final cohort, 272 (64.0%) had appropriate indications for revascularization, while 57 (13.4%) had inappropriate indications, and 96 (22.6%) had uncertain indications respectively. All of the 57 patients who had inappropriate indications had single or double vessel disease without involvement of the LAD and 40.4% were asymptomatic. The majority (51 patients/89.4%) were patients who were receiving minimal or no anti-anginal medications, with low-risk findings on non-invasive testing and were either asymptomatic (n = 17) or minimally symptomatic with CCS 1–2 (n = 34). The remaining 6 inappropriate patients were all asymptomatic, and had either low-risk non-invasive findings and were on maximal anti-anginal medical therapy (n = 4), or intermediate findings with minimal/no medications (n = 2). In the appropriate indication category, 75% of the patients underwent revascularization. In contrast, 53% of the patients with inappropriate indications underwent revascularization. Of the 96 patients with uncertain indications, 62% underwent revascularization.

The baseline characteristics for the cohort are shown on Table 1. Only 19.8% of patients were asymptomatic, with CCS 0 angina. Of the 425 patients in the cohort, 44.2% had single vessel disease, with 31.3% having double vessel disease and 24.6% having either triple vessel or left main artery disease. As expected, there were substantial differences between appropriateness categories in terms of the distribution of symptoms and anatomy, given that these are components of the appropriate use criteria. There were no statistically significant differences in the distribution of LV function. Only 26.1% of the overall

Table 1 Baseline Characteristics

Variable	TOTAL N = 425	Appropriate N = 272	Inappropriate N = 57	Uncertain N = 96	P-value	Medical N = 130	Revascularization N = 295	P-value
Age Mean ± SD	65.34 ± 10.86	66.04 ± 11.04	64.11 ± 10.90	64.09 ± 10.23	0.852	65.52 ± 11.69	65.26 ± 10.49	0.823
Male	79.1%	80.1%	78.9%	76.0%	0.123	84.6%	76.6%	0.155
Diabetes	35.1%	38.2%	21.1%	34.4%	0.047	36.9%	34.2%	0.593
Hypertension	74.8%	75.0%	73.7%	75.0%	0.475	80.8%	72.2%	0.152
Hyperlipidemia	89.9%	89.7%	89.5%	90.6%	0.443	90.8%	89.5%	0.764
Smoking	60.0%	62.1%	52.6%	58.3%	0.409	53.1%	3.1%	0.061
Symptom Severity								
CCS 0	19.8%	12.1%	40.4%	29..2%	<0.001	23.1%	18.3%	0.029
CCS 1-2	48.9%	44.1%	59.6%	56.3%		54.6%	46.4%	
CCS 3-4	31.3%	43.8%	0%	14.6%		22.3%	35.3%	
LV ejection Fraction								
> = 60%	56.0%	54.4%	68.4%	53.1%	0.371	48.5%	59.3%	0.039
40-59%	21.9%	22.4%	14.0%	25.0%		30.0%	18.3%	
20-39%	9.4%	11.0%	8.8%	5.2%		10.0%	9.2%	
<=20%	0.7%	0.7%	0.0%	1.0%		1.5%	0.3%	
NA	12.0%	11.4%	8.8%	15.6%		10.0%	12.9%	
Coronary Anatomy								
1 -or 2 vessel CAD without involvement of proximal LAD	55.1%	40.8%	100.0%	68.8%	<.001	63.8%	51.2%	0.016
Chronic total occlusion of 1 major epicaridial coronary artery without other coronary stenoses	0.5%	0.7%	0.0%	0.0%	0.568	0.0%	0.7%	0.347
1- vessel CAD involving the proximal LAD	8.0%	8.8%	0.0%	10.4%	0.051	4.6%	9.5%	0.088
2-vessel CAD involving the proximal LAD	4.7%	3.7%	0.0%	10.4%	0.005	4.6%	4.7%	0.953
3-vessel CAD (no left main)	18.8%	25.7%	0.0%	10.4%	<.001	17.7%	19.3%	0.692
left main stenosis	13.4%	21.0%	0.0%	0.0%	<.001	9.2%	15.3%	0.093
Previous CABG	16.7%	19.9%	1.8%	16.7%	0.005	28.5%	11.5%	<.001
Previous CHF	6.4%	6.6%	3.5%	7.3%	0.74	12.3%	3.7%	0.003
Previous PCI	29.9%	29.4%	29.8%	31.3%	0.159	34.6%	27.8%	0.11
Prior MI	34.8%	33.8%	28.1%	41.7%	0.236	43.1%	31.2%	0.043
PVD	12.5%	11.8%	12.3%	14.6%	0.806	13.8%	11.9%	0.553
Creatinine Mean ± SD	95.92 ± 68.21	90.89 ± 23.96	94.46 ± 44.47	111.04 ± 132.88	0.221	106.38 ± 106.79	91.31 ± 40.45	0.971
Dialysis	1.4%	0.7%	1.8%	3.1%	0.227	2.3%	1.0%	0.299
Stroke	9.6%	9.9%	14.0%	6.3%	0.351	8.5%	10.2%	0.831

Table 1 Baseline Characteristics *(Continued)*

Dementia	0.7%	0.7%	0.0%	1.0%	0.341	0.8%	0.7%	0.102
Cancer	10.4%	11.8%	8.8%	7.3%	0.703	7.7%	11.5%	0.01
COPD	7.5%	8.8%	7.0%	4.2%	0.327	(4.6%	8.8%	0.131
Medications								
% on Maximal Anti-anginal Therapy	26.1%	32.0%	7.0%	20.8%	<.001	20.8%	28.5%	0.096
ACE inhibitor/ARB	67.5%	66.9%	68.4%	68.8%	0.936	72.3%	65.4%	0.163
Statin	82.1%	83.1%	82.5%	79.2%	0.688	81.5%	82.4%	0.836
B-Blocker	66.4%	68.8%	56.1%	65.6%	0.184	71.5%	64.1%	0.133
Treatment Strategy								
CABG	18.4%	21.7%	14.0%	11.5%	0.002	0.0%	26.4%	<.001
Medical	30.6%	24.6%	47.4%	37.5%		130 100.0%	0.0%	
PCI	51.1%	53.7%	38.6%	51.0%		0.0%	73.6%	
Outcomes								
1- year Mortality	2.6%	2.6%	0.0%	4.2%	0.292	5.4%	1.4%	0.016
1-year Readmission for MI	9.9%	10.3%	7.0%	10.4%	0.738	5.4%	11.9%	0.039
1-year repeat PCI/CABG	10.4%	12.5%	3.5%	8.3%	0.098	5.4%	12.5%	0.026

SD: standard deviation; *CCS*: Canadian Cardiovascular Society; *LV*: left ventricular; *CABG*: coronary artery bypass grafting; *PCI*: percutaneous coronary intervention; *MI*: myocardial infarction; *PVD*: peripheral vascular disease; *COPD*: chronic obstructive lung disease; *CHF*: Congestive heart failure; *ARB*: angiotensin receptor blocker.

cohort were on maximal anti-anginal therapy. The use of statin, β-blockers and ACE inhibitor/ARB medications were high among the cohort, with no differences between appropriateness groups (Table 1). Over a 1- year follow-up period mortality after the index angiogram was 2.6%; 9.9% of the cohort had a repeat MI within 1 year, while 10.4% underwent repeat PCI/CABG within 1 year. There were no differences among the three appropriateness categories in these outcomes; however, patients who were vascularized had a lower unadjusted mortality, but higher rates of both readmission for MI and repeat revascularization.

Quality of life

There was varying degrees of missing data for the six quality of life measures at the two time points of our study. As seen in (Additional file 1: Table S1), only 4.7% (n = 20) of the patients were missing baseline angina frequency scores, but almost 50% were missing angina stability at 1 year. Of the 425 patients, only 113 patients had complete data on all six quality of life measures for both time points. In (Additional file 1: Table S1), the sample size for the primary analyses for each quality indicator is shown. As expected this varied from 252 with complete data on EQ-5D to 213 with complete data on angina stability. Comparison of the patients with missing quality of life measures and those with complete data is found in (Additional file 1: Table S2). The groups were similar with no differences in baseline characteristics. In particular, the proportion of patients that had appropriate, uncertain and inappropriate indications was similar for the complete dataset and that with missing data (Additional file 1: Table S2).

Summary results for our primary analysis on patients with complete data are shown on Figure 1a-f. As is apparent, most quality of life indices had either statistically significant improvements or remained constant over the 1 year, regardless of appropriateness indication or treatment strategy. Indeed, we did not find a gradient between the appropriate, uncertain or inappropriate criteria. The exception was in patients treated medically who had inappropriate indications for revascularization; these patients had a significant worsening in their mean physical limitation scores over the 1 year (Figure 1c). Angina frequency and angina stability improved significantly for all patients, except those who had inappropriate indications and were treated medically (Figure 1a and 1b respectively). Disease perception improved significantly over the course of the 1-year follow-up in all groups (Figure 1d). Treatment satisfaction only improved significantly for patients with appropriate indications who were revascularized. In (Additional file 1: Table S3), we compared the proportion of patients who had substantial improvements (>20 point) over the 1-year of follow-up in the SAQ sub-scales. Patients who were revascularized had a higher proportion of patients with substantial improvements in angina frequency (33.9% vs 15.4%; $p < 0.001$), physical limitation (20% vs 5.4%; $p < 0.001$) and disease perception 31.9% vs 20% $p = 0.012$). However, across the appropriate use criteria, the only difference was in physical limitation (18.0% for appropriate vs 5.3% inappropriate $p = 0.052$).

A comparison of baseline quality of life measures for the patients with complete and missing data, stratified by appropriateness category is found in (Additional file 1: Table S4). There were no significant differences in baseline scores for the five angina specific measures from the SAQ, except for physical limitation where patients with missing values had lower scores. There were also differences in generic quality of life as measured by the EQ-5D. Patients with missing data tended to have lower baseline quality of life as measured in the EQ-5D.

Appropriate indications

In the appropriate category, patients who were treated with revascularization tended to have lower baseline quality of life scores compared to medical therapy patients (Figure 1a-f). However, when comparing risk-adjusted changes over time (Table 2), there were statistically significant differences in the angina stability, physical limitation, disease perception and treatment satisfaction SAQ subcategories, as well as in generic EQ-5D in patients with appropriate indications for revascularization who were revascularized compared to those who were treated medically. In each of these categories, patients who had appropriate indications and were revascularized had incrementally greater improvements in quality of life compared to those who were treated medically.

Inappropriate and uncertain indications

Interestingly, patients who had inappropriate indications for revascularization also had greater improvements in disease perception and physical limitation when treated with revascularization compared to medical therapy (Table 2). Similarly, patients with uncertain indications had greater improvements in physical limitation with revascularization.

Sensitivity analyses

Multiple imputation was used to account for missing data. As seen in the (Additional file 1: Table S5), although there were no qualitative differences in the trend of our results when compared to our primary analysis, the findings were no longer statistically significant.

The risk-adjusted models, stratified by revascularization modality are found in (Additional file 1: Table S6). We found similar findings for patients treated with CABG, as compared to the overall primary results for both patients with appropriate and inappropriate indications. However,

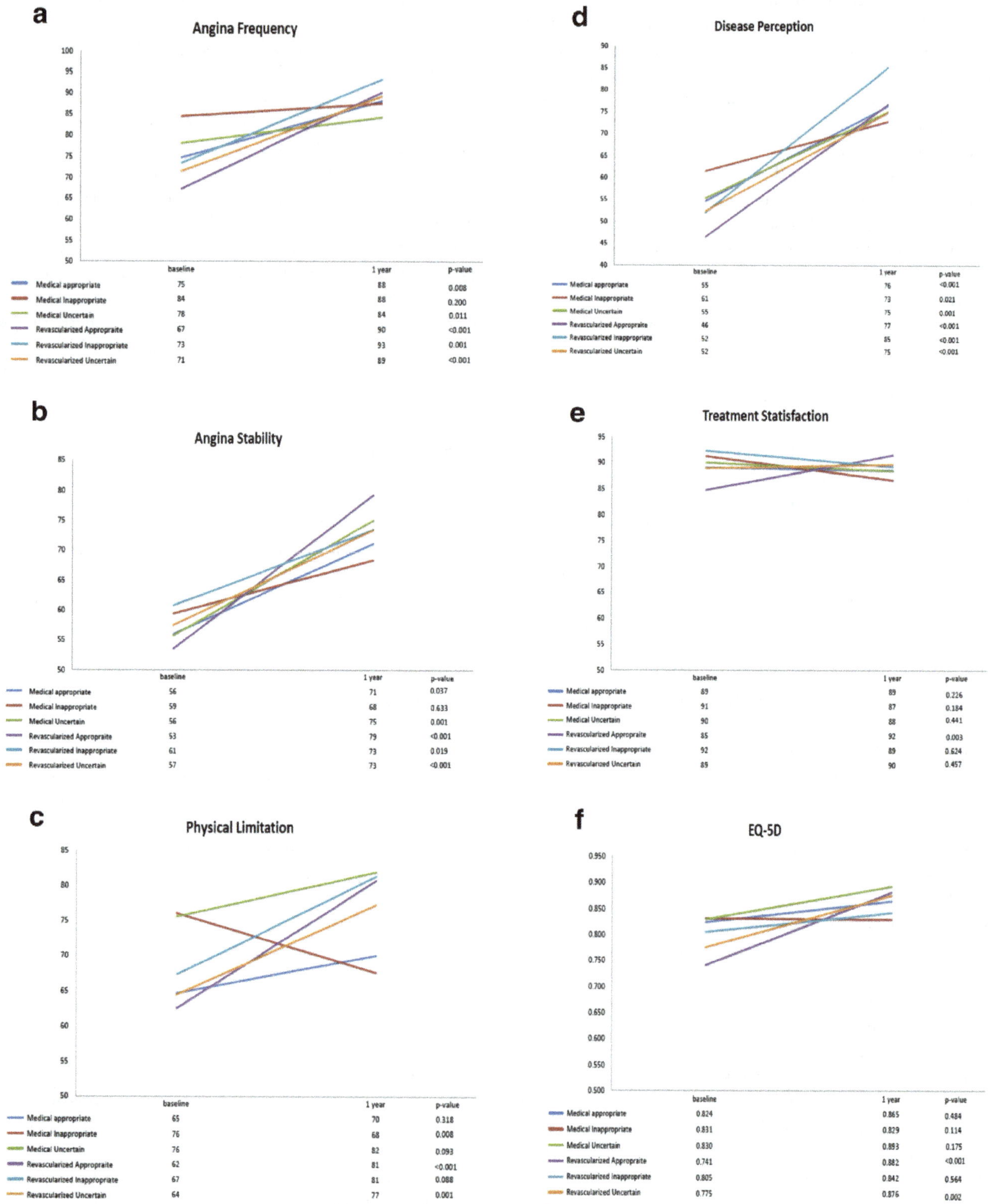

Figure 1 Changes in quality of life from baseline to 1 year. a-f: Changes in quality of life from baseline to 1 year are shown for patients categorized by treatment strategy and appropriateness category. P-values are based on per patient changes over time. For angina frequency (Figure 1a), higher scores represent less frequent angina.

Table 2 Comparisons of Changes in Quality of Life Indices from baseline to 1 year

Comparison		Unadjusted (95% CI)	p-value	Adjusted (95% CI)	p-value
ANGINA FREQUENCY: n = 247					
Indication	*Therapy*				
Appropriate	Revascularization VS medical therapy	10.2 (−0.6,20.9)	0.063	9.8 (−1.6,21.2)	0.093
Inappropriate	Revascularization VS medical therapy	13.6 (−2.1,29.3)	0.090	10.0 (−6.2,26.2)	0.227
Uncertain	Revascularization VS medical therapy	10.6 (−1.7,22.9)	0.09	11.3 (−1.3,24.0)	0.080
ANGINA STABILITY: n = 213					
Indication	*Therapy*				
Appropriate	Revascularization VS medical therapy	14.6 (0.8,28.3)	0.038	14.6 (0.8,28.3)	0.038
Inappropriate	Revascularization VS medical therapy	13.0 (−17.3,43.3)	0.401	9.7 (−20.4,39.7)	0.529
Uncertain	Revascularization VS medical therapy	−9.4 (−35.1,16.3)	0.475	−7.7 (−34.4,19.0)	0.571
PHYSICAL LIMITATION: n = 239					
Indication	*Therapy*				
Appropriate	Revascularization VS medical therapy	10.1 (1.8,18.5)	0.017	9.3 (0.7,17.8)	0.034
Inappropriate	Revascularization VS medical therapy	18.3 (5.8,30.8)	0.004	17.7 (3.9,31.6)	0.012
Uncertain	Revascularization VS medical therapy	19.3 (8.6,29.9)	<0.001	19.2 (8.2,30.1)	<0.001
DISEASE PERCEPTION: n = 243					
Indication	*Therapy*				
Appropriate	Revascularization VS medical therapy	14.4 (5.6,23.1)	0.001	12.7 (4.3,21.1)	0.003
Inappropriate	Revascularization VS medical therapy	26.0 (13.6,38.5)	<0.001	26.9 (13.6,40.3)	<0.001
Uncertain	Revascularization VS medical therapy	7.2 (−4.8,19.1)	0.239	6.5 (−5.7,18.8)	0.294
TREATMENT SATISFACTION: n = 246					
Indication	*Therapy*				
Appropriate	Revascularization VS medical therapy	7.6 (2.1,13.1)	0.007	7.6 (1.9,13.2)	0.009
Inappropriate	Revascularization VS medical therapy	4.5 (−4.1,13.1)	0.302	6.0 (−2.5,14.5)	0.167
Uncertain	Revascularization VS medical therapy	1.2 (−8.4,10.9)	0.802	1.7 (−8.1,11.4)	0.733
EQ_5D: n = 252					
Indication	*Therapy*				
Appropriate	Revascularization VS medical therapy	0.095 (0.024,0.165)	0.008	0.073 (0.003,0.144)	0.040
Inappropriate	Revascularization VS medical therapy	−0.010 (−0.0168,0.148)	0.902	−0.009 (−0.189,0.171)	0.920
Uncertain	Revascularization VS medical therapy	0.062 (−0.012,0.135)	0.099	0.063 (−0.014,0.139)	0.107

for patients treated with PCI who had appropriate indications, improvements in quality of life were limited to treatment satisfaction and disease perception.

Discussion

We found that the majority of patients with significant SIHD who underwent coronary angiography had appropriate indications for revascularization. Approximately three quarters of these patients underwent subsequent revascularization. Most patients had improvements in their self-reported quality of life in the first year after coronary angiography. Although patients with appropriate indications for revascularization derived greater improvements with revascularization compared to medical therapy, improvements were also seen for revascularized patients with uncertain and inappropriate indications, albeit in fewer quality of life sub-categories. However, these findings were not robust in sensitivity analyses that accounted for missing data with multiple imputations, and were most apparent in patients who underwent CABG, as opposed to those who were revascularized with PCI. Although appropriate use criteria appear to identify appropriate candidates for revascularization, our study raises doubts as to the utility of these criteria in excluding patients who are not candidates for revascularization.

There has been substantial interest in the development for appropriate use criteria for diagnostic tests and therapies, particularly in cardiovascular disease [11-13]. These appropriate use criteria are developed through the expert consensus, and as such it is important to evaluate if the criteria translate into improved outcomes. Previous work from our group has validated the appropriateness criteria for revascularization by demonstrating that in SIHD patients who have appropriate indications, medical therapy was associated with worse outcomes when compared to revascularization, with a 39% increased hazard of death or repeat myocardial infarction over 3 years of follow-up [14]. Moreover, we found that revascularization was underutilized, with about 30% of patients with appropriate indications not receiving revascularization [14]. However, we did not find worse outcomes in revascularized patients who had uncertain or inappropriate indications, a finding consistent with other studies [14,15]. We extend this previous work in the current study by evaluating the impact of under and overutilization of coronary revascularization on quality of life.

Quality of life is increasingly used as a patient-centered endpoint in cardiovascular disease studies, especially in SIHD, where invasive therapy is indicated for the relief of symptoms [16,17]. In the landmark Clinical Outcomes Utilizing Revascularization and Aggressive Drug Evaluation (COURAGE) trial, both patients treated with optimal medical therapy and those revascularized with PCI, had marked improvements in their quality of life as measured on the SAQ [18]. Patients who were treated with PCI had small incremental benefits over medical therapy, which was most prominent in the patient subgroup with more severe angina symptoms at baseline [18]. This is consistent with other evidence that has shown that the most important predictor of quality of life improvements post PCI is the severity of baseline angina [19]. Our study adds to these previous findings. Similar to the COURAGE trial, we found that the majority of patients tended to have improvements in quality of life. The greater benefit associated with revascularization compared to medical therapy seen in our study, in contrast to the COURAGE trial, maybe related to the relatively low proportion of patients in our cohort who on maximum anti-anginal therapy.

In patients with appropriate indications, we have reinforced the validation of the appropriate category, given the improved quality of life we observed for patients treated with revascularization who had appropriate indications. In combination with our previous work showing improved clinical outcomes for these patients with revascularization, this supports the use of the appropriate use criteria in identifying suitable candidates for revascularization.

The interpretation of the quality of life changes in the uncertain and inappropriate categories is complex. The rationale underlying the inappropriate indication category is that revascularization in these patients should not be of any benefit at all, and potentially harmful because these patients have minimal chest pain and good baseline function. However, despite the relatively small number of patients in these categories, we found that revascularization in patients with both uncertain and inappropriate criteria appeared to have greater improvements in quality of life in some of the SAQ sub-categories when compared to medical therapy. This suggests the appropriate use criteria may need greater refinement in order to better exclude patients who are indeed poor candidates for revascularization. The lack of discrimination for the appropriateness guidelines for clinical benefit may relate to the inclusion of symptomatic patients in the inappropriate category. Indeed, of the 57 patients with inappropriate indications, 60% had symptoms. Potential refinements may be the inclusion of quality of life as measured on instruments such as the SAQ, as opposed to CCS class, in order to better identify patients with minimal symptoms who would not benefit from revascularization.

Our study must be interpreted in the context of several limitations that merit discussion. First, despite our best efforts, a considerable portion of enrolled patients did not complete all the quality of life surveys. We evaluated the impact of missing data in the sensitivity analyses through multiple imputations. Although it is reassuring that the qualitative direction of our results were maintained, the comparisons between treatment strategies within appropriateness categories were not longer statistically significant. Second, our analysis was restricted to patients who survived at least a year after their index coronary angiogram. This limitation is mitigated by the fact that we were evaluating a SIHD population and therefore, we would not expect a high mortality rate. In addition, it is notable that only approximately a quarter of our patients were on optimal medical therapy, reflecting the inadequacy of routine medical care in real world practice. Our cohort consisted of patients recruited at a single, large tertiary academic hospital in Ontario, Canada. Indeed, previous work from our group suggests that there maybe a higher threshold for invasive testing in Canada, and as such our results may not be generalizable to other jurisdictions or patient populations [4]. We were limited in the anatomical data available to the location of the lesions. Although this was sufficient to assign patients to appropriateness categories, we were not able to account for the complexity of anatomy, such as the presence of calcification or bifurcation status which may have impacted the decision to revascularize. Finally, this is an observational study designed to evaluate associations between treatment strategy, appropriate use criteria and outcomes. We cannot establish causality, and so our work should be considered hypothesis generating and not conclusive. We believe that our results reinforce the need for an adequately powered randomized trial to evaluate the benefit of determining treatment strategy based on appropriate use criteria.

Conclusions

In conclusion, we found that coronary revascularization is associated with greater improvements in quality of life compared to medical therapy, in particular in patients with appropriate indications. However, refinements are needed in the appropriate use criteria to better exclude patients who would not derive benefit from revascularization.

Competing interests

The authors have no relevant relationships with industry to disclose.

Author's contributions

The specific contributions of the authors are outlined below: HCW: 1) conception, design, analysis and interpretation of data; 2) drafting of the manuscript; and 3) final approval of the manuscript submitted. FQ: 1) analysis and interpretation of data; 2) revising the manuscript critically for important intellectual content; and 3) final approval of the manuscript submitted. PF: 1) conception and design; 2) revising the manuscript critically for important intellectual content; and 3) final approval of the manuscript submitted. MCB: 1) analysis and interpretation of data; 2) revising the manuscript critically for important intellectual content; and 3) final approval of the manuscript submitted. PCA: 1) analysis and interpretation of data; 2) revising the manuscript critically for important intellectual content; and 3) final approval of the manuscript submitted. DTK: 1) conception, design, analysis and interpretation of data; 2) revising the manuscript critically for important intellectual content; and 3) final approval of the manuscript submitted.

Acknowledgements

We acknowledge and thank Kimberley Lew and Param Narine for their invaluable assistance.

Funding sources

This work was funded in part by a Canadian Institute of Health Research (CIHR) Operating Grant MOP (102487). Dr H. Wijeysundera is supported by a Distinguished Clinical Scientist Award from the Heart and Stroke Foundation of Canada. Dr. Ko is supported by a Clinician Scientist Phase II personnel award from the Heart and Stroke Foundation, Ontario Provincial Office. Dr Austin is supported in part by a Career Investigator Award from the Heart and Stroke Foundation.

Author details

[1]Schulich Heart Centre, Division of Cardiology, Sunnybrook Health Sciences Centre, University of Toronto, Toronto, Ontario, Canada. [2]Institute of Health Policy, Management and Evaluation, University of Toronto, Toronto, Ontario, Canada. [3]Institute for Clinical Evaluative Sciences (ICES), Toronto, Ontario, Canada. [4]Li Ka Shing Knowledge Institute of St. Michael's Hospital, Toronto, Ontario, Canada. [5]Leviev Heart Center, Sheba Medical Center, Tel Hashomer and Tel Aviv University, Ramat Aviv, Israel.

References

1. Boden WE, O'Rourke RA, Teo KK, Hartigan PM, Maron DJ, Kostuk WJ, Knudtson M, Dada M, Casperson P, Harris CL, Chaitman BR, Shaw L, Gosselin G, Nawaz S, Title LM, Gau G, Blaustein AS, Booth DC, Bates ER, Spertus JA, Berman DS, Mancini GB, Weintraub WS: **Optimal medical therapy with or without PCI for stable coronary disease.** *N Engl J Med* 2007, **356**(15):1503–1516.
2. Bari 2D Study Group, Frye RL, August P, Brooks MM, Hardison RM, Kelsey SF, MacGregor JM, Orchard TJ, Chaitman BR, Genuth SM, Goldberg SH, Hlatky MA, Jones TL, Molitch ME, Nesto RW, Sako EY, Sobel BE: **A randomized trial of therapies for type 2 diabetes and coronary artery disease.** *N Engl J Med* 2009, **360**(24):2503–2515.
3. Trikalinos TA, Alsheikh-Ali AA, Tatsioni A, Nallamothu BK, Kent DM: **Percutaneous coronary interventions for non-acute coronary artery disease: a quantitative 20-year synopsis and a network meta-analysis.** *Lancet* 2009, **373**(9667):911–918.
4. Ko DT, Tu JV, Austin PC, Wijeysundera HC, Samadashvili Z, Guo H, Cantor WJ, Hannan EL: **Prevalence and extent of obstructive coronary artery disease among patients undergoing elective coronary catheterization in New York State and Ontario.** *JAMA* 2013, **310**(2):163–169.
5. Ko DT, Tu JV, Samadashvili Z, Guo H, Alter DA, Cantor WJ, Hannan EL: **Temporal trends in the use of percutaneous coronary intervention and coronary artery bypass surgery in New York State and Ontario.** *Circulation* 2010, **121**(24):2635–2644.
6. Patel MR, Dehmer GJ, Hirshfeld JW, Smith PK, Spertus JA: **ACCF/SCAI/STS/AATS/AHA/ASNC 2009 Appropriateness Criteria for Coronary Revascularization: a report of the American College of Cardiology Foundation appropriateness criteria task force, Society for cardiovascular angiography and interventions, Society of thoracic surgeons, American association for thoracic surgery, American heart association, and the American society of nuclear cardiology: endorsed by the American society of echocardiography, the heart failure society of America, and the society of cardiovascular computed tomography.** *Circulation* 2009, **119**(9):1330–1352.
7. Patel MR, Dehmer GJ, Hirshfeld JW, Smith PK, Spertus JA: **ACCF/SCAI/STS/AATS/AHA/ASNC/HFSA/SCCT 2012 appropriate use criteria for coronary revascularization focused update a report of the American college of cardiology Foundation appropriate use criteria task force, Society for cardiovascular angiography and interventions, Society of thoracic surgeons, American association for thoracic surgery, American heart association, American Society of nuclear cardiology, and the society of cardiovascular computed tomography.** *J Am Coll Cardiol* 2012, **59**(9):857–881.
8. Spertus JA, Winder JA, Dewhurst TA, Deyo RA, Prodzinski J, McDonell M, Fihn SD: **Development and evaluation of the Seattle Angina questionnaire: a new functional status measure for coronary artery disease.** *J Am Coll Cardiol* 1995, **25**(2):333–341.
9. Brooks R: **EuroQol: the current state of play.** *Health Policy* 1996, **37**(1):53–72.
10. Wijeysundera HC, Farshchi-Zarabi S, Witteman W, Bennell MC: **Conversion of the Seattle Angina Questionnaire into EQ-5D utilities for ischemic heart disease: a systematic review and catalog of the literature.** *Clinicoecon Outcomes Res* 2014, **6**:253–268.
11. Brindis RG, Douglas PS, Hendel RC, Peterson ED, Wolk MJ, Allen JM, Patel MR, Raskin IE, Hendel RC, Bateman TM, Cerqueira MD, Gibbons RJ, Gillam LD, Gillespie JA, Hendel RC, Iskandrian AE, Jerome SD, Krumholz HM, Messer JV, Spertus JA, Stowers SA: **ACCF/ASNC appropriateness criteria for single-photon emission computed tomography myocardial perfusion imaging (SPECT MPI): a report of the American College of Cardiology Foundation Quality Strategic Directions Committee Appropriateness Criteria Working Group and the American Society of Nuclear Cardiology endorsed by the American Heart Association.** *J Am Coll Cardiol* 2005, **46**(8):1587–1605.
12. Douglas PS, Khandheria B, Stainback RF, Weissman NJ, Brindis RG, Patel MR, Khandheria B, Alpert JS, Fitzgerald D, Heidenreich P, Martin ET, Messer JV, Miller AB, Picard MH, Raggi P, Reed KD, Rumsfeld JS, Steimle AE, Tonkovic R, Vijayaraghavan K, Weissman NJ, Yeon SB, Brindis RG, Douglas PS, Hendel RC, Patel MR, Peterson E, Wolk MJ, Allen JM: **ACCF/ASE/ACEP/ASNC/SCAI/SCCT/SCMR 2007 appropriateness criteria for transthoracic and transesophageal echocardiography: a report of the American College of Cardiology Foundation Quality Strategic Directions Committee Appropriateness Criteria Working Group, American Society of Echocardiography, American College of Emergency Physicians, American Society of Nuclear Cardiology, Society for Cardiovascular Angiography and Interventions, Society of Cardiovascular Computed Tomography, and the Society for Cardiovascular Magnetic Resonance endorsed by the American College of Chest Physicians and the Society of Critical Care Medicine.** *J Am Coll Cardiol* 2007, **50**(2):187–204.
13. Douglas PS, Khandheria B, Stainback RF, Weissman NJ, Peterson ED, Hendel RC, Stainback RF, Blaivas M, Des Prez RD, Gillam LD, Golash T, Hiratzka LF, Kussmaul WG, Labovitz AJ, Lindenfeld J, Masoudi FA, Mayo PH, Porembka D, Spertus JA, Wann LS, Wiegers SE, Brindis RG, Douglas PS, Hendel RC, Patel MR, Peterson ED, Wolk MJ, Allen JM: **ACCF/ASE/ACEP/AHA/ASNC/SCAI/SCCT/SCMR 2008 appropriateness criteria for stress echocardiography: a report of the American College of Cardiology Foundation Appropriateness Criteria Task Force, American Society of Echocardiography, American College of Emergency Physicians, American Heart Association, American Society of Nuclear Cardiology, Society for Cardiovascular Angiography and Interventions, Society of Cardiovascular Computed Tomography, and Society**

for Cardiovascular Magnetic Resonance endorsed by the Heart Rhythm Society and the Society of Critical Care Medicine. *J Am Coll Cardiol* 2008, **51**(11):1127–1147.

14. Ko DT, Guo H, Wijeysundera HC, Natarajan MK, Nagpal AD, Feindel CM, Kingsbury K, Cohen EA, Tu JV: **Cardiac Care Network of Ontario Variations in Revascularization Practice in Ontario Working G: Assessing the association of appropriateness of coronary revascularization and clinical outcomes for patients with stable coronary artery disease.** *J Am Coll Cardiol* 2012, **60**(19):1876–1884.
15. Bradley SM, Chan PS, Spertus JA, Kennedy KF, Douglas PS, Patel MR, Anderson HV, Ting HH, Rumsfeld JS, Nallamothu BK: **Hospital percutaneous coronary intervention appropriateness and in-hospital procedural outcomes: insights from the NCDR.** *Circ Cardiovasc Qual Outcomes* 2012, **5**(3):290–297.
16. Spertus JA, Bliven BD, Farner M, Gillen A, Hewitt T, Jones P, McCallister BD: **Integrating baseline health status data collection into the process of care.** *Jt Comm J Qual Improv* 2001, **27**(7):369–380.
17. Spertus JA, Winder JA, Dewhurst TA, Deyo RA, Fihn SD: **Monitoring the quality of life in patients with coronary artery disease.** *Am J Cardiol* 1994, **74**(12):1240–1244.
18. Weintraub WS, Spertus JA, Kolm P, Maron DJ, Zhang Z, Jurkovitz C, Zhang W, Hartigan PM, Lewis C, Veledar E, Bowen J, Dunbar SB, Deaton C, Kaufman S, O'Rourke RA, Goeree R, Barnett PG, Teo KK, Boden WE, Mancini GB: **Effect of PCI on quality of life in patients with stable coronary disease.** *N Engl J Med* 2008, **359**(7):677–687.
19. Spertus JA, Salisbury AC, Jones PG, Conaway DG, Thompson RC: **Predictors of quality-of-life benefit after percutaneous coronary intervention.** *Circulation* 2004, **110**(25):3789–3794.

4

Prevalence and characteristics of coronary artery anomalies in an adult population undergoing multidetector-row computed tomography for the evaluation of coronary artery disease

Christos Graidis*, Dimokritos Dimitriadis, Vasileios Karasavvidis, Georgios Dimitriadis, Efstathia Argyropoulou, Fotios Economou, Dadoush George, Antonios Antoniou and Georgios Karakostas

Abstract

Background: Congenital coronary anomalies are uncommon with an incidence ranging from 0.17 % in autopsy cases to 1.2 % in angiographically evaluated cases. The recent development of ECG–gated multi–detector row computed tomography (MDCT) coronary angiography allows accurate and noninvasive depiction of coronary artery anomalies.

Methods: This retrospective study included 2572 patients who underwent coronary 64-slice MDCT coronary angiography from January 2008 to March 2012. Coronary angiographic scans were obtained with injection of 80 ml nonionic contrast medium. Retrospective gating technique was used to synchronize data reconstruction with the ECG signal. Maximum intensity projection, multi-planar reformatted, and volume rendering images were derived from axial scans.

Results: Of the 2572 patients, sixty (2.33 %) were diagnosed with coronary artery anomalies (CAAs), with a mean age of 53.6 ± 11.8 years (range 29–80 years). High take-off of the RCA was seen in 16 patients (0.62 %), of the left main coronary artery (LMCA) in 2 patients (0.08 %) and both of them in 2 patients (0.08 %). Separate origin of the left anterior descending artery (LAD) and left circumflex artery (LCx) from left sinus of Valsalva (LSV) was found in 15 patients (an incidence of 0.58 %). In 9 patients (0.35 %) the right coronary artery (RCA) arose from the opposite sinus of Valsalva with a separate ostium. In 6 patients (0.23 %) an abnormal origin of LCX from the right sinus of Valsalva (RSV) was found with a further posterior course within the atrioventricular groove. A single coronary artery was seen in 3 patients (0.12 %). It originated from the right sinus of Valsalva in one patient and from LSV in two patients. In two other patients (0.08 %) the left coronary trunk originated from the RSV with separate ostium from the RCA. LCA originating from the pulmonary artery was found in one patient (0.04 %). A coronary artery fistula, which is a termination anomaly, was detected in 4 patients (0.15 %).
(Continued on next page)

* Correspondence: dimitriadis1980@gmail.com
Department of Interventional Cardiology, Kyanous Stavros Hospital, Vizyis-Vyzantos 1 Street, Thessaloniki 54636, Greece

(Continued from previous page)

Discussion: Although these anomalies, which are remarkably different from the normal structure, exist as early as birth, they are incidentally encountered during selective angiography or at autopsy. The incidence in reported angiographic series ranges from 0.6 % to 1.3 %. Variations in the frequency of primary congenital coronary anomalies may possibly have a genetic background. The largest angiographic series of 126595 patients, by Yamanaka and Hobbs, reported a 1.3 % incidence of anomalous coronary artery.

Conclusion: The results of this study support the use MDCT coronary angiography as a safe and effective noninvasive imaging modality for defining CAAs in an appropriate clinical setting, providing detailed three-dimensional anatomic information that may be difficult to obtain with invasive angiography.

Keywords: Coronary artery anomalies, Coronary angiography, Multi-detector computed tomography

Background

The anomalous origin of the coronary artery is a rare congenital condition with an incidence ranging from 0.17 % in autopsy cases [1] to 1.2 % in angiographically evaluated cases [2]. About 20 % of coronary anomalies produce life-threatening symptoms, including arrhythmias, syncope, myocardial infarction, or sudden death [3]. Coronary artery anomaly is the second most common cause of sudden cardiac death (SCD) in young athletes [4]. This imaging technique has limitations due to its projectional and invasive nature. The purpose of this study was to retrospectively determine the prevalence of origination, course, and termination anomalies of coronary arteries, CAA in subjects who presented different symptoms and underwent MDCT coronary angiography for the assessment of coronary artery disease.

Methods

Between January 2008 and March 2012 a total number of 2572 consecutive patients were referred to the Euromedica-Kyanous Stavros Hospital, Department of Radiology, Thessaloniki, Greece, for cardiac MDCTA, due to suspicion(atypical stest pain, angina equivalent symptoms or multiple risk factors for cardiovascular disease) or assumed progression of coronary artery disease. Within these patients all datasets were reviewed in search of coronary anomalies of origin and further vessel course. Standardized patient preparation procedure included the administration of beta-blocker prior to the scan in order to stabilize and/or lower their heart rates below 65 beats per minute if needed (patients with HR > 70 bpm, and no contraindications). Additionally, patients sublingually received nitroglycerin immediately before contrast enhanced scan procedure to widen coronary arteries. An 18–20 gauge needle was placed into the antecubital vein, and heart rhythm was monitored by electrocardiography. MDCT coronary angiography was performed by using a 64-slice scanner (LightSpeed VCT 64 GE Healthcare device). The scan parameters were a collimation either 40 × 0.625 mm or 64 × 0.625 mm, rotation time 0.4 seconds, tube voltage 120 kV, and mAs 500–700. A bolus tracking technique was used to synchronise the arrival of contrast at the level of the coronary arteries at the beginning of acquisition. The images of the entire heart were acquired during apnea of 6 to 8 seconds, with intravenous infusion of 80 to 90 mL of iodinated contrast material, in infusion pump flow of 5 mL/s. A 30-mL bolus of normal saline was given after administering the contrast material to decrease the number of artifacts from the contrast material in the right heart. Two-dimensional maximum intensity projection, multiplanar reformatted and 3-D volume rendering images were produced throughout thin axial scans and then the coronary anatomy and arteries were evaluated. In all patients, images were reconstructed in end diastole (75 % of the R-R interval) and image quality was evaluated on a per segment basis. Where images were judged to be suboptimal, additional reconstruction windows (35 %, 65 % and 85 %) were explored in order to achieve optimal quality images. All analyses were performed on a dedicated workstation (Brilliance Workspace, GE Healthcare). All coronary MDCT coronary angiography images were assessed by an experienced radiologist who was blinded to the study and the whole data, figure and picture processing were approved by the Scientific Counsil of our hospital (reference number 13709).

Results

Between January 2008 and March 2012 a total number of 2572 consecutive patients were referred for evaluation by MDCT coronary angiography. The patients were being tested for stent occlusion, for screening due to the presence of multiple risk factors, or due to chest pain, equivalent symptoms or inconclusive stress tests. Of the 2572 patients, sixty (2.33 %) were diagnosed with coronary artery anomalies, with a mean age of 53.6 ± 11.8 years (range 29–80 years), of which fifty (83.3 %) were males. The details of these coronary artery anomalies are summarized in the Table 1.

High take-off of the right coronary artery (RCA) was seen in 16 patients (0.62 %), of the left main

Table 1 Coronary artery anomalies encountered in our series

Type of anomaly	Number Of patients	Incidence (%)	Anomalies (%)
High "take-off"	20	0.78	33.3
Separate ostia for LAD and Cx inside the left SoV	15	0.58	25
RCA from LSV	9	0.35	15
Cx originating from the right SoV or RCA	6	0.23	10
Single coronary artery	3	0.12	5
LCA from RSoV	2	0.08	3.3
LCA from PA (ALCAPA)	1	0,04	1.7
Coronary artery fistulae	4	0.15	6.7
Total	60	2.33	

LAD left anterior descending, *Cx* circumflex, *RCA* right coronary artery, *LCA* left coronary artery, *SoV* sinus of Valsalva, *PA* pulmonary artery

coronary artery (LMCA) in 2 patients (0.08 %) and both of them in 2 patients (0.08 %) (Fig 1). Separate origin of the left anterior descending artery (LAD) and left circumflex artery (LCx) from left sinus of Valsalva (LSV) was found in 15 patients (an incidence of 0.58 % or 25 % of all coronary anomalies) (Fig 2). In 9 patients (0.35 %) the right coronary artery (RCA) arose from the opposite sinus of Valsalva with a separate ostium for RCA and LM. In two patients the anomalous RCA had a malignant inter-arterial course (Fig 3). In 6 patients (0.23 % or 10 % of all anomalies) an abnormal origin of LCX from the right sinus of Valsalva (RSV) was found with a further posterior course within the atrioventricular groove (Fig 4). Termination of LCx was normal in all patients.

A single coronary artery was seen in 3 patients (0.12 % or 5 % of anomalies). It originated from the RSV in one patient and from LSV in two patients. A 58-year-old man with positive exercise test was found to have a single coronary artery originating from the right sinus of Valsalva (Fig 5). The RCA gave rise to the LMCA, which had a course between the aorta and the right ventricular outflow tract (RVOT). In a 49-year-old man MDCTA revealed a single coronary artery arising from the left sinus of Valsalva (Fig 6). The right coronary artery ostium was congenitally absent. The LCx was markedly dominant and continued beyond the crux into the atrioventricular groove and provided branches to the right ventricle and atrium. In a 48-year-old man with history of syncope MDCT coronary angiography demonstrated a single coronary artery arising from the left coronary sinus, where the LMCA gave rise to the right coronary artery (RCA). The RCA had a malignant course between the pulmonary artery (PA) and the aorta (Fig 7).

In 2 patients (0.08 % or 3.3 % of all anomalies) the left coronary trunk originated from the RSV with separate ostium from the RCA. In a 62-year-old woman the entire coronary system arose from right sinus of Valsalva from three separate ostia (Fig 8). The LAD passed anteriorly to the right ventricular outflow tract. The LCx passed posteriorly between left atrium and aortic root to resume its normal position in left atrioventricular groove. The RCA had normal anatomical apperance. A 49-year-old man with atypical chest pain was found to have anomalous origin of the left coronary system from the right coronary cusp (separate ostium), (Fig 9). LMCA from the pulmonary artery (ALCAPA) was seen in one patient (0.04 %). A 44-year old male with symptoms of heart failure was referred to our hospital for evaluation. MDCT coronary angiography demonstrated anomalous origin of the LMCA from the pulmonary artery and a dilated, tortuous and dominant RCA from the right aortic sinus, with profuse collateral channels feeding the left coronary system (Fig 10).

A coronary artery fistula, which is a termination anomaly, was detected in 4 patients (0.15 % or 6.7 % of all coronary anomalies). Three patients had coronary artery fistula between the left anterior descending artery and the pulmonary artery (Fig 11). In one patient the coronary artery fistula was located between the right coronary artery and the pulmonary artery.

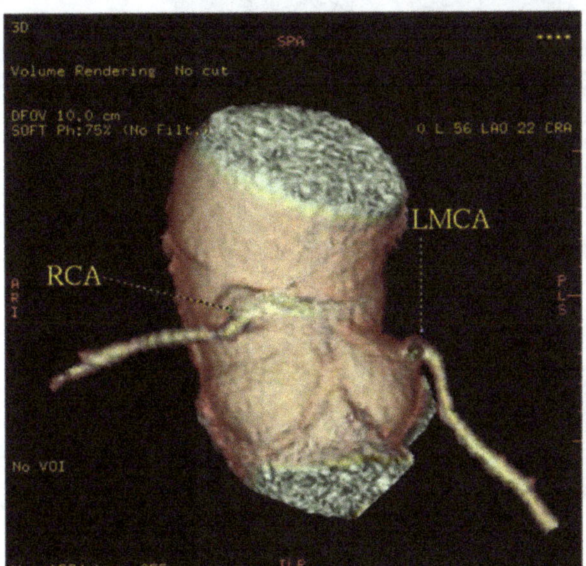

Fig. 1 Volume-rendered image show high take-off of the right coronary artery (RCA) above the sinotubular junction

Discussion

Although these anomalies, which are remarkably different from the normal structure, exist as early as birth, they are

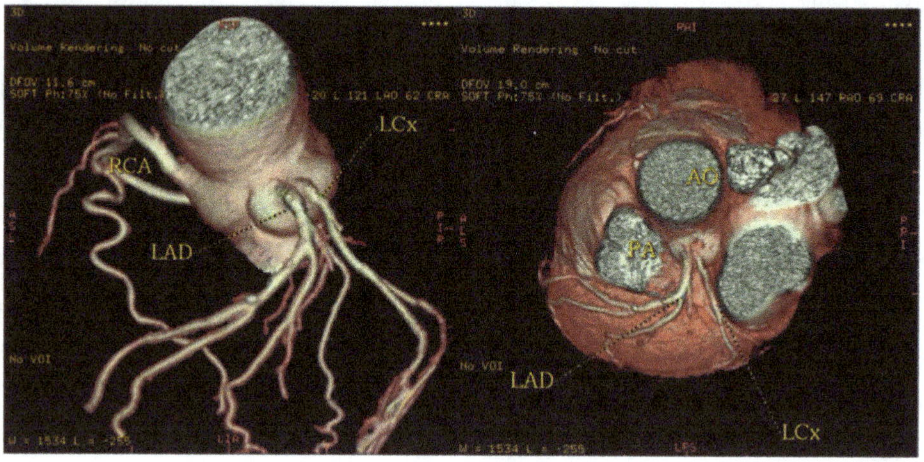

Fig. 2 Volume-rendered images show the absence of the left main coronary artery, with separate ostia of the LAD and LCX arteries from the left sinus of Valsalva (LSV). A = aorta

incidentally encountered during selective angiography or at autopsy. The incidence in reported angiographic series ranges from 0.6 % to 1.3 %. Variations in the frequency of primary congenital coronary anomalies may possibly have a genetic background [5–10]. The largest angiographic series of 126595 patients, by Yamanaka and Hobbs, reported a 1.3 % incidence of anomalous coronary artery (8).

In our study, an overall of 60 patients (2.33 %) with CAAs were identified using MDCT coronary angiography.

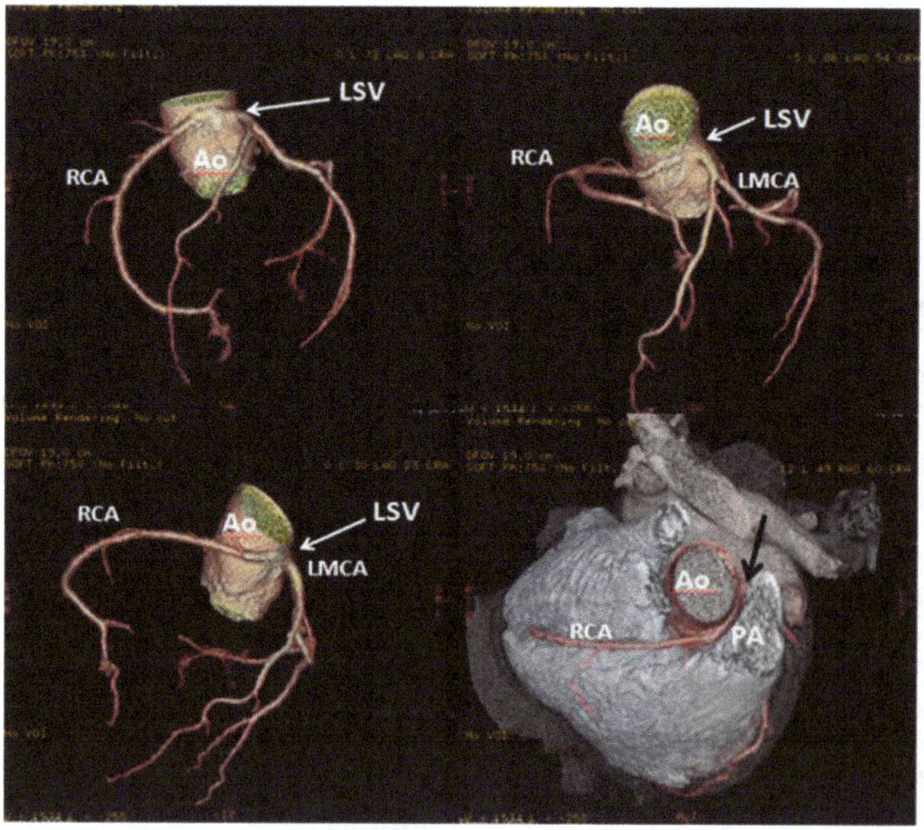

Fig. 3 Three-dimensional volume-rendered image shows the RCA arising from the left coronary sinus and with a malignant inter-arterial course between the pulmonary artery (PA) and the aorta (Ao)

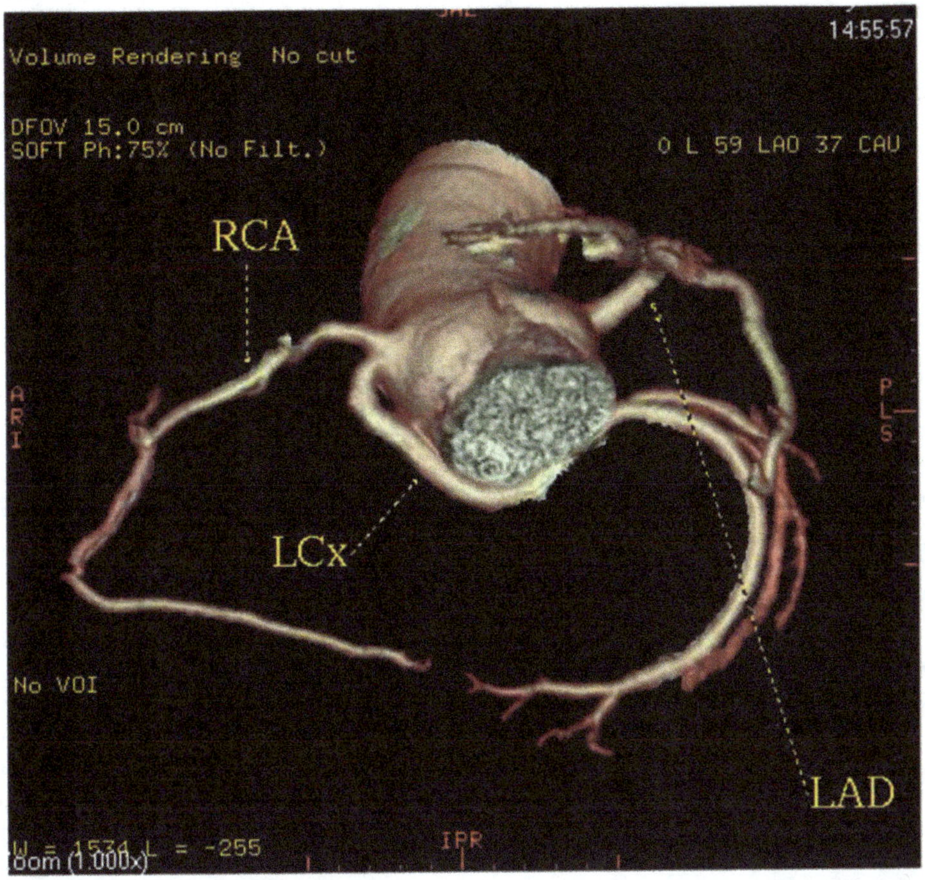

Fig. 4 A patient with a left circumflex artery (LCX) anomalous origin. Three-dimensional volume-rendered image shows the LCX arising separately close to the origin of the right coronary artery (RCA) from the right coronary sinus and coursing below and behind the aortic root

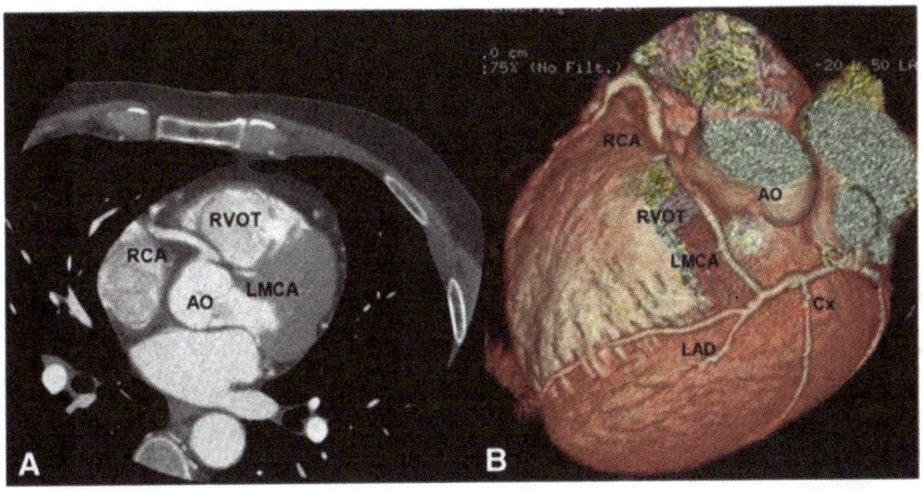

Fig. 5 A patient with a single coronary artery originating from the right sinus of Valsalva. **a** Axial image demonstrating the left main coronary artery travelling between the aorta (AO) and the right ventricular outflow tract (**b**). Cardiac transparency image shows the anomalous origin of the LM, its course and the detailed anatomic relationship

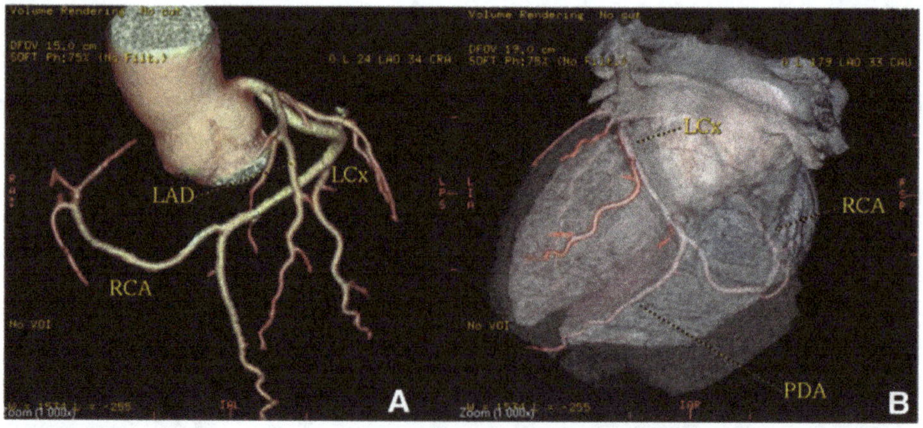

Fig. 6 A patient with a single coronary artery. Volume-rendered and cardiac transparency images reveals a SCA arising from the left sinus of Valsalva and gives off the left anterior descending (LAD) and circumflex (LCx) branches. The right coronary artery ostium was congenitally absent (Panel **A**). The LCx is markedly dominant and continues beyond the crux into the atrioventricular groove and provides branches to the right ventricle and atrium (Panel **B**)

However there is a wide variety in the reported prevalence rate of CAAs [9–13]. De Jonge and co-workers also describe a prevalence of 7 % of CAAs including coronary fistulas [9] in their patient population. In one study the authors report a prevalence of coronary anomalies of origin and further course of 7.9 % in mainly symptomatic patients [10]. Very similarly, Shi et al. [11] demonstrated CTA to outperform invasive angiography for identifying the origin of anomalous coronary arteries and for confirming their anatomic course in relation to the great vessels. Of 240 patients, 16 (6.6 %) with anomalous coronary arteries were detected. In one study [12], anomalies were found in 44 (2.5 %) of 1,758 individuals undergoing MDCT coronary angiography. Recently, Srinivasan et al. [13] assessed 1495 patients using MDCT coronary angiography for the evaluation of coronary artery disease and found the prevalence to be 0.8 %. These discrepancies in reported prevalence might be caused by referral bias and lack of clear diagnostic criteria, which both are prerequisites for defining the true prevalence in a general population. Some of these patients with CAAs might have been or were referred because of known presence of CAAs and not because of unrelated factors as in the general population. In our study CAAs appear to be more common in men ($n = 50$; 83.3 %) than in women ($n =$

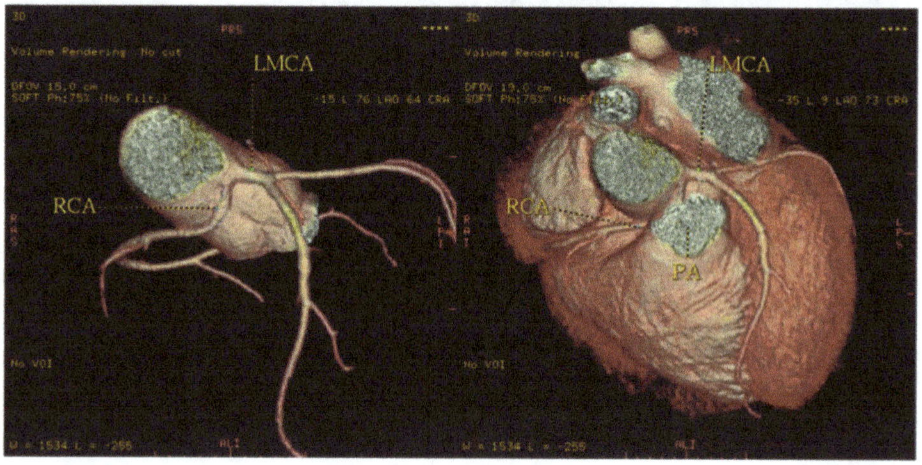

Fig. 7 3-D volume-rendered images of the coronary tree showing a single coronary artery arising from the left coronary sinus, where the left main artery (LM) gives rise to the right coronary artery (RCA) as shown by the black arrow. The RCA runs a malignant course between the pulmonary artery (PA) and the aorta

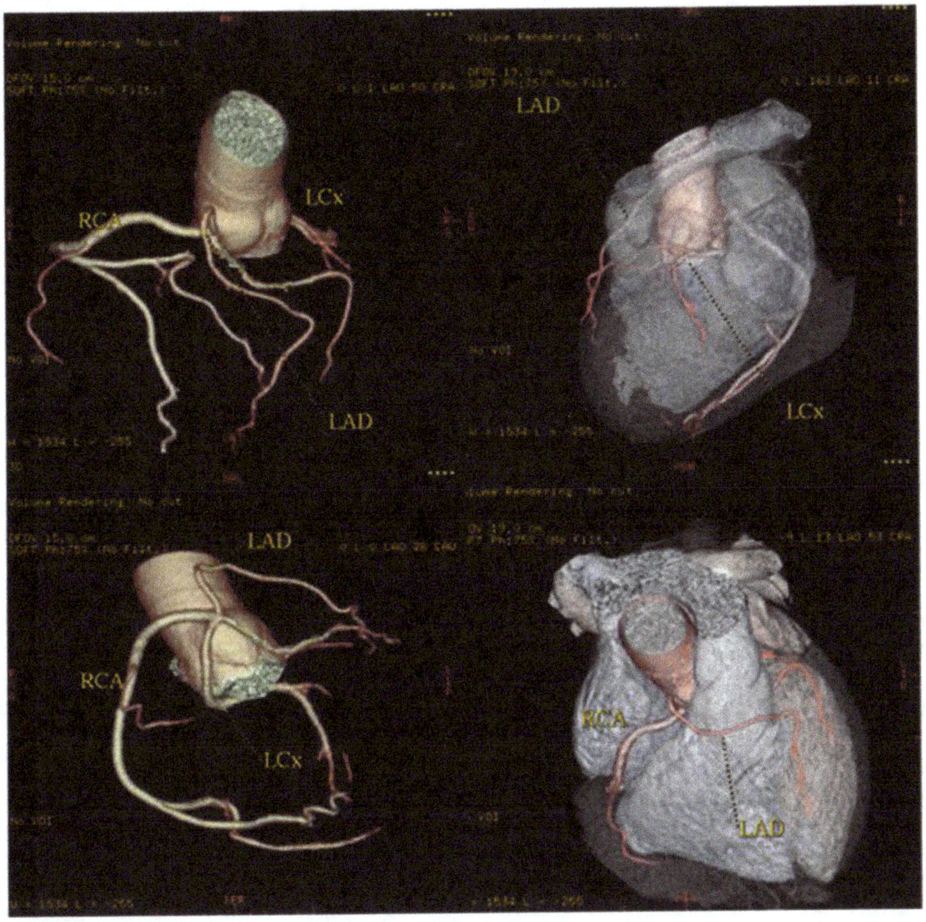

Fig. 8 3-D Volume-rendered images, shows the entire coronary system originating from right sinus of Valsalva from three separate ostia. Left anterior descending coronary artery passes anterior to the right ventricular outflow tract. Circumflex artery passes posteriorly between the left atrium and the aortic root to resume its normal position in left atrioventricular groove. The Right coronary artery has normal configuration

10; 16.7 %). This was also shown in previous reports although such a finding may reflect the selective nature of referral for cardiac MDCTA.

High take-off of coronary arteries was the most commonly seen coronary artery anomaly in this study (0.78 %). "High take-off" refers to an unusually high origin of either the RCA or the LMCA artery from the ascending aorta at a point above the junctional zone between its sinus and the tubular part [14]. The most common is a high origin of the RCA above the sinotubular junction. Rarely, the coronary artery can arise from the aortic arch, the brachiocephalic artery, the internal mammary, bronchial, or subclavian arteries, or even the descending aorta. High take-off positions are without any haemodynamic significance, well tolerated and asymptomatic, but they may lead to unexpected angiographic problems while localizing and engaging the orifices. High take-off is better represented on the angiographic view or volume-rendered reformatted images [15]. It is important for cardiac surgeons to be aware of this anomaly, because during cardiac bypass surgery when the aorta is cross-clamped, high cannulation is needed to avoid accidental cross-clamping or transection of the RCA.

The LAD and LCX arteries may arise separately from the left sinus of Valsalva (LSV) with an absence of the LMCA. (Estimated to be seen in 0.5 % to 8 % of population). This anomaly was the second most common anomaly in our series and was found in 15 patients (an incidence of 0.58 % or 25 % of all coronary anomalies). Multiple ostia [16] usually present no major clinical problems, but they may cause difficulty in cannulating the vessels during invasive coronary angiography.

With a prevalence ranging from 0.2 to 1.0 % [17], the anomalous origination of a coronary artery from the opposite sinus of Valsalva (ACAOS), represent a common cause of sudden cardiac death in the young population, particularly in individuals that undergo strenuous exercise [18]. In our series, similar to previous reports [6,

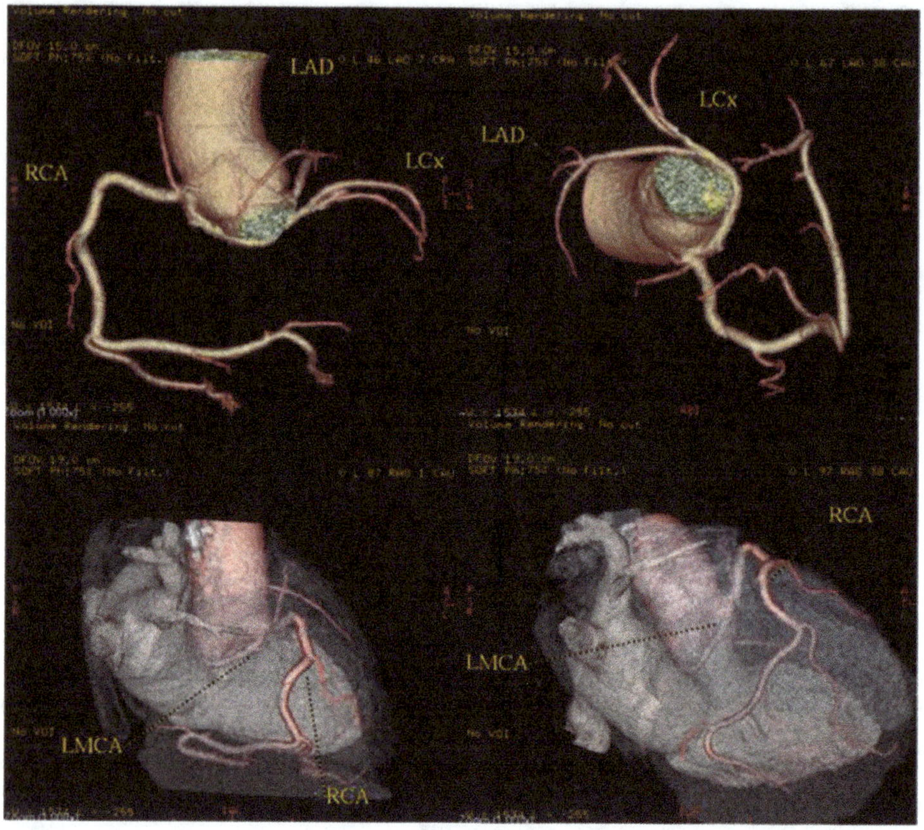

Fig. 9 A patient with anomalous origin of the left coronary system from the right coronary cusp (separate ostium). 3-D volume-rendered and images show the anomalous origin of the LM, its course and the detailed anatomic relationship

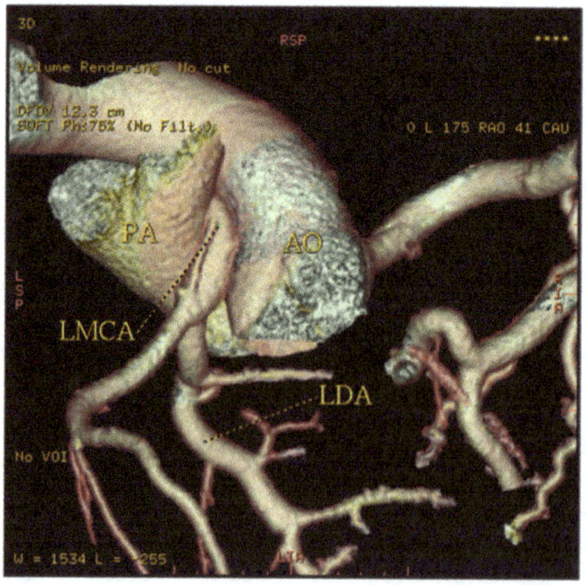

Fig. 10 Three-dimensional volume-rendered image shows the dilated RCA from the aorta (Ao), the anomalous origin of the LMCA from pulmonary artery (PA), along with their anatomical relationship with surrounding structures. Rich collateral channels between RCA and LCA are shown

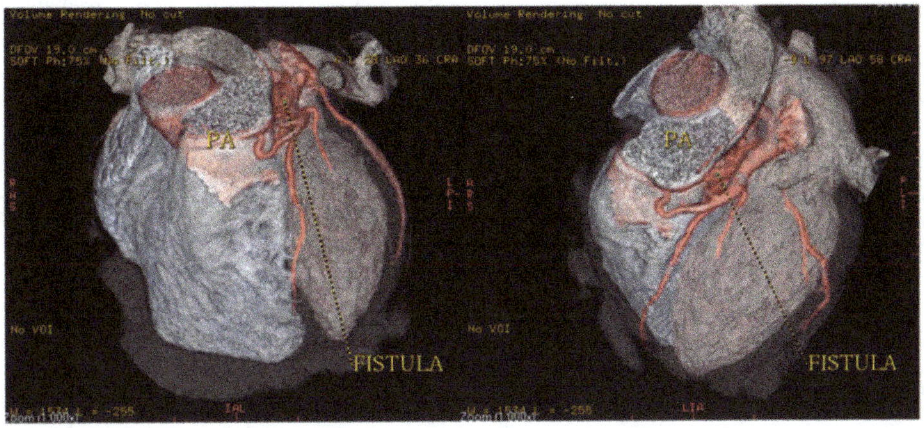

Fig. 11 3-D volume rendering images showing the coronary fistula located between the left anterior descending (LAD) artery and the pulmonary artery

10], the prevalence of ACAOS was 0.78 % (33.3 % of all coronary anomalies), and 18 out of 20 patients were male. MDCTA allowed the identification of the ostium and proximal course of the anomalous coronary arteries and in addition, we were able to differentiate between high (i.e. interarterial) and low (i.e. retro-aortic) risk ACAOS. In our study a total of 6 patients with malignant inter-arterial course of the anomalous artery was found, either of the RCA ($n = 4$) or the left coronary artery ($n = 2$).

One of the most common coronary anomalies in our patient population was an anomalous RCA arising with separate ostium from the opposite sinus of Valsalva ($n = 9$, 0.35 %). Less often the RCA arises entirely from a single ostium in left coronary sinus (Fig. 7). The most common course of an anomalous RCA arising from the left sinus of Valsalva is interarterial [8]; this variant can be associated with sudden cardiac death in up to 30 % of patients [18]. In our series, four patients were found to have a malignant inter-arterial course of the anomalous RCA (Fig 3).

In this study, we report an incidence of 0.23 % for anomalous LCX, which account for a 10 % of the overall incidence of congenital coronary anomalies. The anomalous LCX artery always coursed posterior to the aorta to reach its normal distribution and its course was typical in all our patients. This anomaly alone causes no functional impairment of the myocardium, and it is therefore considered benign [19].

The single coronary artery refers to the origination of both the left and right coronary arteries from a single aortic ostium. In this study we observed three patients with single left coronary artery (0.12 % or 5 % of anomalies). It originated from the right Sinus of Valsalva in one patient and from LSV in two patients (in two patients, the anomalous artery had a malignant course between the pulmonary artery and the aorta).

Anomalous Origin of the Coronary Artery from the Pulmonary Artery is one of the most serious congenital coronary artery anomalies. In our study LCA originating from the pulmonary artery was seen in one patient (0.04 %). In rare instances the LCX or both the RCA and the LCA can originate from the pulmonary artery. Coronary artery origin from the pulmonary artery can occur as an isolated finding, though an associated cardiac abnormality, such as ASD, VSD, tetralogy of Fallot, aortic coarctation, double outlet right ventricle, and patent ductus arteriosus, can be seen in 5 % of cases [20, 21]. Extensive inter-coronary collaterals develop that are often dilated and tortuous. Symptoms usually occur due to coronary steal phenomenon caused by the flow of blood from the higher pressure coronary arterial system to the lower pressure pulmonary arteries. Surgical treatment is usually recommended for this anomalies [22].

A coronary artery fistula is an abnormal connection between one of the coronary arteries and another structure, most commonly a venous structure or a chamber on the right side of the heart. The prevalence is reported to be 0.002 % [23].

Conclusions

The results of this study suggest that CT is a viable noninvasive modality for delineating coronary arterial anomalies. Knowledge of the CT appearances of various coronary artery anomalies and an understanding of the clinical significance of these anomalies are essential in making a correct diagnosis and planning patient treatment.

Competing interests

The authors declare that they have no competing interests.

Authors' contribution

"GrCh had a substantial contribution in drafting the manuscript, performing, analysis and interpretation of the coronary angiography data; DD made substantial contributions to the conception, design, drafting, and critical revision of the manuscript. He gave final approval for publication. KV analysed and interpreted the data regarding hospital admittance. He had substantial contribution to conception, in drafting the manuscript and revising it critically along with analysis and interpretation of MDCT data; DG had substantial contribution in drafting the manuscript, performing, analysis and interpretation of computed angiography data; AE and OF showed substantial contribution in collection and acquisition of data, drafting the manuscript. KG had contribution in drafting and revising the manuscript; DG and AA made substantial contributions to conception and design, acquisition of data, analysis and interpretation of data. He was involved in revising the manuscript critically and gave final approval for publication." All authors read and approved the final manuscript.

Authors' information

Not applicable.

Acknowledgements

There are not any acknowledgements.

References

1. Alexander RW, Griffith GC. Anomalies of the coronary arteries and their clinical significance. Circulation. 1956;14:800–5.
2. Engel HJ, Torres C, Page HL. Major variations in anatomical origin of the coronary arteries: angiographic observations in 4250 patients without congenital heart disease. Cathet Cardiovasc Diagn. 1975;1:157–69.
3. Datta J, White CS, Gilkeson RC, Meyer CA, Kansal S, Jani ML, et al. Anomalous coronary arteries in adults: Depiction at multidetector row CT angiography. Radiology. 2005;235(3):812–8. Epub 2005 Apr 15.
4. Maron BJ. Sudden death in young athletes. N Engl J Med. 2003;349:1064–75.
5. Kaku B, Shimizu M, Yoshio H, Ino H, Mizuno S, Kanaya H, et al. Clinical features of prognosis of Japanese patients with anomalous origin of the coronary artery. Jpn Circ J. 1996; 60:731–41.
6. Kardos A, Babai L, Rudas L, Gaál T, Horváth T, Tálosi L, et al. Epidemiology of congenital coronary artery anomalies: a coronary arteriography study on a central European population. Cathet Cardiovasc Diagn. 1997;42:270–5.
7. Harikrishnan S, Jacob SP, Tharakan J, Titus T, Kumar VK, Bhat A, et al. Congenital coronary anomalies of origin and distribution in adults: a coronary arteriographic study. Indian Heart J. 2002;54:271–5.
8. Yamanaka O, Hobbs RE. Coronary artery anomalies in 126,595 patients undergoing coronary arteriography. Cathet Cardiovasc Diagn. 1990;21:28–40.
9. de Jonge GJ, van Ooijen PM, Piers LH, Dikkers R, Tio RA, Willems TP, et al. Visualization of anomalous coronary arteries on dual-source computed tomography. Eur Radiol. 2008;18:2425–32.
10. Cademartiri F, La Grutta L, Malagò R, Alberghina F, Meijboom WB, Pugliese F, et al. Prevalence of anatomical variants and coronary anomalies in 543 consecutive patients studied with 64-slice CT coronary angiography. Eur Radiol. 2008;18:781–91.
11. Shi H, Aschoff AJ, Brambs HJ, Hoffmann MH. Multislice CT imaging of anomalous coronary arteries. Eur Radiol. 2004;14(12):2172–81. Epub 2004 Oct 15.
12. Schmitt R, Froehner S, Brunn J, Wagner M, Brunner H, Cherevatyy O, et al. Congenital anomalies of the coronary arteries: Imaging with contrast-enhanced, multidetector computed tomography. Eur Radiol. 2005;15(6):1110–21. Epub 2005 Mar 9.
13. Srinivasan KG, Gaikwad A, Kannan BR, Ritesh K, Ushanandini KP. Congenital coronary artery anomalies: diagnosis with 64 slice multidetector row computed tomography coronary angiography: a single-centre study. J Med Imaging Radiat Oncol. 2008;52:148–54.
14. Kim SY, Seo JB, Do KH, Heo JN, Lee JS, Song JW, et al. Coronary artery anomalies: classification and ecg-gated multi–detector row CT findings with angiographic correlation. Radiographics. 2006;26:317–33.
15. Dodd JD, Ferencik M, Liberthson RR, Cury RC, Hoffmann U, Brady TJ, et al. Congenital anomalies of coronary artery origin in adults: 64-MDCT appearance. AJR Am J Roentgenol. 2007;188:138–46.
16. Vilallonga JR. Anatomical variations of the coronary arteries: the most frequent variations. Eur J Anat. 2003;1:29–41.
17. Roberts WC, Siegel RJ, Zipes DP. Origin of the right coronary artery from the left sinus of Valsalva and its functional consequences: analysis of 10 necropsy patients. Am J Cardiol. 1982;49:863–8.
18. Basso C, Maron BJ, Corrado D, Thiene G. Clinical profile of congenital coronary artery anomalies with origin from the wrong aortic sinus leading to sudden death in young competitive athletes. J Am Coll Cardiol. 2000;35:1493–501.
19. Cieslinski G, Rapprich B, Kober G. Coronary anomalies: Incidence and importance. Clin Cardiol. 1993;16:711–5.
20. Montaudon M, Latrabe V, Iriart X, et al. Congenital coronary arteries anomalies: Review of the literature and multidetector computed tomography (MDCT)-appearance. Surg Radiol Anat. 2007;29:343–55.
21. Angeli E, Napoleone CP, Oppido G, Martìn-Suàrez S, Gargiulo G. Anomalous origin of additional coronary artery arising from the pulmonary artery in complex congenital heart disease. Cardiovasc Pathol. 2008;17:190–1.
22. Dodge-Khatami A, Mavroudis C, Backer CL. Anomalous origin of the left coronary artery from the pulmonary artery: collective review of surgical therapy. Ann Thorac Surg. 2002;74:946–55.
23. Mavroudis C, Backer CL, Rocchini AP, Muster AJ, Gevitz M. Coronary artery fistulas in infants and children: A surgical review and discussion of coil embolization. Ann Thorac Surg. 1997;63:1235–42.

5

Screening for asymptomatic coronary artery disease in patients with diabetes mellitus

Christophe Bauters[1,2,3,4*] and Gilles Lemesle[1,3,4]

Abstract

Background: Screening diabetic patients for the presence of asymptomatic coronary artery disease (CAD) may potentially impact therapeutic management and outcome. We performed a systematic review and meta-analysis of randomized trials addressing this question.

Methods: We searched the PubMed database for studies reporting a randomized comparison of systematic screening for CAD in diabetic patients versus no systematic screening. The screening protocols were variable with the use of exercise electrocardiogram test, or stress echocardiography, or nuclear test, or coronary computed tomography angiography.

Results: The final analysis included 5 randomized studies and 3,314 patients altogether. The screening strategy had no detectable impact on outcome with odds ratios (OR) [95 % confidence interval (CI)] of 1.00 [0.67–1.50], 0.72 [0.33–1.57], 0.71 [0.40–1.27], and 0.60 [0.23–1.52] for all-cause death, cardiovascular death, non-fatal myocardial infarction, and the composite cardiovascular death or non-fatal myocardial infarction, respectively. Protocol-related coronary procedures were relatively infrequent in screened patients: coronary angiography was performed in 8 % of the cases, percutaneous coronary intervention in 2.5 %, and coronary artery bypass surgery in 1.5 %. There was no evidence for an effect of screening on the use of statins (OR = 1.19 [0.94–1.51]), aspirin (OR = 1.02 [0.83–1.25]), or angiotensin-converting enzyme inhibitors/angiotensin receptor blockers (OR = 0.97 [0.79–1.19]).

Conclusion: The present analysis shows no evidence for a benefit of screening diabetic patients for the presence of asymptomatic CAD. The proportion of patients who undergo myocardial revascularization as a consequence of screening was low.

Keywords: Diabetes mellitus, Coronary artery disease, Screening, Randomized study, Stress test, Coronary angiography, Percutaneous coronary intervention, Coronary artery bypass surgery

Background

Diabetes mellitus (DM) is a major risk factor for the development of coronary artery disease (CAD) [1]. CAD is frequently asymptomatic in diabetic patients and is often diagnosed when an acute myocardial infarction (MI) occurs [2]; these acute events are frequently responsible of irreversible myocardial damage, even when modern therapeutic strategies are used [3]. Moreover, when the diagnosis of CAD is made, the prognosis of diabetic patients is worse than that of non-diabetic patients [4–7]. Since an early detection of the disease may potentially impact therapeutic strategies and prevent cardiac events, there has for long been interest in the screening of diabetic patients for the presence of asymptomatic CAD [8, 9]. In 2009 however, the report of the Detection of Ischemia in Asymptomatic Diabetics (DIAD) study has modified the perception of the benefit of this approach by showing

* Correspondence: christophe.bauters@chru-lille.fr
[1]Centre Hospitalier Régional et Universitaire de Lille, Lille, France
[2]Inserm U1167, Institut Pasteur de Lille, Université Lille Nord de France, Lille, France
Full list of author information is available at the end of the article

similar rates of cardiac events in the screening and the control groups [10]. Although DIAD was a breakthrough study with rapid incorporation into the guidelines, it was acknowledged that, due to the low rate of events overall, the power of the study to exclude a difference in outcome was limited. Since then, several other studies randomizing screening strategies in diabetic populations have been published, including very recently [11]. In the present paper, our aim was to perform a systematic review and meta-analysis of randomized trials that addressed this question.

Methods

Search strategy

The PubMed database was searched for eligible studies with no restriction of time in January 2016 by using the terms « (((diabetes) AND coronary) AND screening) AND "randomized controlled trial" [Publication Type] » and the filters « Humans » and « English ». Two investigators (CB and GL) independently checked retrieved titles and abstracts for eligibility and relevant full texts were systematically retrieved for further detailed assessment. The search procedure was repeated in Science Direct and ISI Web of Knowledge (All databases). Major reviews regarding screening for CAD in diabetic patients were also hand-searched. Cross-references and quoted papers were checked to identify other relevant studies. The retrieved studies were examined to exclude overlapping data. Unpublished data and meeting abstracts were not considered for the present analysis because they could not provide adequately detailed data and their results might not be final.

Study eligibility

Studies were eligible only if they reported a randomized comparison of systematic screening for CAD in diabetic patients versus no systematic screening. Inclusion criteria were: *(i)* prospective randomized study; *(ii)* comparison of screening for CAD with exercise electrocardiogram test (ETT), or stress echocardiography, or nuclear stress test, or coronary computed tomography angiography (CCTA), versus no screening; *(iii)* in asymptomatic diabetic patients with no evidence of CAD; *(iv)* with a follow-up > 1 year; *(v)* with availability of at least one of the following events at follow-up: all-cause death, cardiovascular death, non-fatal MI, the composite of cardiovascular death or non-fatal MI. Exclusion criteria were: *(i)* cohort studies; *(ii)* studies performed in patients with prior CAD; *(iii)* studies with overlapping data; *(iv)* studies performed in animals; *(v)* studies performed without final report and only abstracts available.

Data extraction

The following information was extracted from each study: study name and first author; number of patients; monocentric or multicentric study; geographic area; period of inclusion; duration of follow-up; inclusion criteria; exclusion criteria; screening protocol; treatment plan if screening test was abnormal; baseline characteristics of the patients for the different studies (age, body-mass index, gender, smoking, systolic and diastolic blood pressure, low-density lipoprotein cholesterol, high-density lipoprotein cholesterol, triglycerides, type of DM, duration of DM, insulin treatment, levels of glycated hemoglobin, retinopathy, peripheral vascular disease, statin use at baseline, aspirin use at baseline, angiotensin-converting enzyme inhibitor/angiotensin receptor blocker (ACE/ARB) use at baseline); number of patients with all-cause death, cardiovascular death, non-fatal MI, the composite of cardiovascular death or non-fatal MI, in the screening groups versus the control groups at follow-up; number of patients receiving statins, aspirin, ACE/ARB in the screening groups versus the control groups at follow-up; number of patients with abnormal screening; number of patients with protocol-related coronary procedures (coronary angiography, percutaneous coronary intervention (PCI), coronary artery bypass surgery (CABG)) in the screening group.

Data synthesis and statistical analysis

Statistical analysis was performed using STATA version 14.0, StataCorps, College Station, Texas. Odds ratios (ORs) and 95 % confidence intervals (CI) of all-cause death, cardiovascular death, non-fatal MI, cardiovascular death or non-fatal MI, statin use, aspirin use, ACE/ARB use were calculated using the *metan* command. Overall estimates of effect were calculated with a random-effects model. Between-study statistical heterogeneity was assessed by using the Cochran Q chi-square and the I^2 test. Small-study effect was assessed visually by examining funnel plots of each trial effect size against the standard error.

Results

Search results and study selection

We found 926 citations in PubMed. Among 21 potentially relevant studies for which a detailed assessment of the full-text was performed, 16 were excluded. The reasons for exclusion were: studies not focusing on screening for CAD in diabetic patients ($n = 4$), non randomized studies ($n = 3$), studies comparing two screening strategies with no control group ($n = 1$), studies comparing 2 treatment strategies after systematic screening ($n = 2$), and studies with overlapping data ($n = 6$). We finally included 5 randomized comparisons of systematic screening for CAD in asymptomatic diabetic patients versus no systematic screening: the Faglia et al. study [12], the DIAD study [10], the Do You Need to Assess Myocardial Ischemia in Type-2 diabetes? (DYNAMIT) study [13], the FACTOR-64 study [14], and the Does coronary

Atherosclerosis Deserve to be Diagnosed earlY in Diabetic patients? (DADDY-D) study [11]. The search procedure was repeated in ScienceDirect and ISI Web of Knowledge; we found no additional studies that met our inclusion criteria. Further searches using cross-references and quoted papers as well as analyses of review papers on screening for CAD in diabetic patients did not identify other studies. The study selection process is summarized in Fig. 1.

Studies and patients characteristics

Table 1 shows the characteristics of the five included studies. The number of patients ranged from 141 to 1,123 (total = 3,314). All studies were randomized; recruitment was monocentric in the Faglia et al. and in the DADDY-D studies, and multicentric in DIAD, DYNAMIT, and FACTOR-64. Overall, the inclusion periods varied from 1998 to 2013 and the follow-up time was in the 3 to 5-year range. With the exception of FACTOR-64 in which there was a small proportion (12 %) of patients with type 1 DM, inclusion was limited to patients with type 2 DM. Inclusion criteria are summarized in Table 1. The Faglia et al. and DYNAMIT studies focused on diabetic patients with other risk factors; DADDY-D included diabetic patients with high cardiovascular risk score. The screening protocols were variable with the use of ETT, stress echocardiography, or nuclear stress test to detect myocardial ischemia; in the Faglia at al. study, two tests were used; in FACTOR-64, CCTA was used to directly test for the presence of coronary atherosclerosis rather than assessing ischemia. Treatment plans in case of abnormal screening test were also variable. In Faglia et al., FACTOR-64 and DADDY-D, coronary angiography was recommended, while in DIAD and DYNAMIT, subsequent investigations were left at the decision of the physician or cardiologist. The overall quality assessment of the different studies was good (Additional file 1: Table S1).

As shown in Table 2, the mean age varied between 58 and 64 years and the proportion of women varied between 20 % and 48 %. The mean duration of DM ranged from 8 to 13 years and the mean HbA1c from 7.0 to 8.7 %. The distribution of other coronary risk factors among studies is summarized in Table 2 as well as the use of insulin, statins, aspirin and ACE/ARB prior to randomization.

Effect of screening on clinical events during follow-up

Follow-up data were available in 4 studies for all-cause death, cardiovascular death, and non-fatal MI, and in three studies for the combined endpoint of cardiovascular death or non-fatal MI. The proportion of patients with events during follow-up were 3.5, 1.5, 2.4, and 3.9 %, for all-cause death, cardiovascular death, non-fatal MI, and the composite cardiovascular death or non-fatal MI, respectively. Figure 2 shows forest plots for the effect of screening on clinical events. In the pooled analysis, there was no impact of screening on all-cause death (OR = 1.00 [0.67–1.50], P = 0.996), cardiovascular death (OR = 0.72 [0.33–1.57], P = 0.407), non-fatal MI (OR = 0.71 [0.40–1.27], P = 0.246), and the composite cardiovascular death or non-fatal MI (OR = 0.60 [0.23–1.52], P = 0.280). The funnel plots

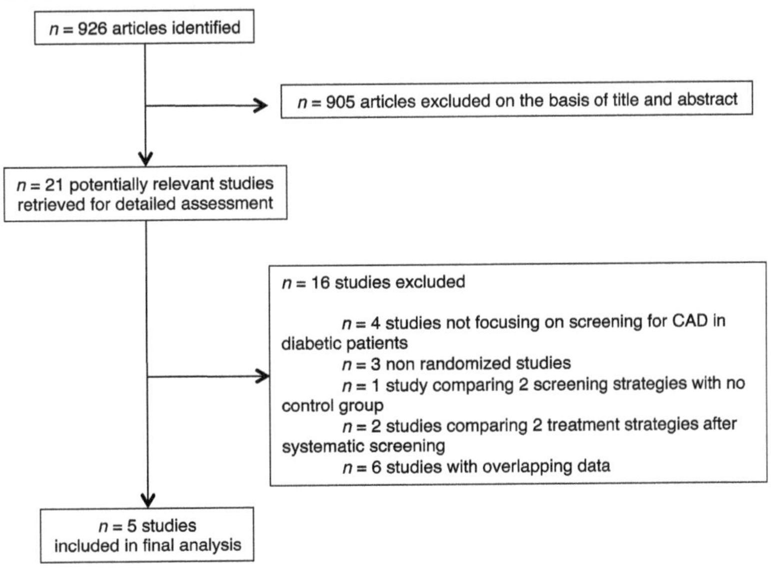

Fig. 1 Flow chart of the study selection process

Table 1 Description of the studies included in the meta-analysis

	Faglia et al. (2005)	DIAD (2009)	DYNAMIT (2011)	FACTOR-64 (2014)	DADDY-D (2015)
Number of patients	141	1123	631	899	520
Design	Randomized	Randomized	Randomized	Randomized	Randomized
	Monocenter	Multicenter	Multicenter	Multicenter	Monocenter
	Italy	USA and Canada	France	USA	Italy
Period of inclusion	July 1998 to July 1999	July 2000 to August 2002	December 2000 to June 2003	July 2007 to May 2013	September 2007 to May 2012
Follow-up	4.3 years	5 years	3.5 years	4 years	3.6 years
Inclusion criteria	- Type 2 DM - 45–75 years - At least 2 of the following: 1. total cholesterol ≥240 mg/dL or HDL-cholesterol ≤35 mg/dL or pharmacological therapy 2. blood pressure >140–90 mmHg or pharmacological therapy 3. active smoking 4. albumin excretion >30 mg/24 h 5. family history of CAD	- Type 2 DM occurring at age 30 years or older with no history of ketoacidosis - 50–75 years	- Type 2 DM - 55–75 years - At least 2 of the following: 1. albumin excretion >30mg/L or >30 mg/24 h 2. treated or untreated hypertension 3. treated or untreated lipid abnormality 4. peripheral arterial disease 5. prior transient ischemic accident 6. smoking 7. family history of CAD	- Type 1 or type 2 DM - Men ≥50 years or women ≥55 years with DM documented for ≥3 years, or men ≥40 years or women ≥45 years with DM documented for ≥5 years - Use of antidiabetic medication for ≥1 year prior to enrollment	- Type 2 DM documented for ≥1 year - 50–70 years - Normal sinus rhythm on ECG - Cardiovascular risk score ≥10 % according to Italian risk chart [11] - Ability to exercise
Exclusion criteria	- Dialysis - Leg amputation - Poor-prognostic disease	- Angina pectoris or chest discomfort - Stress test or coronary angiography within the prior 3 years - History of MI, heart failure, or coronary revascularization - Abnormal results of rest ECG - Any clinical indication for stress testing - Active bronchospasm precluding the use of adenosine - Limited life expectancy due to cancer or end-stage renal or liver disease	- History of MI, CAD, or stroke - Previous positive stress test or myocardial perfusion imaging - Previous negative stress test or myocardial perfusion imaging within the last 3 years	- Any documented atherosclerotic cardiovascular disease - Treatment with an investigational drug within 30 days - Therapy or condition posing a risk for adherence to study requirements - Pregnancy, lactation, or childbearing potential without effective contraception - Limited life expectancy or comorbidity making primary screening and treatment inappropriate	- Prior CAD or heart failure - ETT or other stress testing or coronary angiography performed within 1 year - ECG showing left bundle branch block or ST depression >1 mm or a Q wave - Glomerular filtration rate <40 ml/min/1.73 m^2 - Contraindication to double antiplatelet agent treatment - Life-threatening condition or major psychiatric disorder or active drug abuse

Table 1 Description of the studies included in the meta-analysis *(Continued)*

Screening protocol	ETT and dipyridamole stress echography.	Adenosine Tc-99 m sestamibi myocardial perfusion imaging.	ETT or dipyridamole SPECT in patients unable to perform the exercise test, with a sub-maximal negative exercise test result or with ECG abnormalities impairing the interpretation of the exercise test.	CCTA screening. If the serum creatinine level was 2.0 mg/dL or greater for men or 1.8 mg/dL or greater for women, or if some other contraindication to performing CCTA was present, screening was performed without contrast, and only a CAC score was obtained.	ETT.
Treatment plan if screening test abnormal	All subjects with ≥1 test positive were advised to undergo coronary angiography. All subjects with positive screening had to undergo cardiological consultation and follow-up. All the subjects with negative screening and the subjects in the control arm did not undergo any cardiological workup in the absence of any cardiac symptoms.	None. The results of the screening test were communicated to the participants and their personal physicians.	None. Subsequent investigations (such as coronary angiography) and treatments (such as revascularization procedures) were left at the cardiologist's decision.	Based on CCTA results, patients with severe stenosis were recommended to undergo coronary angiography; patients with moderate stenosis were recommended to receive stress cardiac imaging. Standard medical management was recommended to patients of the control group and to patients with normal CCTA. Patients with abnormal CCTA or a CAC score >10 were recommended to begin aggressive care to reduce risk factors [14].	Coronary angiography was proposed to all patients with positive ETT.

CAC coronary artery calcium, *CAD* coronary artery disease, *CCTA* coronary computed tomography angiography, *DM* diabetes mellitus, *ECG* electrocardiogram, *ETT* exercise electrocardiogram test, *HDL* high-density lipoprotein, *MI* myocardial infarction, *SPECT* single photon emission computed tomography

Table 2 Description of the baseline characteristics of the patients in the different studies included in the meta-analysis

	Faglia et al. (2005)	DIAD (2009)	DYNAMIT (2011)	FACTOR-64 (2014)	DADDY-D (2015)
Number of patients					
- Screening	71	561	316	452	262
- Control	70	562	315	447	258
Age, y ± SD					
- Screening	58.7 ± 8.3	60.7 ± 6.7	64.1 ± 6.4	61.5 ± 7.9	61.9 ± 4.8
- Control	61.5 ± 8.1	60.8 ± 6.4	63.7 ± 6.4	61.6 ± 8.4	62.0 ± 5.1
BMI, kg/m^2 ± SD					
- Screening	27.2 ± 5.1	31.1 ± 6.5	30.4 + 4.7	32.9 ± 6.8	29.6 ± 4.9
- Control	28.3 ± 4.6	31.0 + 6.1	30.8 ± 5.3	33.4 ± 7.1	30.6 ± 7.2
Women					
- Screening	39 %	48 %	45 %	48 %	20 %
- Control	47 %	45 %	46 %	47 %	20 %
Smokers[a]					
- Screening	65 %	10 %	17 %	17 %	40 %
- Control	79 %	9 %	15 %	15 %	38 %
Systolic BP, mmHg ± SD					
- Screening	143 ± 19	133 ± 17	–	129 ± 12	140 ± 15
- Control	142 ± 17	132 ± 16	–	131 ± 11	141 ± 15
Diastolic BP, mmHg ± SD					
- Screening	86 ± 11	80 ± 9	–	74 ± 8	82 ± 7
- Control	84 ± 10	79 ± 8	–	74 ± 8	81 ± 7
LDL-C, mg/dL ± SD					
- Screening	–	114 ± 32	–	86 ± 29	125 ± 37
- Control	–	114 ± 33	–	88 ± 33	119 ± 33
HDL-C, mg/dL ± SD					
- Screening	49 ± 15	50 ± 15	–	45 ± 14	42 ± 11
- Control	46 ± 15	49 ± 15	–	45 ± 13	42 ± 12
Triglycerides, mg/dL ± SD or [95 % CI]					
- Screening	154 ± 105	172 ± 118	–	144 [99–201]	163 ± 140
- Control	161 ± 88	168 ± 101	–	132 [92–198]	161 ± 96
Type 2 diabetes					
- Screening	100 %	100 %	100 %	88 %	100 %
- Control	100 %	100 %	100 %	88 %	100 %
Duration of DM, y ± SD					
- Screening	11.6 ± 10.6	8.2 ± 7.1	–	12.3 ± 9.2	9.9 ± 6.7
- Control	11.3 ± 10.3	8.9 ± 6.9	–	13.5 ± 10.7	10.0 ± 6.2
Insulin					
- Screening	11 %	24 %	–	43 %	23 %
- Control	14 %	22 %	–	43 %	21 %
HbA1c, % ± SD					
- Screening	8.6 ± 2.3	7.2 ± 1.6	8.6 ± 2.2	7.4 ± 1.4	7.7 ± 1.4
- Control	8.4 ± 1.9	7.0 ± 1.5	8.7 ± 2.0	7.5 ± 1.4	7.8 ± 3.1
Retinopathy					
- Screening	56 %	14 %	–	–	14 %

Table 2 Description of the baseline characteristics of the patients in the different studies included in the meta-analysis *(Continued)*

- Control	59 %	16 %	–	–	17 %
Peripheral vascular disease					
- Screening	–	9 %	14 %	–	5 %
- Control	–	9 %	14 %	–	7 %
Statins use (baseline)					
- Screening	39 %	37 %	–	77 %	49 %
- Control	30 %	41 %	–	72 %	44 %
Aspirin use (baseline)					
- Screening	13 %	43 %	–	43 %	29 %
- Control	17 %	46 %	–	41 %	26 %
ACE/ARB use (baseline)					
- Screening	14 %	37 %	–	–	62 %
- Control	14 %	41 %	–	–	65 %

ACE/ARB angiotensin-converting enzyme inhibitors/angiotensin receptor blockers, *BMI* body-mass index, *BP* blood pressure, *CI* confidence interval, *DM* diabetes mellitus, *HbA1c* glycated hemoglobin, *HDL-C* high-density lipoprotein cholesterol, *LDL-C* low-density lipoprotein cholesterol

[a]data are for smokers in Faglia et al. and DYNAMIT, current smokers in DIAD and DADDY-D, former or current smokers in FACTOR-64

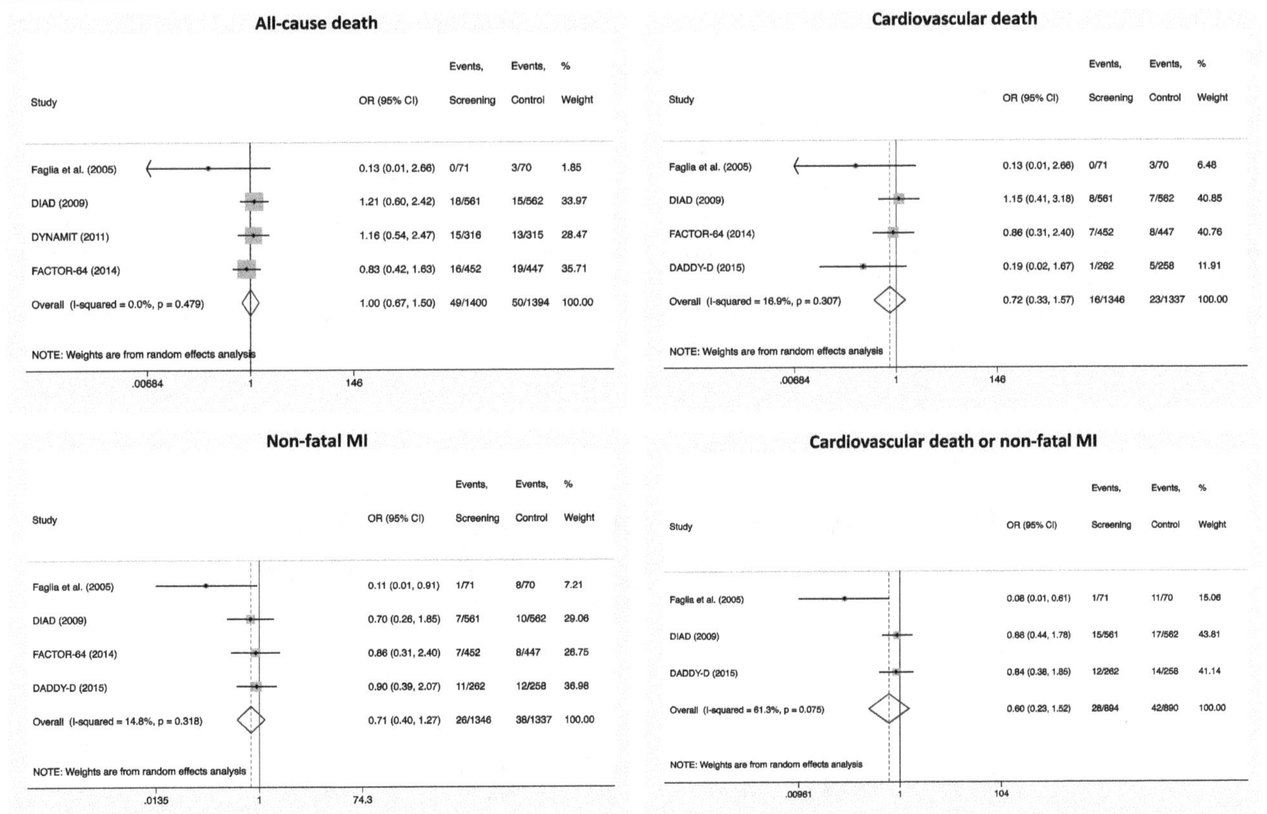

Fig. 2 Effect of screening on all-cause death, cardiovascular death, non-fatal myocarial infarction (MI), the composite of cardiovascular death or non-fatal MI. Odds ratios (OR) with 95 % confidence intervals (CI). For each study, the area of the box represents its contribution to the meta-analysis (weight). Numbers of events are shown in the screening group and in the control group. Overall estimates of effects were calculated with a random effect model

Table 3 Results of the screening procedures for the different studies included in the meta-analysis

	Faglia et al. (2005)	DIAD (2009)	DYNAMIT (2011)	FACTOR-64 (2014)	DADDY-D (2015)
Number of patients in the screening arm	71	561	316	452	262
Patients with positive screening, n (%)	15 (21 %)	83 (15 %)	–	76 (17 %)[a]	20 (8 %)
Patients with abnormal[b] screening, n (%)	15 (21 %)	113 (20 %)	68 (22 %)	76 (17 %)	20 (8 %)
Coronary angiography related to abnormal screening, n (%)	14 (20 %)	25 (4 %)	38 (12 %)	36 (8 %)	17 (6 %)
Proportion of patients with abnormal screening who underwent coronary angiography	14/15 = 93 %	25/113 = 22 %	38/68 = 56 %	36/76 = 47 %	17/20 = 85 %
Patients with significant CAD on coronary angiography performed subsequently to the initial screening, n (%)	9 (13 %)	9 (2 %)	–	–	12 (5 %)
Proportion of patients with coronary angiography who had significant CAD	9/14 = 64 %	9/25 = 36 %	–	–	12/17 = 71 %

[a]moderate to severe coronary stenosis by CCTA

[b]abnormal screening included patients with positive screening and patients with non-perfusion abnormality (ischemic ECG changes, transient left ventricle dilation, or baseline left ventricle dysfunction) in the DIAD study; patients with positive screening and SPECT results showing small defects (uncertain results) in the DYNAMIT study

(Additional file 2: Figure S1) suggested asymmetry along the treatment effect, indicating possible small-study effect.

Coronary angiography and revascularization

The results of the screening and the early protocol-related coronary procedures in the screening groups are summarized in Table 3 and Fig. 3. The number of patients with abnormal screening varied between 8 % and 21 %. The proportion of patients with abnormal screening who underwent coronary angiography varied between 22 % and 93 % (Table 3). Overall, coronary angiography related to a positive screening was performed in 130 patients out of the 1,662 patients randomized to screening (8 %). Among the 130 patients with angiography, half underwent myocardial revascularization, 40 by PCI and 25 by CABG, representing 2.5 % and 1.5 % of the total number of screened patients, respectively (Fig. 3).

Impact of screening on statin, aspirin and ACE/ARB use

Information on statins use after screening was available in all five studies. As shown in Fig. 4, there was no evidence in the pooled analysis for an increased use of statins in screened patients (OR = 1.19 [0.94–1.51]) (P = 0.158). Information on aspirin use after screening was available in 4 studies. Likewise, as shown in Fig. 4, there

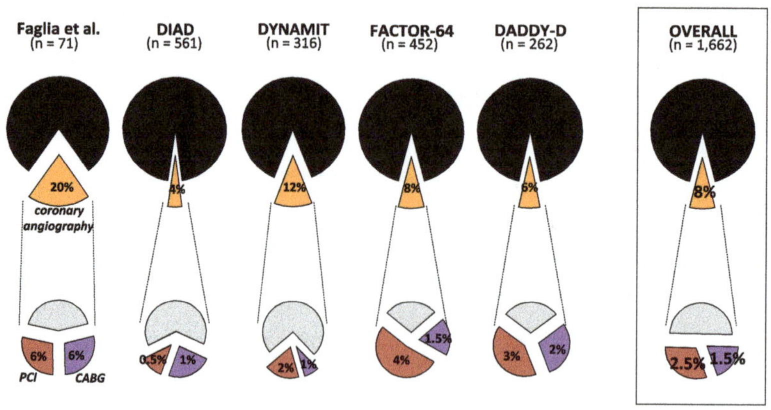

Fig. 3 Coronary angiography and revascularization procedures in the screening arms of the 5 studies and in the pooled analysis. The proportions of coronary angiography, PCI (percutaneous coronary interventions) and CABG (coronary artery bypass surgery) are expressed relative to the number of patients undergoing screening

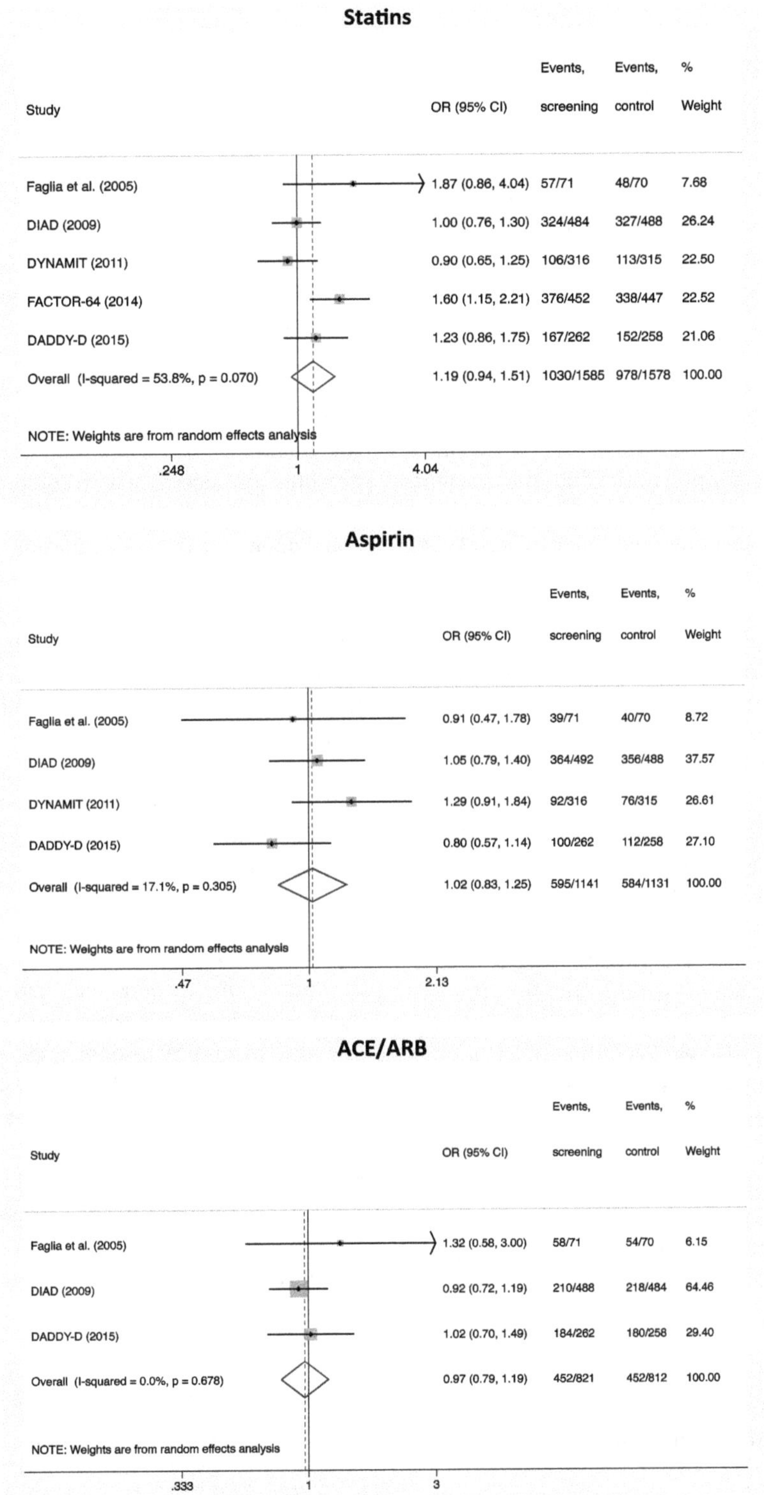

Fig. 4 Effect of screening on statin, aspirin and angiotensin-converting enzyme inhibitor/angiotensin receptor blocker (ACE/ARB) use

was no evidence for an increased use of aspirin in screened patients (OR = 1.02 [0.83–1.25] ($P = 0.837$). Information on ACE/ARB use after screening was available in three studies. Likewise, as shown in Fig. 4, there was no evidence for an increased use of ACE/ARB in screened patients (OR = 0.97 [0.79–1.19] ($P = 0.780$).

Discussion

A significant proportion of the diabetic patients with no clinical evidence for CAD have abnormal stress tests [8, 9, 15] and are at greater risk for cardiovascular events [16]. Screening for asymptomatic CAD in these patients is intuitively attractive as this could potentially lead to additional therapies (coronary revascularization, intensification of preventive medications) and closer follow-up. Several randomized trials have been performed to answer to this clinical question [10–14]. However, the cardiac event rates were significantly lower than originally anticipated when these studies were designed [10, 13, 14] and whether the strategy of systematic screening may improve outcome is still a matter of debate [17, 18].

The present pooled analysis shows that systematic coronary screening of asymptomatic diabetic patients has no detectable impact on the subsequent risk of all-cause death, cardiovascular death, non-fatal MI, and the composite of cardiovascular death or non-fatal MI.

In screened diabetic patients, protocol-related coronary angiographies were relatively infrequent (8 %) and myocardial revascularization was only performed in one half of this group. Although revascularization has not been shown to be superior to optimal medical therapy in the overall population of stable CAD patients with DM [19, 20], it has been suggested that the subgroup with the most severe disease may benefit from CABG [20, 21]. However, even if beneficial for some individuals, CABG in this population is very rare and its impact is unlikely to be detectable in the overall screened group. In the present analysis, CABG was performed in 1.5 % of the screened patients, a figure very similar to the 1 % rate reported in a recent prospective cohort [16].

As far as medical prevention therapy is concerned, our results show that statin, aspirin and ACE/ARB use did not differ in the screening and control groups at follow-up. This is probably related to the fact that, nowadays, diabetic patients have a good background of medical prevention irrespective of CAD diagnosis. Indeed, it is generally accepted that patients with DM have a risk approaching that of CAD patients [22] and aggressive risk factor reduction is recommended for these patients [23]. The reduced plaque burden may consequently decrease the risk of events [24].

The present study has several limitations. Firstly, even in the pooled analysis, the number of events was low and the power to exclude a difference between groups is limited. However, this demonstrates the reasonably good prognosis of asymptomatic diabetic patients candidate to screening, a useful information in clinical practice. Secondly, the study protocols differed widely. Although all included studies were designed as comparisons of screening for CAD versus no screening, the screening methods were variable (ETT, stress echocardiography, nuclear stress test, or CCTA) and have different sensitivities, specificities, and predictive values for the detection of CAD. The screening methods also provide different information for physicians (indicators of myocardial ischemia, anatomical information). It should thus be acknowledged that this is a limitation of our study, and that - if realized in the future - an adequately powered study specifically focusing on one screening method may be positive. In addition, some studies included a treatment plan in case of abnormal screening while, in other studies, the results of the screening were communicated to the personal physician or cardiologist who decided if subsequent investigations and treatments were needed. As a consequence, the rate of coronary angiography in case of positive screening varied from nearly 100 % (when indicated by the protocol) to only 20 % (when left at the physician's decision). Regarding medical prevention, the recommendation to provide aggressive care to reduce risk factors in patients with abnormal CCTA or CAC score in FACTOR-64 is probably the explanation for the increased statin use at follow-up which was solely observed in this study (Fig. 4). Finally, the limited number of studies precluded to analyze how study-level covariates may impact on the benefit of screening.

Conclusions

In conclusion, diabetic patients included in randomized comparisons of CAD screening versus no screening have a low risk of clinical events during follow-up. The present analysis shows no evidence for a benefit of screening in term of outcome. The proportion of patients who undergo myocardial revascularization as a consequence of screening is low; the percentage of patients undergoing CABG is in the 1 % range. Overall, screening has no detectable impact on the prescription of preventive medications including statins, aspirin and ACE/ARB.

Abbreviations

ACE: angiotensin-converting enzyme inhibitor; ARB: angiotensin receptor blocker; BMI: body-mass index; BP: blood pressure; CABG: coronary bypass surgery; CAC: coronary artery calcium; CAD: coronary artery disease; CCTA: coronary computed tomography angiography; CI: confidence interval; DM: diabetes mellitus; ECG: electrocardiogram; ETT: exercise electrocardiogram test; HbA1c: glycated hemoglobin; HDL-C: high-density lipoprotein cholesterol; LDL-C: low-density lipoprotein cholesterol; MI: myocardial infarction; OR: odds ratio; PCI: percutaneous coronary intervention; SPECT: single photon emission computed tomography.

Competing interests

The authors declare that they have no competing interests.

Authors'contributions
C.B., conception and design of the study, analysis and interpretation of data, drafting of the article; G.L., analysis and interpretation of data, critical revision for important intellectual content. All authors read and approved the final manuscript.

Funding
None.

Author details
[1]Centre Hospitalier Régional et Universitaire de Lille, Lille, France. [2]Inserm U1167, Institut Pasteur de Lille, Université Lille Nord de France, Lille, France. [3]Faculté de Médecine de Lille, Lille, France. [4]Hôpital Cardiologique, CHRU de Lille, Boul. Prof. Leclercq, 59037 Lille Cedex, France.

References

1. Grundy SM, Benjamin IJ, Burke GL, Chait A, Eckel RH, Howard BV, Mitch W, Smith SC, Jr., Sowers JR. Diabetes and cardiovascular disease: a statement for healthcare professionals from the American Heart Association. Circulation. 1999;100(10):1134–46.
2. Jacoby RM, Nesto RW. Acute myocardial infarction in the diabetic patient: pathophysiology, clinical course and prognosis. J Am Coll Cardiol. 1992; 20(3):736–44.
3. Savoye C, Equine O, Tricot O, Nugue O, Segrestin B, Sautiere K, Elkohen M, Pretorian EM, Taghipour K, Philias A, Aumegeat V, Decoulx E, Ennezat PV, Bauters C. Left ventricular remodeling after anterior wall acute myocardial infarction in modern clinical practice (from the REmodelage VEntriculaire [REVE] study group). Am J Cardiol. 2006;98(9):1144–9.
4. Malmberg K, Ryden L. Myocardial infarction in patients with diabetes mellitus. Eur Heart J. 1988;9(3):259–64.
5. Bauters C, Lamblin N, Mc Fadden EP, Van Belle E, Millaire A, de Groote P. Influence of diabetes mellitus on heart failure risk and outcome. Cardiovasc Diabetol. 2003;2:1.
6. De Groote P, Lamblin N, Mouquet F, Plichon D, McFadden E, Van Belle E, Bauters C. Impact of diabetes mellitus on long-term survival in patients with congestive heart failure. Eur Heart J. 2004;25(8):656–62.
7. Bauters C, Deneve M, Tricot O, Meurice T, Lamblin N. Prognosis of patients with stable coronary artery disease (from the CORONOR study). Am J Cardiol. 2014;113(7):1142–5.
8. Koistinen MJ. Prevalence of asymptomatic myocardial ischaemia in diabetic subjects. BMJ. 1990;301(6743):92–5.
9. Langer A, Freeman MR, Josse RG, Steiner G, Armstrong PW. Detection of silent myocardial ischemia in diabetes mellitus. Am J Cardiol. 1991;67(13):1073–8.
10. Young LH, Wackers FJ, Chyun DA, Davey JA, Barrett EJ, Taillefer R, Heller GV, Iskandrian AE, Wittlin SD, Filipchuk N, Ratner RE, Inzucchi SE, for the DIAD Investigators. Cardiac outcomes after screening for asymptomatic coronary artery disease in patients with type 2 diabetes: the DIAD study: a randomized controlled trial. JAMA. 2009;301(15):1547–55.
11. Turrini F, Scarlini S, Mannucci C, Messora R, Giovanardi P, Magnavacchi P, Cappelli C, Evandri V, Zanasi A, Romano S, Cavani R, Ghidoni I, Tondi S, Bondi M. Does coronary Atherosclerosis Deserve to be Diagnosed earlY in Diabetic patients? The DADDY-D trial. Screening diabetic patients for unknown coronary disease. Eur J Intern Med. 2015;26(6):407–13.
12. Faglia E, Manuela M, Antonella Q, Michela G, Vincenzo C, Maurizio C, Roberto M, Alberto M. Risk reduction of cardiac events by screening of unknown asymptomatic coronary artery disease in subjects with type 2 diabetes mellitus at high cardiovascular risk: an open-label randomized pilot study. Am Heart J. 2005;149(2):e1–6.
13. Lievre MM, Moulin P, Thivolet C, Rodier M, Rigalleau V, Penfornis A, Pradignac A, Ovize M. Detection of silent myocardial ischemia in asymptomatic patients with diabetes: results of a randomized trial and meta-analysis assessing the effectiveness of systematic screening. Trials. 2011;12:23.
14. Muhlestein JB, Lappe DL, Lima JA, Rosen BD, May HT, Knight S, Bluemke DA, Towner SR, Le V, Bair TL, Vavere AL, Anderson JL. Effect of screening for coronary artery disease using CT angiography on mortality and cardiac events in high-risk patients with diabetes: the FACTOR-64 randomized clinical trial. JAMA. 2014;312(21):2234–43.
15. Miller TD, Rajagopalan N, Hodge DO, Frye RL, Gibbons RJ. Yield of stress single-photon emission computed tomography in asymptomatic patients with diabetes. Am Heart J. 2004;147(5):890–6.
16. Cosson E, Nguyen MT, Chanu B, Banu I, Chiheb S, Balta C, Takbou K, Valensi P. Cardiovascular risk prediction is improved by adding asymptomatic coronary status to routine risk assessment in type 2 diabetic patients. Diabetes Care. 2011;34(9):2101–7.
17. Petretta M, Cuocolo A. Screening asymptomatic patients with type 2 diabetes is recommended: Pro. J Nucl Cardiol. 2015;22(6):1225–8.
18. Gibbons RJ. Screening asymptomatic patients with type 2 diabetes is recommended-Con. J Nucl Cardiol. 2015;22(6):1229–32.
19. Boden WE, O'Rourke RA, Teo KK, Hartigan PM, Maron DJ, Kostuk WJ, Knudtson M, Dada M, Casperson P, Harris CL, Chaitman BR, Shaw L, Gosselin G, Nawaz S, Title LM, Gau G, Blaustein AS, Booth DC, Bates ER, Spertus JA, Berman DS, Mancini GB, Weintraub WS. Optimal medical therapy with or without PCI for stable coronary disease. N Engl J Med. 2007;356(15):1503–16.
20. Frye RL, August P, Brooks MM, Hardison RM, Kelsey SF, MacGregor JM, Orchard TJ, Chaitman BR, Genuth SM, Goldberg SH, Hlatky MA, Jones TL, Molitch ME, Nesto RW, Sako EY, Sobel BE. A randomized trial of therapies for type 2 diabetes and coronary artery disease. N Engl J Med. 2009;360(24): 2503–15.
21. Sorajja P, Chareonthaitawee P, Rajagopalan N, Miller TD, Frye RL, Hodge DO, Gibbons RJ. Improved survival in asymptomatic diabetic patients with high-risk SPECT imaging treated with coronary artery bypass grafting. Circulation. 2005;112(9 Suppl):I311–6.
22. Haffner SM, Lehto S, Ronnemaa T, Pyorala K, Laakso M. Mortality from coronary heart disease in subjects with type 2 diabetes and in nondiabetic subjects with and without prior myocardial infarction. N Engl J Med. 1998;339(4):229–34.
23. Ryden L, Grant PJ, Anker SD, Berne C, Cosentino F, Danchin N, Deaton C, Escaned J, Hammes HP, Huikuri H, Marre M, Marx N, Mellbin L, Ostergren J, Patrono C, Seferovic P, Uva MS, Taskinen MR, Tendera M, Tuomilehto J, Valensi P, Zamorano JL. ESC Guidelines on diabetes, pre-diabetes, and cardiovascular diseases developed in collaboration with the EASD: the Task Force on diabetes, pre-diabetes, and cardiovascular diseases of the European Society of Cardiology (ESC) and developed in collaboration with the European Association for the Study of Diabetes (EASD). Eur Heart J. 2013;34(39):3035–87.
24. D'Ascenzo F, Agostoni P, Abbate A, Castagno D, Lipinski MJ, Vetrovec GW, Frati G, Presutti DG, Quadri G, Moretti C, Gaita F, Zoccai GB. Atherosclerotic coronary plaque regression and the risk of adverse cardiovascular events: a meta-regression of randomized clinical trials. Atherosclerosis. 2013;226(1):178–85.

Genetic deletion in uncoupling protein 3 augments ^{18}F-fluorodeoxyglucose cardiac uptake in the ischemic heart

Sara Gargiulo[1,2,3†], Maria Piera Petretta[1†], Adelaide Greco[1,2], Mariarosaria Panico[3], Michele Larobina[3], Matteo Gramanzini[1,2,3], Gabriele G Schiattarella[1], Giovanni Esposito[1], Mario Petretta[4], Arturo Brunetti[1,2] and Alberto Cuocolo[1*]

Abstract

Background: We investigated the effects of uncoupling protein 3 (UCP3) genetic deletion on ^{18}F-fluorodeoxyglucose (FDG) cardiac uptake by positron emission tomography (PET)/computed tomography (CT) dedicated animal system after permanent coronary artery ligation.

Methods: Cardiac ^{18}F-FDG PET/CT was performed in UCP3 knockout (UCP3$^{-/-}$) and wild-type (WT) mice one week after induction of myocardial infarction or sham procedure.

Results: In sham-operated mice no difference in left ventricular (LV) volume was detectable between WT and UCP3$^{-/-}$. After myocardial infarction, LV volume was higher in both WT and UCP3$^{-/-}$ compared to sham animals, with a significant interaction ($p < 0.05$) between genotype and myocardial infarction. In sham-operated animals no difference in FDG standardized uptake value (SUV) was detectable between WT (1.8 ± 0.6) and UCP3$^{-/-}$ (1.8 ± 0.6). After myocardial infarction SUV was significantly higher in remote areas than in infarcted territories in both UCP3–/– and WT mice (both $p < 0.01$). Moreover, in remote areas, SUV was significantly higher ($p < 0.001$) in UCP3–/– as compared to WT, while in the infarcted territory SUV was comparable ($p = 0.29$). A significant relationship ($r = 0.68$, $p < 0.001$) between LV volume and SUV was found.

Conclusions: In a mice model of permanent coronary occlusion, UCP3 deficiency results in a metabolic shift that favored glycolytic metabolism and increased FDG uptake in remote areas.

Keywords: Uncoupling protein, Myocardial infarction, Glucose metabolism, Positron emission tomography

Background

The family of mitochondrial uncoupling proteins (UCP) has been recognized as being important in the regulation of mitochondrial function and reactive oxygen species (ROS) production [1]. In mitochondria from skeletal muscle, UCP3 was found to be necessary for the fasting-induced enhancement of fatty acid oxidation rate and capacity, possibly via mitigated mitochondrial oxidative stress [2]. Moderate physiological induction of UCP3 protein expression in muscle cells results in increased fatty acid oxidation in the absence of uncoupling, leading to the possibility that it may be involved in protection from lipotoxicity in muscle [3].

In the mammalian heart, UCP2 and UCP3 are the predominant isoforms [4] and have a protective effect in ischemia-reperfusion injury [5,6]. However, the role of UCP3 in cardiac muscle remains relatively unexplored and it is still controversial [7,8]. Animal models over- or under-expressing UCP3, evaluated by ex vivo genomic or proteomic analysis, did not provide uniform answers. Essop et al. [9] demonstrated a marked reduction in left ventricular (LV) UCP3 mitochondrial gene expression following experimental chronic hypoxia in association with metabolic switch from fatty acid to glucose utilization, resulting in an increased reliance on anaerobic glycolysis

* Correspondence: cuocolo@unina.it
†Equal contributors
[1]Department of Advanced Biomedical Sciences, University Federico II, Via Pansini 5, 80131 Naples, Italy
Full list of author information is available at the end of the article

by cardiomyocytes. More recent evidences suggest that UCP3 genetic deletion promotes mitochondrial dysfunction, and increases ROS production and apoptotic cell death after myocardial infarction in mice, enlarging infarct size and accelerating heart failure [10]. However, the effects of UCP3 deletion on glucose metabolism after permanent coronary artery ligation have never been tested. In this study we measured in vivo ^{18}F-fluorodeoxyglucose (FDG) cardiac uptake by high-resolution positron emission tomography (PET)/computed tomography (CT) in a mouse model lacking UCP3 after permanent coronary artery ligation to highlight possible alterations in myocardial energetic metabolism.

Methods

Animal studies

Animal experiments conformed to the "Guide for the Care and Use of Laboratory Animals" published by the US National Institutes of Health (NIH Publication No. 85–23, revised 1996) and were approved by the animal welfare regulation of University Federico II of Naples, Italy. Mice were purchased from the Jackson Laboratory (genetic background-strain: 129S4/SvJae). The UCP3 knockout (UCP3$^{-/-}$) mice were obtained as previously described [11]. Male adult UCP3$^{-/-}$ (aged 8 to 9 weeks, n = 17) and wild-type (WT) mice (aged 8 to 9 weeks, n = 14) were included in the study and maintained under identical conditions of temperature (21 ± 1°C), humidity (60 ± 5%), and light–dark cycle and had free access to normal mouse chow.

Mouse model of myocardial infarction

Myocardial infarction was induced in UCP3$^{-/-}$ (n = 8) and WT mice (n = 8) by permanent ligation of the left coronary artery. Sham-operated animals underwent the same procedure without ligation of the coronary artery at the same time (sham: UCP3$^{-/-}$, n = 9 and WT, n = 6). Permanent ligation of left coronary artery was performed as previously described [12] using a surgical microscope to clearly detect and ligate the small vessel, dedicated microsurgical instruments, thin sutures and needles, and a customized mouse ventilator (Harvard Apparatus, March-Hugstetten, Germany). Briefly, mice were anesthetized with 2.4% sevofluorane plus oxygen, fixed in a supine position on a heating table to prevent hypothermia, intubated and ventilated with a tidal volume of 200 μl and a respiratory rate of about 110 breaths/min. The thoracotomy was performed by a transverse 5 mm incision of the left fifth intercostal space, 2 mm away from the left sternal border, then the pericardial sac was opened and the left anterior descending coronary artery was occluded 2–3 mm distal to the tip of the left auricle using a 7.0 silk suture.

Trans-thoracic echocardiography

Trans-thoracic echocardiography was performed 7 days (range 5–8) after surgery in both myocardial infarction and sham groups using the Vevo 770 high-resolution imaging system (VisualSonics), as previously described [13]. Briefly, the mice were anesthetized with an intramuscular injection of ketamine 100 mg/kg and xylazine 2.5 mg/kg, and echocardiograms were performed with a 30-MHz RMV-707B scanning head. Cardiac function was evaluated by measuring LV fractional shortening [13].

PET/CT imaging

The same day of echocardiography, PET/CT was performed in all mice using a dedicated animal scanner (eXplore Vista, GE Healthcare, Milwaukee, WI, USA). The scanner has a PET spatial resolution of 1.6 mm full-width at half maximum and a CT spatial resolution of 200 μm. The animals had unrestricted access to water and their normal food before scanning. Prior to imaging, mice were warmed for 15 minutes with an infrared lamp to induce vasodilatation of the lateral tail vein. Mice were then anesthetized with a mixture of isoflurane 4% and oxygen 1 L/minute for 5 minutes and positioned in the mouse restrainer. A dose of 300 MBq/kg of ^{18}F-FDG was administrated as a bolus in the lateral tail vein by a 30-gauge needle (injection volume, 100 μL). Animals were maintained at a temperature of 23°C during the biodistribution of FDG. This standardized protocol safeguarded animal welfare and optimized the PET scan with FDG, i.e., avoiding stress for restrain or cold to reduce interscapular brown fat uptake and improve the uptake in the target structure. In addition, it minimizes the risk of motion artifacts during acquisition. After 40 minutes, mice were anesthetized with ketamine 100 mg/kg and xylazine 10 mg/kg (injection volume, 100 μL/10 g). Thereafter, the mice, with the heart centered in the tomograph, were symmetrically positioned on a warm bed with micropore tape, and a 15-minute static PET (single bed position with an axial field-of-view of 4.8 cm; energy window 250–700 keV) scan was performed, followed by a 7-minute CT scan.

PET/CT images were processed as previously described [14]. PET data were reconstructed using a 3D-FORE/2D-OSEM iterative algorithm (16 subsets, 2 iterations, matrix size 175 × 175, voxel size of 0.3875 × 0.3875 × 0.7750 mm^3) including random, scatter correction, dead time, decay, and attenuation correction using CT data. Reconstructed images were reoriented to obtain axial sections perpendicular to the LV long axis and the whole ventricle wall was manually segmented tracing a region of interest in each slice (eXplore Vista Software). FDG uptake was measured in the LV wall volume and expressed as standardized uptake value (SUV): tissue activity (MBq/cc)/[injected dose (MBq)/body weight (g)]). Ellipsoidal regions of interest were also drawn on the right lobe of the liver and on the left triceps brachii muscle and FDG uptake was expressed as average SUV. In UCP3$^{-/-}$ and WT mice with myocardial infarction, SUV was also measured separately in the infarcted territory and in remote areas. Automated image analysis software (MunichHeart) was used to measure LV volume and infarct size on the basis of volumetric sampling of tracer uptake [15,16]. This software allowed long-axis definition, volumetric polar map calculation, and report page generation for the database. Each polar map was normalized to its maximum uptake value. Extent of infarct was expressed in percentage value (% defect area/LV area) by counting the elements in the polar map with an activity below a threshold (50% of the maximum) and relating this value to the total number of polar map elements. The reproducibility and accuracy of this approach for measurement of infarct size in a mice model of permanent coronary occlusion have been documented [14].

Statistical analysis

All data were expressed as mean ± standard deviation. Comparisons between two groups were performed using the unpaired Student *t* test. Two-way analysis of variance was performed to analyze differences by genotype and myocardial infarction among the four groups, including a Tukey post-hoc analysis if a significant F test occurred. Linear regression analysis was performed to evaluate the relationship between LV volume and SUV. A p value < 0.05 was considered statistically significant.

Results

Individual values of LV volume in the four groups of mice are illustrated in Figure 1. In sham-operated mice no difference was detectable between WT (56.1 ± 6.1 µl) and UCP3$^{-/-}$ (58.7 ± 5.1 µl). After myocardial infarction, LV volume was higher in both WT (59.9 ± 9.3 µl) and UCP3$^{-/-}$ (75.5 ± 10.8 µl) as compared to sham animals, with UCP3$^{-/-}$ mice showing the highest values. At two-way analysis of variance a significant interaction ($p < 0.05$) between genotype and myocardial infarction was found (Table 1).

Table 1 Effects of genotype and myocardial infarction and their interaction on left ventricular volume at two-way analysis of variance

	Sum of square	Degree of freedom	Mean square	F-value	p-value
Model	1782	3	594	8.78	0.0003
Genotype	627	1	627	9.27	0.005
Myocardial infarction	805	1	805	11.9	0.002
Genotype/myocardial infarction	323	1	323	4.78	0.04
Residual	1826	27	68		
Total	3608	30	120		

At trans-thoracic echocardiography, sham-operated UCP3$^{-/-}$ mice showed LV fractional shortening comparable to WT (56.5 ± 4.6% and 54.1 ± 4.2%, respectively, p = NS). After myocardial infarction, LV fractional shortening was significantly lower ($p < 0.05$) in both WT (42.7 ± 3.1%) and UCP3$^{-/-}$ (24.4 ± 2.5%) mice compared to sham-operated animals. UCP3$^{-/-}$ mice displayed a significant worsening in cardiac function after coronary artery ligation compared with WT ($p < 0.05$). Furthermore, UCP3 genetic deletion increased infarct size after coronary artery ligation as compared to WT (44 ± 9% vs. 29 ± 7%, $p < 0.005$). Vertical long-axis, horizontal long-axis, and short-axis slices and the resulting polar map in a WT mouse and an UCP3$^{-/-}$ mouse after myocardial infarction are illustrated in Figure 2.

Figure 3 shows individual values of SUV in the four groups of mice. In sham-operated animals no difference was detectable between WT (1.8 ± 0.6) and UCP3$^{-/-}$ (1.8 ± 0.6). After myocardial infarction, SUV was higher in both WT (2.2 ± 0.6) and UCP3$^{-/-}$ (4.0 ± 0.9) compared to sham animals, with UCP3$^{-/-}$ mice showing the highest

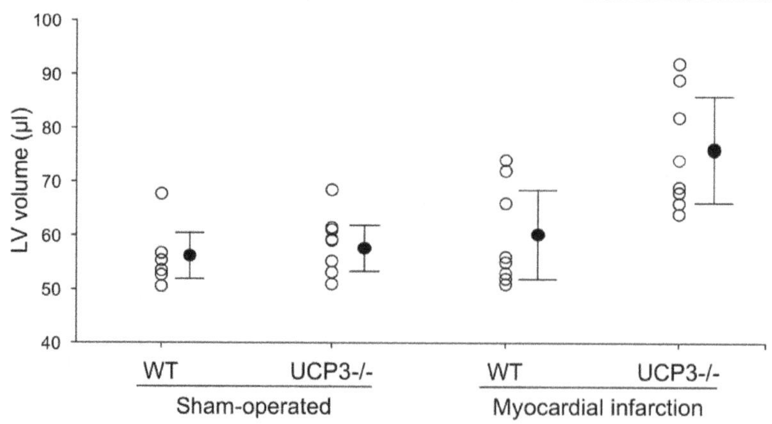

Figure 1 Individual values for LV volume in sham-operated and myocardial infarction WT and UCP3$^{-/-}$ mice. Closed circles indicate mean ± standard deviation.

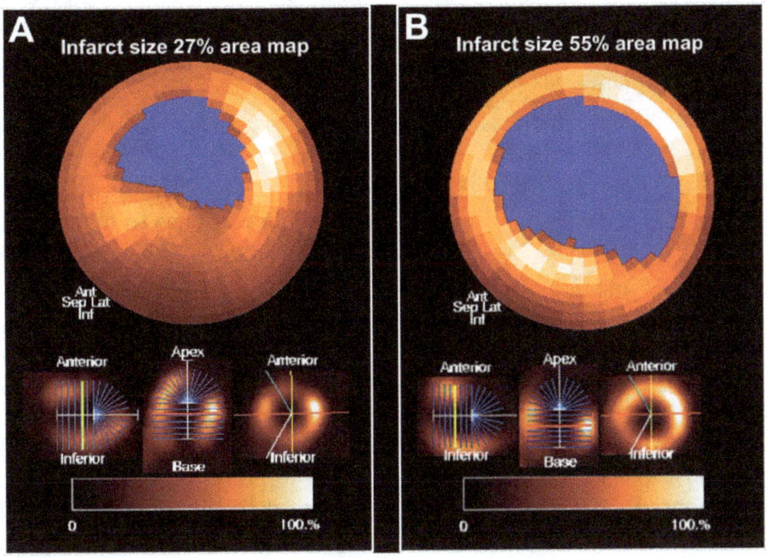

Figure 2 Vertical long-axis, horizontal long-axis, and short-axis slices (on the bottom) and the resulting polar map (on the top) in a WT mouse (A) and an UCP3$^{-/-}$ mouse (B) after myocardial infarction.

values. The results of two-way analysis of variance are reported in Table 2. As shown, a significant interaction ($p < 0.005$) between genotype and myocardial infarction was found. At linear regression analysis a significant relationship ($r = 0.68$, $p < 0.001$) between LV volume and SUV was found (Figure 4). At separate analysis, after myocardial infarction SUV was significantly higher in remote areas than in infarcted territories in both UCP3$^{-/-}$ and WT mice (Table 3). In remote areas, SUV was significantly higher ($p < 0.001$) in UCP3$^{-/-}$ as compared to WT, while in the infarcted territory SUV was comparable ($p = 0.29$) in the two groups of mice. Finally, in non-cardiac tissue (liver and muscles) SUV was independent from UCP deletion and myocardial infarction (Table 4).

Discussion

This study demonstrates that after permanent coronary artery ligation UCP3 genetic deletion is associated with larger infarct size and remodeling and higher cardiac FDG uptake in remote areas as compared to WT mice. These findings suggest that UCP3 deletion induces a metabolic shift that favored glycolytic metabolism. Moreover, the larger area of necrosis and remodeling in response to ischemia in mice leaking UCP3 confirms the cardioprotective role of this protein.

The physiological function of UCP3 is as yet unknown. It has been hypothesized that UCP3 facilitate high rates of fatty acid oxidation [17]. UCP3 is proposed to export the potentially detrimental fatty acid anions to the intermembrane

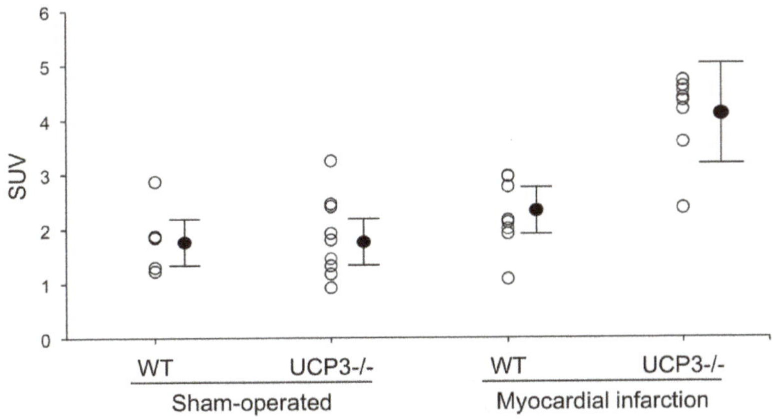

Figure 3 Individual values for SUV in sham-operated and myocardial infarction WT and UCP3$^{-/-}$ mice. Closed circles indicate mean ± standard deviation.

Table 2 Effects of genotype and myocardial infarction and their interaction on SUV at two-way analysis of variance

	Sum of square	Degree of freedom	Mean square	F-value	p-value
Model	24	3	8.0	14.4	0.0001
Genotype	5.8	1	5.8	10.3	0.003
Myocardial infarction	12	1	12	21.6	0.0001
Genotype/myocardial infarction	5.4	1	5.4	9.79	0.004
Residual	15	27	0.56		
Total	39	30	1.30		

Table 3 SUV values in infarcted territory and remote areas in WT and UCP3$^{-/-}$ mice after myocardial infarction

	Infarcted territory	Remote areas	p-value
WT	1.3 ± 0.3	2.5 ± 0.7	<0.01
UCP3$^{-/-}$	1.7 ± 0.9	4.3 ± 1.0*	<0.01

*p < 0.001 WT vs. UCP3$^{-/-}$.

space and cytosol where they can be re-esterified for subsequent use in other pathways. This hypothesis was supported by MacLellan et al. [3] who observed an increased fatty acid oxidation due to augmented UCP3 expression. These results are consistent with the clinical findings of Argyropoulos et al. [18] who demonstrated decreased fat oxidation by indirect calorimetry in a population of Gullah-speaking African Americans with an exon six-splice donor single nucleotide polymorphism in the UCP3 gene. Decreased fat oxidation has also been documented through indirect calorimetry in UCP3$^{-/-}$ mice [19]. These findings support and extend the latter and provide a potential mechanism for the detrimental effects of decreased UCP3 expression in muscle with regard to the development of lipotoxicity and insulin resistance in muscle. Seifert et al. [2] also indicated a role for UCP3 in the adaptation of fatty acid oxidation capacity to fasting and possibly more broadly to perturbed energy balance. In addition, Essop et al. [9] demonstrated a decrease of UCP3 gene expression in rat heart during hypoxia, associated with reduced fatty acid oxidation and increased reliance on glucose metabolism. These data support an overall reduction in the dependence on mitochondrial oxidative phosphorylation in the left ventricle for ATP production in response to hypobaric hypoxia. However, more recent studies have shown that UCP3 is robustly upregulated in skeletal muscle in response to hypoxia [20]. Therefore, the effect of hypoxia on UCP3 expression is still unclear.

UCP3 is expressed in response to reperfusion after ischemia and, activating a mechanism cytoprotective antioxidant, it is capable of reducing the production of ROS and subsequent reperfusion injury [21,22]. In rats it has been shown that the expression of UCP3 is inversely associated with infarct size, probably by activating a protective mechanism to prevent the death of cardiomyocytes in the tissue surrounding the infarcted area [23]. An increased UCP3 expression after ischemia-reperfusion has been demonstrated also in the isolated mouse heart [24] and in the mouse heart in vivo [25]. Therefore, this protein might be a potential therapeutic target for the management of cardiac ischemic disease. During myocardial ischemia, impairment of the energetic activity of the heart is associated with increased level of circulating free fatty acids [26]. However, it has been demonstrated that muscle mitochondrial fatty acid oxidation is decreased in UCP3$^{-/-}$ as compared to WT mice [27]. Thus, it is conceivable that also in the heart the reduced UCP3 levels may lead to a reduction in capacity to oxidize lipids and to in increased glucose consumption. Our data indicate that this metabolic shift is present in remote myocardium where SUV was significantly higher in UCP3$^{-/-}$ than in WT mice (Table 3), indicating the presence of signaling mechanisms between ischemic/necrotic and control remote tissue.

In this study we found that after permanent coronary artery ligation, infarct size and LV volume were significantly greater in UCP3$^{-/-}$ group compared to WT mice. Infarct size is one of the major determinants of post-ischemic cardiac remodeling and adverse outcome. To evaluate cardiac

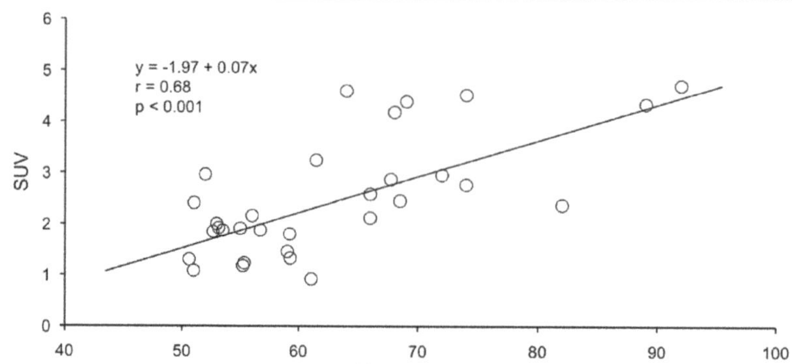

Figure 4 Relationship between LV volume and SUV at linear regression analysis.

Table 4 Liver and muscle SUV values for sham-operated and myocardial infarction WT and UCP3$^{-/-}$ mice

	Sham-operated		Myocardial infarction			
	WT	UCP3$^{-/-}$	WT	UCP3$^{-/-}$	F-value	p-value
Liver	0.42 ± 0.12	0.39 ± 0.18	0.46 ± 0.15	0.38 ± 0.12	0.48	0.69
Muscle	0.78 ± 0.28	0.79 ± 0.24	0.76 ± 0.27	0.75 ± 0.41	0.03	0.99

function in WT and UCP3$^{-/-}$ mice after myocardial infarction, transthoracic echocardiography was performed in all experimental groups. Sham-operated UCP3$^{-/-}$ mice showed LV fractional shortening comparable to WT. After myocardial infarction, LV fractional shortening was significantly lower compared to sham-operated mice in both WT and UCP3$^{-/-}$ mice. Moreover, UCP3$^{-/-}$ mice displayed a significant worsening in cardiac function after coronary artery ligation compared with WT.

Mailloux et al. [28] demonstrated that deficiency in UCP3 resulted in a metabolic shift in skeletal muscles that favored glycolytic metabolism, increased glucose uptake and increased sensitivity to oxidative challenge and these findings were confirmed by FDG uptake at PET imaging. To explore whether this metabolic shift towards glycolysis is present also in cardiac muscle, we measured glucose uptake by monitoring myocardial FDG activity in UCP3$^{-/-}$ and in WT mice with and without coronary artery ligation. Our results show no differences in sham-operated animals between WT and UCP3$^{-/-}$. On the other hand, after myocardial infarction SUV in remote areas was higher in both WT and UCP3$^{-/-}$ compared to sham animals. Noteworthy, UCP3$^{-/-}$ mice showed the highest value of SUV and the results of two-way analysis of variance demonstrated a significant interaction between genotype and myocardial infarction. Finally, we found a significant relationship between LV volume and SUV. This finding indicates that adverse remodeling and metabolic derangement are direct related and that UCP3 deletion has an unfavorable impact on both parameters.

This study has some limitations. First, serum glucose levels were not available at time of imaging. In addition, no dynamic acquisition was performed and cardiac glucose metabolism was indexed by SUV. This approach might have been hampered by the systemic effect of UCP3 deletion on glycolytic flux in the whole body tissues. However, in non-cardiac tissue SUV was independent from UCP deletion and myocardial infarction (Table 4), indicating that blood tracer availability for myocardial uptake was not altered in UCP3$^{-/-}$ mice.

Conclusions

In this study we demonstrate for the first time that, in a mice model of permanent coronary occlusion, UCP3 deficiency results in a metabolic shift that favored glycolytic metabolism and increased FDG uptake in remote areas. We also found a negative remodeling of the left ventricle in response to ischemia in mice leaking UCP3, confirming the cardioprotective role of this protein.

Abbreviations

UCP: Uncoupling proteins; ROS: Reactive oxygen species; LV: Left ventricular; FDG: Fluorodeoxyglucose; PET: Positron emission tomography; CT: Computed tomography; WT: Wild-type; SUV: Standardized uptake value.

Competing interests

The authors declare that they have no competing interests.

Authors' contributions

SG and MPP performed the statistical analysis and drafted the manuscript. GGS made substantial contribution with statistical analysis. GE, MPe, AB and AC contributed with the conception and design of the study. AG, MPa, ML and MG analyzed the collected data. GE, MPe, AB and AC participated in the study design and interpretation and revised the manuscript critically for important intellectual content. All authors read and approved the final manuscript.

Acknowledgements

The authors do not have someone to acknowledge.

Author details

[1]Department of Advanced Biomedical Sciences, University Federico II, Via Pansini 5, 80131 Naples, Italy. [2]CEINGE Scarl, Naples, Italy. [3]Institute of Biostructure and Bioimaging, National Council of Research, Naples, Italy. [4]Department of Translational Medical Sciences, University Federico II, Naples, Italy.

References

1. Mailloux RJ, Harper ME: **Uncoupling proteins and the control of mitochondrial reactive oxygen species production.** *Free Radic Biol Med* 2011, **51**:1106–1115.
2. Seifert EL, Bézaire V, Estey C, Harper ME: **Essential role for uncoupling protein-3 in mitochondrial adaptation to fasting but not in fatty acid oxidation or fatty acid anion export.** *J Biol Chem* 2008, **283**:25124–25131.
3. MacLellan JD, Gerrits MF, Gowing A, Smith PJ, Wheeler MB, Harper ME: **Physiological increases in uncoupling protein 3 augment fatty acid oxidation and decrease reactive oxygen species production without uncoupling respiration in muscle cells.** *Diabetes* 2005, **54**:2343–2350.
4. Bezaire V, Seifert EL, Harper ME: **Uncoupling protein-3: clues in an ongoing mitochondrial mystery.** *FASEB J* 2007, **21**:312–324.
5. Sack MN: **Mitochondrial depolarization and the role of uncoupling proteins in ischemia tolerance.** *Cardiovasc Res* 2006, **72**:210–219.
6. Bodyak N, Rigor DL, Chen YS, Han Y, Bisping E, Pu WT, Kang PM: **Uncoupling protein 2 modulates cell viability in adult rat cardiomyocytes.** *Am J Physiol Heart Circ Physiol* 2007, **293**:H829–H835.
7. Ljubicic V, Adhihetty PJ, Hood DA: **Role of UCP3 in state 4 respiration during contractile activity-induced mitochondrial biogenesis.** *J Appl Physiol* 2004, **97**:976–983.
8. Nabben M, Hoeks J: **Mitochondrial uncoupling protein 3 and its role in cardiac- and skeletal muscle metabolism.** *Physiol Behav* 2008, **94**:259–269.
9. Essop MF, Razeghi P, McLeod C, Young ME, Taegtmeyer H, Sack MN: **Hypoxia-induced decrease of UCP3 gene expression in rat heart parallels metabolic gene switching but fails to affect mitochondrial respiratory coupling.** *Biochem Biophys Res Commun* 2004, **314**:561–564.
10. Perrino C, Schiattarella GG, Sannino A, Pironti G, Petretta MP, Cannavo A, Gargiulo G, Ilardi F, Magliulo F, Franzone A, Carotenuto G, Serino F, Altobelli GG, Cimini V, Cuocolo A, Lombardi A, Goglia F, Indolfi C, Trimarco B, Esposito G: **Genetic deletion of uncoupling protein 3 exaggerates apoptotic cell death in the ischemic heart leading to heart failure.** *J Am Heart Assoc* 2013, **2**:e000086.
11. Vidal-Puig AJ, Grujic D, Zhang CY, Hagen T, Boss O, Ido Y, Szczepanik A, Wade J, Mootha V, Cortright R, Muoio DM, Lowell BB: **Energy metabolism**

in uncoupling protein 3 gene knockout mice. *J Biol Chem* 2000, **275:**16258–16266.

12. Curcio A, Noma T, Naga Prasad SV, Wolf MJ, Lemaire A, Perrino C, Mao L, Rockman HA: **Competitive displacement of phosphoinositide 3-kinase from beta-adrenergic receptor kinase-1 improves postinfarction adverse myocardial remodeling.** *Am J Physiol Heart Circ Physiol* 2006, **291:**H1754–H1760.
13. Esposito G, Perrino C, Cannavo A, Schiattarella GG, Borgia F, Sannino A, Pironti G, Gargiulo G, Di Serafino L, Franzone A, Scudiero L, Grieco P, Indolfi C, Chiariello M: **EGFR trans-activation by urotensin II receptor is mediated by beta-arrestin recruitment and confers cardioprotection in pressure overload induced cardiac hypertrophy.** *Basic Res Cardiol* 2011, **106:**577–589.
14. Greco A, Petretta MP, Larobina M, Gargiulo S, Panico M, Nekolla SG, Esposito G, Petretta M, Brunetti A, Cuocolo A: **Reproducibility and accuracy of noninvasive measurement of infarct size in mice with high-resolution PET/CT.** *J Nucl Cardiol* 2012, **19:**492–499.
15. Higuchi T, Nekolla SG, Jankaukas A, Weber AW, Huisman MC, Reder S, Ziegler SI, Schwaiger M, Bengel FM: **Characterization of normal and infarcted rat myocardium using a combination of small-animal PET and clinical MRI.** *J Nucl Med* 2007, **48:**288–294.
16. Nekolla SG, Miethaner C, Nguyen N, Ziegler SI, Schwaiger M: **Reproducibility of polar map generation and assessment of defect severity and extent assessment in myocardial perfusion imaging using positron emission tomography.** *Eur J Nucl Med* 1998, **25:**1313–1321.
17. Himms-Hagen J, Harper ME: **Physiological role of UCP3 may be export of fatty acids from mitochondria when fatty acid oxidation predominates: an hypothesis.** *Exp Biol Med* 2001, **226:**78–84.
18. Argyropoulos G, Brown AM, Willi SM, Zhu J, He Y, Reitman M, Gevao SM, Spruill I, Garvey WT: **Effects of mutations in the human uncoupling protein 3 gene on the respiratory quotient and fat oxidation in severe obesity and type 2 diabetes.** *J Clin Invest* 1998, **102:**1345–1351.
19. Bezaire V, Hofmann W, Kramer JK, Kozak LP, Harper ME: **Effects of fasting on muscle mitochondrial energetics and fatty acid metabolism in Ucp3$^{-/-}$ and wild-type mice.** *Am J Physiol Endocrinol Metab* 2001, **281:**E975–E982.
20. Lu Z, Sack MN: **ATF-1 is a hypoxia-responsive transcriptional activator of skeletal muscle mitochondrial-uncoupling protein 3.** *J Biol Chem* 2008, **283:**23410–23418.
21. Cadenas S, Aragonés J, Landàzuri MO: **Mitochondrial reprogramming through cardiac oxygen sensor in ischemic heart disease.** *Cardiovasc Res* 2010, **88:**219–228.
22. Safari F, Anvari Z, Moshtaghioun S, Javan M, Bayat G, Forosh SS, Hekmatimoghaddam S: **Differential expression of cardiac uncoupling proteins 2 and 3 in response to myocardial ischemia-reperfusion in rats.** *Life Sci* 2014, **98:**68–74.
23. Laskowski KR, Russell RR 3rd: **Uncoupling proteins in heart failure.** *Curr Heart Fail Rep* 2008, **5:**75–79.
24. Anedda A, López-Bernardo E, Acosta-Iborra B, Saadeh Suleiman M, Landázuri MO, Cadenas S: **The transcription factor Nrf2 promotes survival by enhancing the expression of uncoupling protein 3 under conditions of oxidative stress.** *Free Radic Biol Med* 2013, **61C:**395–407.
25. Ozcan C, Palmeri M, Horvath TL, Russell KS, Russell RR 3rd: **Role of uncoupling protein 3 in ischemia-reperfusion injury, arrhythmias, and preconditioning.** *Am J Physiol Heart Circ Physiol* 2013, **304:**H1192–H1200.
26. Lopaschuk G: **The role of fatty acid oxidation in cardiac ischemia and reperfusion.** *Adv Stud Med* 2004, **4:**S803–S807.
27. Senese R, Valli V, Moreno M, Lombardi A, Busiello RA, Cioffi F, Silvestri E, Goglia F, Lanni A, de Lange P: **Uncoupling protein 3 expression levels influence insulin sensitivity, fatty acid oxidation, and related signaling pathways.** *Pflugers Arch* 2011, **461:**153–164.
28. Mailloux RJ, Dumouchel T, Aguer C, de Kemp R, Beanlands R, Harper ME: **Hexokinase II acts through UCP3 to suppress mitochondrial reactive oxygen species production and maintain aerobic respiration.** *Biochem J* 2011, **437:**301–311.

7

Atherosclerotic and thrombotic genetic and environmental determinants in Egyptian coronary artery disease patients

Manal S. Fawzy[1*], Eman A. Toraih[2*], Nagwa M. Aly[1], Abeer Fakhr-Eldeen[3], Dahlia I. Badran[1] and Mohammad H. Hussein[4]

Abstract

Background: Coronary artery disease (CAD) is the leading cause of morbidity and mortality worldwide. Multiple genetic variants in combination with various environmental risk factors have been implicated. This study aimed to investigate the association of twelve thrombotic and atherosclerotic gene variants in combination with other environmental risk factors with CAD risk in a preliminary sample of Egyptian CAD patients.

Methods: Twenty three consecutive CAD patients undergoing diagnostic coronary angiography and 34 unrelated controls, have been enrolled in the study. Genotyping was based on polymerase chain reaction and reverse multiplex hybridization. Five genetic association models were tested. Data distribution and variance homogeneity have been checked by Shapiro-Wilk test and Levene test, respectively; then the appropriate comparison test was applied. Spearman's rank correlation coefficient was used for correlation analysis and logistic regression has been performed to adjust for significant risk factors. Clustering the study participants according to gene-gene and gene-environment interaction has been done by Detrended Correspondence Analysis (DCA).

Results: The univariate analysis indicated that the five variants; rs1800595 (*FVR2;* factor 5), rs1801133 (*MTHFR*; 5,10-methylenetetrahydrofolate reductase), rs5918 (*HPA-1;* human platelet antigen 1), rs1799752 (*ACE;* angiotensin-converting enzyme), and rs7412 and rs429358 (*ApoE;* apolipoprotein E) were significantly associated with CAD susceptibility under different genetic models. Multivariate analysis revealed clustering of the study population into three patient groups (P) and one control group. *FVR*2 was the most variant associated with CAD patients, combined with the factor V Leiden (*FVL*) variant in P1 cluster and with both *ACE* and *MTHFR* 667C > T in P2. Whereas, P3 was mostly affected by both *MTHFR* 667C > T and *FXIII* (factor 13) V89L mutations. When combined with traditional risk factors, P1 was mostly affected by dyslipidemia, smoking and hypertension, while P2 was mostly affected by their fasting blood sugar levels and *ApoE* variant.

Conclusions: Taken together, these preliminary results could have predictive value to be applied in refining a risk profile for our CAD patients, in order to implement early preventive interventions including specific antithrombotic therapy. Further large scale and follow-up studies are highly recommended to confirm the study findings.

Keywords: Coronary artery disease, Gene variants, Gene-disease interactions, Polymorphism

* Correspondence: manal2_khashana@ymail.com; emantoraih@gmail.com
[1]Department of Medical Biochemistry, Faculty of Medicine, Suez Canal University, Ismailia, Egypt
[2]Department of Histology and Cell Biology (Genetics Unit), Faculty of Medicine, Suez Canal University, Ismailia, Egypt
Full list of author information is available at the end of the article

Background

Coronary artery disease (CAD) is the leading cause of morbidity and mortality worldwide [1]. In Egypt it is responsible for 21% of deaths [2] and reported a prevalence of 8.3% [3]. It is one of the complex diseases that are multifactorial or polygenic disorders, caused by multiple genetic variants with low penetrance in combination with various environmental and lifestyle factors [4]. CAD is characterized by long-term atheromatous plaque formation which culminates into atherothrombotic obstructive lesions leading to tissue damage [5]. Atherosclerosis and thrombosis are the two manifestations underlying CAD. It is known that events such as endothelial dysfunction, inflammation, abnormal lipoprotein and homocysteine metabolism, as well as dysfunctional coagulation and fibrinolysis play a key role in the pathogenesis of CAD [6]. In recent years, several genetic variants robustly associated with CAD have been detected by genome-wide association studies (GWAS), mainly in people of European descent [7]. In order to unravel the genetic profile of a sample of the Egyptian CAD patients with respect to these susceptibility loci, twelve variants were analyzed; Additional file 1: Table S1.

Seven polymorphisms associated with thrombotic risk; (i) Factor V (*FV*): FV Leiden G1691A (R534Q), leads to activated protein C (APC) resistance on the cleavage of factor V and occurs in 20–50% of patients with venous thromboembolism (VTE). It represents one of the most important genetic risk factors for inherited thrombophilia that increases in homozygous state. The contribution of this polymorphism to the pathogenesis of CAD remains controversial [8, 9] (ii) *FVR2* haplotype A4070G (H1299R) was found to be in complete linkage disequilibrium with Factor V Leiden and may confer mild APC resistance. When interacting with the Factor V Leiden mutation could produce a more severe APC resistance phenotype and increased the risk for VTE associated with Factor V Leiden by approximately 3-fold [10]. (iii) Prothrombin, (*PTH*; Factor II) G20210A; the A allele was previously shown to be associated with increased prothrombin levels due to an alteration in the mRNA processing. Its presence with a hypercoagulable state, imply a moderate association with a higher CAD risk [11, 12]. In addition, A allele carriers had about 3-fold elevated risk for cerebral and deep vein thrombosis. This risk increased significantly when combined with FV Leiden [13]. (iv) Factor XIII (*FXIII*) 163G > T (V34L); most of clinical studies have demonstrated a lower incidence of both venous and arterial thrombosis in carriers of the mutant allele (34Leu) compared to Val/Val carriers [14]. This could be explained by lower plasma level of FXIII in carriers of L34 with increased its activation that result in less stabilized and thinner fibrin clot due to easy dissociation of its 2A and 2B subunits [15] (v) 5,10-Methylenetetrahydrofolate Reductase (*MTHFR*) C677T and (vi) *MTHFR* A1298C. The 677TT homozygosity and 677CT/1298 AC compound heterozygote genotypes have been shown to have decreased *MTHFR* activity and higher predisposition to arterial and venous thrombosis in the presence of additional risk factors [16, 17]. (vii) Plasminogen Activator Inhibitor 1 (*PAI-1*, Serpin E1) 4G/5G; the 4G allele was previously found to be associated with higher *PAI-1* transcription rates and considered to be a mild risk factor for VTE and myocardial infarction (MI) [18].

Other five variants associated with atherosclerosis; (viii) Beta-Fibrinogen (*FGB*) -455G > A; confers elevated β-fibrinogen plasma levels, which are directly related to increase the risk of acute coronary syndromes (ACS) [19], premature MI [20] and ischemic stroke [21]. However controversial findings of some researchers that show a protective role of this polymorphism against non-fatal acute MI [22] still present. (ix) Human Platelet Antigen 1 (*HPA-1*; Gp IIIa; integrin b3) L33P (1a/b); studies have shown that, in the normal population, the *HPA-1*b phenotype results in increased platelet aggregation and fibrinogen binding, thus enhancing the risk of MI [23, 24]. (x) Angiotensin-Converting Enzyme (*ACE*) 287 bp insertion/deletion (I/D): D allele has been associated with the elevated *ACE* activity and plasma levels; thereby represents a risk factor for MI in older patients and in smokers [25].)xi) Apolipoprotein B (*Apo B*) R3500Q, that is considered one of the most common single site mutations in the human *ApoB* gene; results in mild to severe hypercholesterolaemia and an increased risk for early onset atherosclerosis [26]. (xii) Apolipoprotein E (*Apo E*) E2/E3/E4; an important predictor of the plasma lipid profile with E2 shows the lowest and E4 shows the highest LDL (low density lipoprotein) and total cholesterol levels; E4 allele was associated with increased susceptibility to early-onset MI, particularly in smokers [27].

Taken together, this study aimed to assess the presence of previously mentioned mutations and polymorphisms in a sample of Egyptian CAD patients and to correlate the co-existence and combination of these variants with the clinical and laboratory risk factors in attempt to be helpful in refining a risk profile for our CAD patients, in order to determine the need for and the intensity of follow-up or to influence decisions about staged implementation of preventive interventions with behavioral or drug therapy.

Methods

Study participants

The current observational case-control study included consecutive 23 unrelated Egyptian stable CAD patients undergoing diagnostic coronary angiography and 34 controls. Patients were recruited from the Cardiology Department, Suez Canal University (SCU) Hospital, Ismailia, Egypt, during the period between October 2015 and February 2016. Diagnosis of CAD was based on detailed history taking via a structured interview, thorough clinical examination, resting electrocardiography and echocardiography, followed by coronary angiography. Patients with congenital heart disease or non-atherosclerotic coronary artery disease were excluded. Unrelated healthy blood donors were included as controls. They had no past history of cardiovascular problems and had a normal resting ECG. They were included irrespective of concomitant risk factors for CAD such as obesity, family history of CAD, hypertension, diabetes mellitus, etc. Selective coronary angiography was not performed for controls following our institutional ethical guidelines that do not permit to apply invasive procedures for controls in research work. The study was conducted in accordance with the guidelines in the Declaration of Helsinki and approved by the Medical Research Ethics Committee of SCU (approval no. 2734). Written informed consent was obtained from all participants.

Cardiovascular disease (CVD) risk assessment

Cardiovascular risk factors were recorded as described previously [28]. Hypertension was defined if the patient was receiving anti-hypertensive drugs or blood pressure exceeded 140/90 mmHg in repeated measurements. Diabetes was considered as a blood sugar ≥ 200 mg/dl on admission, fasting glycemia ≥ 126 mg/dl in two determinants or prior prescription of hypoglycemic drugs. Dyslipidemia was identified if had at least one of the following; triglycerides (TG) ≥ 150 mg/dl, total cholesterol (TC) >200 mg/dl, high density lipoprotein (HDL) <40 mg/dl in males and <50 mg/dl in females or receiving lipid-lowering drugs. Height and weight were measured in all participants and the body mass index (BMI) was calculated. BMI >25 and >30 were considered overweight and obesity, respectively. Individuals who smoked regularly during the previous 12 months were classified as smokers. Other risk factors as lack of exercise and family history of premature CAD (first degree male relatives <55 years or females <65 years) were documented [29].

Multiple methods were used for risk assessment: (1) A qualitative individual risk factor approach in which the sum of risk factors was counted using risk factor categories [30]. (2) A quantitative estimate; "Global CAD risk model" using gender-specific coronary disease prediction algorithm which estimates multivariable CAD risk based on the magnitude or degree of the risk factors [31]. The researchers tried to follow the GRIPS (genetic risk prediction studies) guidelines in reporting the current studied data [32], although our study is not a predictive one, but is considered as a preliminary step in risk assessment in our CAD population.

Echocardiography

A two-dimensional conventional echocardiographic study was performed on all patients using the standard views to exclude the presence of structural heart disease using a commercially available system (General Electric Healthcare Company, Vivid seven Dimensions Vingmed and Horten- Norway) with a 2.5-MHz phased array probe. All echocardiographic data [i.e. the systolic (ejection fraction) and diastolic (grade) functions] were interpreted by two independent experts in echocardiography.

Coronary angiography

Selective coronary cineangiography was performed for all patients using standard, modified Seldinger's technique [33, 34]. Significant obstructive lesions were diagnosed by visual estimation as the presence of ≥ 50% luminal diameter stenosis in at least one major epicardial coronary artery; left main coronary artery (LMCA), left anterior descending (LAD) coronary artery, right coronary artery (RCA), and circumflex coronary artery (Cx) [35]. Basal angiographic characteristics of patients, such as the location and number of diseased vessels were documented [36]. Multivessel disease (MVD) was defined if ≥ 50% luminal narrowing extended to involve two or three major coronary arteries. Vessel scores ranged from 0 to 3, depending on the number of involved vessels.

A modified Gensini score; a quantitative scoring system applied in our hospital protocols, was used to assess CAD extent and severity from coronary angiograms, taking into account the vessel affected and lesion location, the cumulative effect of multiple lesions, the degree of stenosis, and the influence of collaterals [34, 37]. Each item was assigned a number of points. The score for each vessel was calculated separately, and eventually all are added up to give the total score. The following equation was used: severity score x the segment location multiplying factor x collateral adjustment factor [37]. Scores were determined and interpreted by two independent angiographers who were blinded to the clinical data. A Gensini score value greater than 20 was defined as a high Gensini score [38].

Specimen collection and the laboratory investigations

Five milliliter overnight fasting blood samples were collected on both trisodium EDTA (1 mg/ml) tubes for subsequent genetic analysis study and Serum Separator Vacutainer Tubes II (Becton Dickinson Plymouth). After blood clotting, the latter tubes were centrifuged immediately at 2500 rpm for 20 min and the separated serum were aliquoted into eppendorfs (1 ml per aliquot) and stored at -20 °C for subsequent biochemical assay. Fasting blood glucose (FBG), serum total cholesterol (TC), high density lipoprotein cholesterol (HDL-c) and serum triglycerides (TG) were determined by the enzymatic method using Hitachi 912 automated chemistry analyzer (Roche Diagnostics Co, Mannheim, Germany). Low density lipoprotein-cholesterol (LDL-c) value was calculated by the Friedewald's equation [39] as all the study serum TG samples were < 400 mg/dl.

DNA extraction and In vitro amplification

DNA was isolated from whole blood within 2 h from collection using ABIOpureTM Total DNA (version 2.0) (AllianceBio, Catalog no. M501DP100) following the protocol supplied by the manufacturer. DNA concentration and purity at the absorbance ratio 260/280 nm were determined by NanoDrop ND-1000 spectrophotometer (NanoDrop Tech., Inc. Wilmington, DE, USA). Amplification was performed using biotinylated ready-made primers enclosed in CVD StripAssay kit (ViennaLab Labordiagnostika GmbH, Vienna, Austria) [40]; Fig. 1. Polymerase chain reaction (PCR) was performed in a 25-μl reaction volume containing 15 μl amplification mix, 5 μl of Taq DNA polymerase (0.2 U/μl) in the Taq dilution buffer, and 200 ng DNA template. It was carried out in a T-Professional Basic, Biometra PCR System (Biometra, Goettingen, Germeny) at 94 °C for 2 min as pre-PCR, then thermocycling at 94 °C for 15 s, 58 °C for 30 s, and 72 °C for 30 s (35 cycles), with subsequent final extension at 72 °C for 3 min and hold at 4 °C. Amplification products were analyzed by gel electrophoresis (2.5% agarose gel). The following fragment lengths were detected: 134, 165, 173, 202, 223, 254, 283, 324 bp.

Reverse multiplex hybridization

Hybridization of amplification products with saline sodium phosphate EDTA (SSPE) buffer containing 0.5% sodium dodecyl sulfate (SDS) for 30 min was performed to the test strips containing allele-specific oligonucleotide probes immobilized as an array of parallel lines. The strip assays cover 12 variants in the following order: *FV* 1691G > A (Leiden), *FV* H1299R (R2), *Prothrombin*

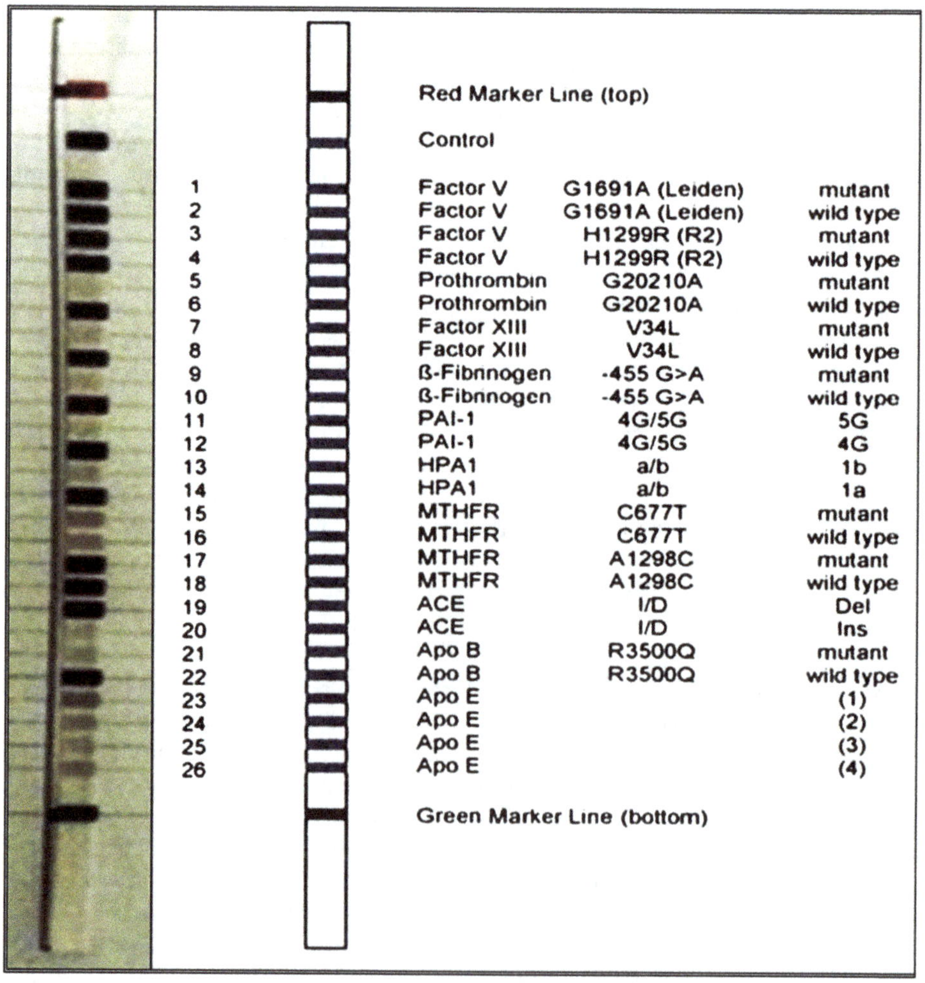

Fig. 1 Design of CVD strip assay test used in the current study (Ref 4-240). The left strip represents an example of the genotype results of a case in the current study

20210G > A, *Factor XIII* V34L, *β-fibrinogeen* -455G > A, *PAI-1* 4G/5G, *HPA1* a/b, *MTHFR* 677C > T, *MTHFR* 1298A > C, *ACE* I/D, *Apo B* R3500Q, *Apo E* ε1/ε2/ε3/ε4, Fig. 1. Following hybridization steps, the bounded biotinylated sequences on the strips were washed with pre-warmed Stringent Wash Solution A (SSPE buffer containing 0.1% SDS) in a microplate thermo-shaker (PST-60HL, Biosan, Riga, Latvia). Then incubated with a conjugate solution containing streptavidin-alkaline phosphatase at room temperature for 15 min. Repeated washing steps with Wash Solution B containing 0.05% sodium azide (NaN_3) was done. Finally color development was performed using color substrates containing nitro blue tetrazolium (NBT) and 5-bromo-4-chloro-3-indolyl phosphate (BCIP) in the dark. Genotype interpretation was determined using the enclosed Collector™ sheet with certain scale. Positive and negative control lines were checked for strip validation; Fig. 1. Positively stained lines were visually noted for each polymorphic position by two independent coauthors and signal pattern of bands were translated into schematic results using stripassay® online calculator [41]; (Additional file 2: Figure S1).

Statistical analysis

Data were managed using the "Statistical Package for the Social Sciences (SPSS) for windows" software (version 20.0) with the aid of Deducer for R-2.15.0 and Microsoft excel 2016. Hardy-Weinberg equilibrium in patients and controls was estimated using the Online Encyclopedia for Genetic Epidemiology (OEGE) software [42]. Pairwise linkage disequilibrium (LD) based on the genotyping data was computed using Haploview software version 4.1. Five genetic association models were used; allelic model, homozygote and heterozygote comparison, dominant and recessive models [43]. Categorical variables were compared using the chi-square ($\chi 2$) or Fisher's exact tests where appropriate, while the Student s t test was used to compare continuous variables between two groups in case the data distribution was concordant with normal distribution (Shapiro-Wilk test) and after checking variance homogeneity (Levene test). If the data did not meet the criteria mentioned above, the non-parametric Mann Whitney-U (MW) and Kruskal-Wallis tests were applied. Spearman's rank correlation coefficient was used for correlation analysis. A two-tailed p-value of < 0.05 was considered statistically significant. Logistic regression has been performed to adjust for significant risk factors using the backward method. For clustering the study participants according to gene-gene and gene-environment interaction, Detrended Correspondence Analysis (DCA) was implemented in PC-ORD version 5, using the default number of segments 26 and rescaling axes [44].

Results

Baseline characteristics of the study population

The general clinical and biochemical characteristics of the study groups are shown in Table 1. A total of 23 patients (17 men and 6 women) had undergone coronary angiography, while 34 apparently healthy subjects were assigned to the control group. There was no significant difference in the frequency of traditional risk factors of cardiovascular disease between patients and controls (as gender, obesity, family history of CAD, and diabetes mellitus). None of the controls were smokers or hypertensive. However, CAD patients had significantly higher glucose levels and worse lipid profile than controls ($p \leq 0.001$). A higher proportion of patients had significantly over three traditional risk factors compared to controls (60.9 and 5.9%, respectively). Coronary angiography revealed that fifth of patients (21.7%) had no occlusion and only 15 out of 23 patients had significant stenosis (≥50% occlusion); 40% (6/15) of whom had complete luminal occlusion. In addition, nearly two-thirds (10/18) of patients with luminal occlusion, had multivessel disease.

Genotype analysis of thrombotic and atherosclerotic variants

The observed genotype distribution of thrombotic and atherosclerotic genes were in agreement with Hardy-Weinberg equilibrium in both patients and controls ($p > 0.05$). However, genotype frequencies of *MTHFR* 667C > T in the CAD group and *ACE* I/D in the control group deviated significantly from the HWE ($p = 0.041$ and 0.001, respectively), possibly due to low sample size.

Among the studied genes, both coagulation factor II (rs1799963) and ApoB100 (rs5742904) variants were normal in all patients and controls, thus they were excluded from further analyses. As shown in Tables 2 and 3, the univariate model indicated that the 5 SNPs (1) rs1800595 (*FVR*), (2) rs1801133 (*MTHFR*), (3) rs5918 (*HPA-1*), (4) rs1799752 (*ACE*), and (5) rs7412 and rs429358 (*ApoE*) were significantly associated with CAD disease under different genetic association models. The heterozygote genotype of *FVR* 4070A > G was significantly higher in patients than controls ($p = 0.024$) with OR (95% CI) of 4.8 (1.2 to 18.3) and 3.8 (1.12–13.5) under heterozygote comparison and allelic models, respectively. The mutant homozygote TT genotype of *MTHFR* 667C > T also showed higher liability of CAD under homozygote comparison and allelic models. Carriers of the *HPA-1* b allele were more frequent among patients (0.26) compared to control group (0.12), ($p = 0.048$). *ACE* D/D genotype and D allele were more prevalent in CAD patients with OR showing higher susceptibility to develop CAD. Whereas, *ApoE* E2 variant showed protection against developing CAD (0.32 in controls compared to 0.13 in patients group, $p = 0.004$), while E3 and E4 individuals were >3 times more liable

Table 1 Clinical and biochemical characteristics of CAD patients and controls

Characteristics	Controls ($n = 34$)	Patients ($n = 23$)	p value	OR (95% CI)
Age, mean (y)	54.7 ± 10.1	54.0 ± 10.1	0.810	
Gender				
Females	16 (47.1)	6 (26.1)	0.166	*Reference*
Males	18 (52.9)	17 (73.9)		2.51 (0.79–7.94)
BMI, kg/m^2	27.7 ± 1.86	28.1 ± 2.07	0.435	
Obesity	6 (17.6)	5 (21.7)	0.742	1.29 (0.34–4.88)
Smoking	–	13 (56.5)		
FH CAD	12 (35.3)	6 (26.1)	0.567	0.64 (0.20–2.07)
Hypertension	–	10 (43.5)		
Diabetes	12 (35.3)	7 (30.4)	0.780	0.82 (0.25–2.49)
Dyslipidemia	–	19 (82.6)		
Biochemical data				
FBS (mg/dl)	99.4 ± 25.7	145.6 ± 62.2	**<0.001**	
TC (mg/dl)	170 ± 18.4	207 ± 61.5	**0.001**	
TG (mg/dl)	103 ± 33.1	155 ± 54.4	**<0.001**	
LDL-c (mg/dl)	74.9 ± 12.6	147 ± 66.3	**<0.001**	
HDL-c (mg/dl)	48.6 ± 8.3	37.8 ± 11.4	**<0.001**	
No of risk factors				
≤ 3	32 (94.1)	9 (39.1)	**<0.001**	*Reference*
> 3	2 (5.9)	14 (60.9)		**24.8 (4.75–130)**
Premature CAD	–	9 (39.1)		
Previous events	–	18 (78.3)		
Stroke	–	1 (4.3)		
Lesion type				
100% Normal	–	5 (21.7)		
< 50% Occlusion	–	3 (13.0)		
50- 99% Occlusion	–	9 (39.2)		
100% Occlusion	–	6 (26.1)		
Lesion site				
Single VD	–	8 (34.8)		
Two VD	–	4 (17.4)		
Three VD	–	6 (26.1)		
CAD severity				
Gensini score	–	14 (1.5–62)		
Vessel score	–	1.0 (0.0–3.0)		
Echo findings				
Ejection fraction	–	57.4 ± 7.98		
Mild DD	–	20 (87.0)		
SWMA	–	9 (39.1)		

Values are shown as a number (percentage), mean ± standard deviation, or median (quartiles). *CAD* coronary artery disease; *OR (95% CI)*, Odds ratio (95% confidence interval); *FH* family history, *FBS* fasting blood sugar, *TC* total cholesterol, *TG* triglycerides, *LDL-c* low density lipoprotein-cholesterol, *HDL-c* high density lipoprotein-cholesterol; Risk factors, Age (men ≥ 45 y and women ≥ 55 y), family history of premature coronary artery disease, hypertension, cigarette smoking, diabetes, hypercholesterolemia, low HDL cholesterol <40 mg/dl, hypertriglyceridemia > 200 mg/dl, and obesity; Premature coronary artery disease, <55 years in males and <65 years in females; previous events, previous acute coronary ischemic events; *VD* vessel disease (defined as luminal narrowing of > 70%); Gensini score to asses disease severity; *DD* diastolic dysfunction; *SWMA*, systolic wall motion abnormalities. *P* value was generated by using Fisher's exact test, and Student's t tests. The bold data are statistically significant at $p < 0.05$

Table 2 Genotype and allele frequencies of thrombotic gene variants in the study population

SNP	Genotypes	Controls ($n = 34$)	Patients ($n = 23$)	*P* values	Crude OR (95% CI)	Adjusted OR (95% CI)
FV: Leiden	Normal	32 (94.1)	20 (87.0)	0.384	1.0	1.0
1691G > A	Hetero	2 (5.9)	3 (13.0)		2.4 (0.3–15.6)	3.08 (0.3–26.3)
	p HWE	0.859	0.737			
	MAF (A)	0.03	0.07	0.359	0.4 (0.05–3.1)	
FV: R2	Normal	30 (8 8.2)	14 (60.9)	**0.024**	1.0	1.0
H1299R	Hetero	4 (11.8)	9 (39.1)		**4.8 (1.2–18.3)**	**7.1 (1.49–33.6)**
4070A > G	*p* HWE	0.715	0.243			
	MAF (G)	0.06	0.20	**0.024**	**3.8 (1.12–13.5)**	
FII: PTH	Normal	34 (100)	23 (100)	NA	NA	
20210G > A	*p* HWE	NA	NA			
FXIII	Normal	30 (88.2)	17 (73.9)	0.287	1.0	1.0
V34L	Hetero	4 (11.8)	6 (26.1)		2.6 (0.6–10.7)	2.29 (0.48–1.5)
	p HWE	0.715	0.471			
	MAF (T)	0.06	0.13	0.185	0.4 (0.09–1.6)	
MTHFR	Normal	22 (64.7)	12 (52.2)	**0.017**	1.0	1.0
677C > T	Hetero	12 (35.3)	6 (26.1)		0.9 (0.2–3.1)	0.82 (0.21–3.3)
	Homo	0 (0.0)	5 (21.7)		**19 (1.0–388)**	
	Dominant model	12 (35.3)	11 (47.8)		1.6 (0.5–4.9)	
	p HWE	0.211	**0.041**			
	MAF (T)	0.18	0.35	**0.037**	**2.4 (1.04–5.9)**	
MTHFR	Normal	10 (29.4)	8 (34.8)	0.648	1.0	1.0
1298A > C	Hetero	16 (47.1)	8 (34.8)		0.6 (0.1–2.2)	0.87 (0.21–3.6)
	Homo	8 (23.5)	7 (30.4)		1.1 (0.2–4.3)	1.46 (0.33–6.4)
	Dominant model	24 (70.6)	15 (65.2)		0.7 (0.2–2.4)	
	p HWE	0.745	0.146			
	MAF (C)	0.47	0.48	0.935	0.9 (0.4–2.1)	
PAI-1	4G/4G	10 (29.4)	7 (30.4)	0.698	1.0	1.0
4G/5G	4G/5G	18 (52.9)	10 (43.5)		0.7 (0.2–2.7)	1.15 (0.24–5.3)
	5G/5G	6 (17.6)	6 (26.1)		1.4 (0.3–6.3)	1.36 (0.27–6.8)
	Dominant model	24 (70.5)	16 (69.6)		0.9 (0.3–3.0)	
	p HWE	0.667	0.536			
	MAF (5G)	0.44	0.48	0.696	0.8 (0.4–1.8)	

FV coagulation factor 5, *PTH* Prothrombin, *FXIII* coagulation factor 13, *MTHFR* Methylenetetrahydrofolate reductase, *PAI-1* plasminogen activator inhibitor-1
Fisher's Exact and Chi-square tests were used; adjusted by potential confounders (gender, age, BMI, FH, DM, obesity). Bold values indicate statistically significant at $p < 0.05$

to have the disease compared to E2 carriers. The adjusted odds ratio for conventional risk factors (gender, age, BMI, family history of heart disease, diabetes, and obesity) further demonstrated that *FVR**AG, *HPA-1* b/b, and *ACE** DD genotypes are independent risk factors for occurrence of CAD.

Among the studied genes, four polymorphisms are located on chromosome 1: *FVL* (rs6025), *FVR* (rs1800595), *MTHFR* (rs1801133), and *MTHFR* (rs1801131). Haplotype analysis showed the presence of two blocks; block 1 included 667C > T and 1298A > C SNPs of *MTHFR* gene and block 2 involving *F5: Leiden* 1691G > A and *F5: R2* 4070A > G. The marker locations and LD block structure of the haplotype blocks are shown in Fig. 2. Our analysis revealed a significant difference in the distribution of GA haplotype in block 2 between cases and controls ($p = 0.039$), Table 4.

Interaction of both gene variants and traditional risk factors with disease risk

Genotype frequencies of variants in patients and controls stratified by cardiovascular risk factors are

Table 3 Genotype and allele frequencies of atherosclerotic gene variants in the study population

SNP	Genotypes	Controls ($n = 34$)	Patients ($n = 23$)	*P* values	Crude OR (95% CI)	Adjusted OR (95% CI)
FGB	Normal	22 (64.7)	12 (52.2)	0.636	1.0	1.0
-455G > A	Hetero	10 (29.4)	9 (39.1)		1.6 (0.5–5.2)	0.28 (0.02–3.1)
	Homo	2 (5.9)	2 (8.7)		1.8 (0.2–14.7)	1.65 (0.1–20.2)
	Dominant model	12 (35.3)	11 (47.8)		1.6 (0.5–4.9)	
	p HWE	0.557	0.866			
	MAF (A)	0.21	0.28	0.344	1.5 (0.6–3.6)	
HPA-1	a/a	26 (76.5)	13 (56.5)	0.112	1.0	1.0
a/b	a/b	8 (23.5)	8 (34.8)		2.0 (0.6–6.5)	
	b/b	0 (0.0)	2 (8.7)		9.8 (0.4–21.9)	**4.0 (1.4–6.4)**
	Dominant model	8 (23.5)	10 (43.5)		2.5 (0.7–7.8)	
	p HWE	0.436	0.638			
	MAF (b)	0.12	0.26	**0.048**	2.6 (0.9–7.1)	
ACE	I/I	6 (17.6)	2 (8.7)	**<0.001**	1.0	1.0
I/D	I/D	26 (76.5)	9 (39.1)		1.0 (0.1–6.1)	2.79 (0.3–29.7)
	D/D	2 (5.9)	12 (52.2)		**18 (2.0–161)**	**88.3 (4.3–179)**
	Dominant model	28 (82.4)	21 (91.3)		2.3 (0.4–12.2)	
	p HWE	0.001	0.866			
	MAF (D)	0.44	0.72	**0.003**	**3.2 (1.4–7.1)**	
ApoB	Normal	34 (100)	23 (100)	NA	NA	
R3500Q	*p* HWE	NA	NA			
ApoE	E2/E2	0 (0.0)	1 (4.3)	**0.009**	1.0	
E2/E3/E4	E2/E4	2 (5.9)	1 (4.3)		0.2 (0.0–8.8)	
	E2/E3	20 (58.8)	3 (13.0)		0.05 (0.0–1.6)	
	E3/E3	10 (29.4)	15 (65.2)		0.4 (0.01–13.2)	
	E3/E4	2 (5.9)	3 (13.0)		0.4 (0.01–16.8)	
	p HWE[a]	0.060	0.550			
	E3	0.61	0.78	**0.004**	1.0	
	E2	0.32	0.13		**0.08 (0.04–0.18)**	
	E4 (MAF)	0.06	0.09		0.61 (0.2–1.87)	

FGB fibrinogen beta polypeptide chain, *HPA-1* human platelet antigen 1, *ACE* angiotensin converting enzyme, *ApoB* Apolipoprotein B-100, *ApoE* apolipotprotein E, [a]The number of degrees of freedom for the chi-square is equal to 3 for three allele systems and 1 for two allele systems. *MAF* minor allele frequency. Fisher's Exact and Chi-square tests were used. Adjusted OR by potential confounders (gender, age, BMI, FH, DM, obesity). Bold values indicate statistically significant at $p < 0.05$

illustrated in Additional file 1: Tables S2 and S3. Significant difference of frequencies of SNPs was observed with gender, obesity and diabetes. Multivariate analysis using an ordination method was used for data clustering, Fig. 3. Analysis of the whole gene variants showed a tendency of the studied population to cluster into 4 groups; one control and three patient groups. Among patients' clusters, *FVR* was the most effective associated gene variant in most of our CAD patients, combined with the *FVL* variant in P1 cluster and with both *ACE* and *MTHFR* 667C > T in P2 cluster. Whereas, the third patient group (P3) was mostly affected by both *MTHFR* 667C > T and *F13* V89L mutations, Fig. 3a. With the intersection of genes with confounders and traditional risk factors, more discrimination between patients and controls was revealed in Fig. 3b. HDL and family history were the most prominent factors in the control group. Patients were clustered into two groups showing more effect of traditional risk factors than genes; P1 group was mostly affected by dyslipidemia, LDL, total triglyceride, total cholesterol, smoking, and hypertension, with little contributing effect of gene variants (*HPA-1, ACE, ApoE,* and *MTHFR*1), while P2 cluster was mostly affected by their fasting blood sugar levels and *ApoE* variant.

Correlation analysis between gene variants and risk factors supported the association between these genes and lipid profile, Additional file 1: Table S4. Four thrombotic and four atherosclerotic gene variants were

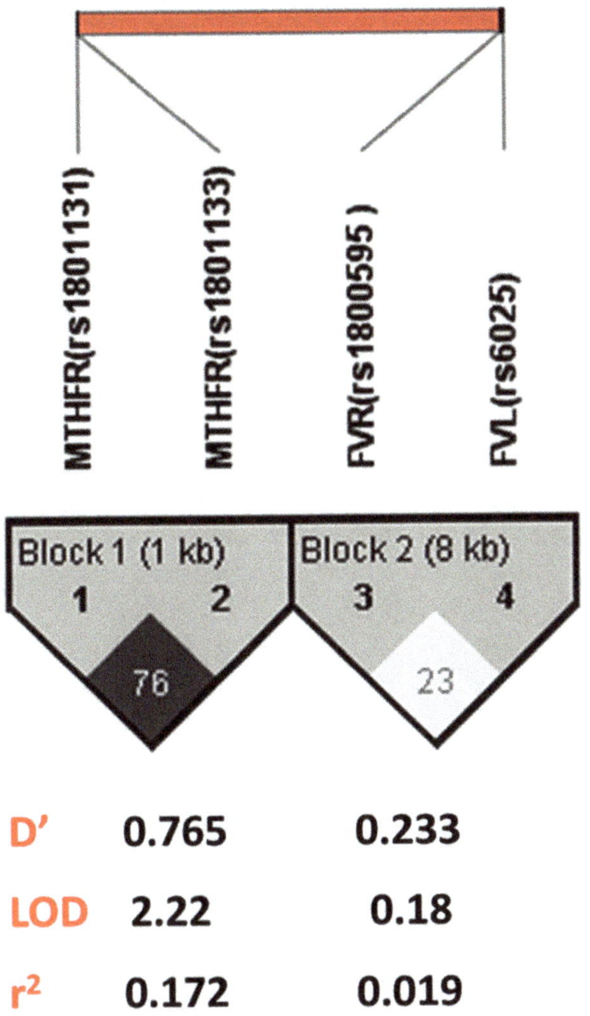

Fig. 2 Estimated linkage disequilibrium and location of haplotype blocks. LD plots with 1 Kb and 8 Kb between marks are contained within black triangles in the figure, and markers order are outside these triangles. Evidence for LD is shown as different shades (white for low D' and dark gray for high D'). The haploblocks were identified using a confidence interval algorithm in haploview program version 4.1

significantly associated with dyslipidemia and lipid profile; *FVR* (4070A > G) with higher total triglyceride (p = 0.004) and lower HDL (p = 0.030), *F13A1* (V35L) and *HPA-1* (a/b) with higher LDL (p = 0.047 and 0.024, respectively), *MTHFR* (667C > T) with total cholesterol (p = 0.004), and *ApoE* with triglyceride (p = 0.002) and LDL (p = 0.017). In addition, similar to DCA plot results, *ApoE* was also positively correlated with fasting blood sugar levels (r = 0.267, p = 0.044). However, *HPA-1* (a/b) variant showed significant association with patients' age (r = -0.352, p = 0.007); youngest age (35.5 ± 10.6) in mutant homozygote individuals, intermediate age (51.3 ± 9.5) in heterozygotes, and later age at onset (56.7 ± 9.0) in normal homozygote carriers (p = 0.016).

Association of traditional risk factors with disease phenotype

Multivessel disease was more frequent among males (p = 0.043) and smokers (p = 0.020). Males also had a higher gensini score (p = 0.048) with OR (95% CI) of 15 (1.2–18.5). CAD patients who had experienced previous acute coronary ischemic events were two times more likely to have significant occlusion >50% (p = 0.033). No association was observed between other traditional risk factors and the degree of CAD at coronary angiography, Table 5. In addition, none of the risk factors showed association with any other clinical characteristics as premature CAD, previous acute coronary ischemic events, echocardiography findings (ejection fraction, diastolic dysfunction, and systolic wall motion abnormalities) in CAD patients (data not shown).

Association of gene variants with disease phenotype

As shown in Table 6, CAD patients carrying mutant allele of *FVR* polymorphism had a lower genseni score (p = 0.04) with OR (95% CI) of 0.09 (0.009–0.96) (r = -0.460, p = 0.027), and lower risk of significant occlusion ≥ 50% (p = 0.023) with OR (95% CI) of 0.08 (0.01–0.64) (r = -0.536, p = 0008). In addition, *MTHFR* 1298A > C mutant homozygotes had a better genseni score (p = 0.035).

Association analysis of gene variants with other clinical characteristics and echocardiography parameters showed *FVR* polymorphism to be inversely related to systolic wall motion abnormalities (r = -0.416, p = 0.048) and *F13A1* (V35L) SNP to be associated with lower ejection fraction in heterozygote compared to normal homozygote (p = 0.020) with moderate inverse correlation (r = -0.50, p = 0.015) (data not shown).

Discussion

To our knowledge, this is the first study conducted to investigate the interaction between twelve atherosclerosis and thrombosis related gene variants and the environmental risk factors that could increase the susceptibility to coronary artery disease in Egyptian CAD patients. The previous studies have confirmed that understanding the gene–environment interactions is very important for the development of novel preventive and therapeutic approaches to reduce the risk of CAD [45–47].

In the current study *FVR* was the most variant associated with CAD patients, combined with the *FVL* variant to increase CAD risk in one of the patient clusters and with both *ACE* and *MTHFR* 667C > T in the second cluster. Because CAD is a multifactorial disorder, its genetic components may be a combined effect of a number of genes with each playing only a small role. Butt et al. [48] have reported that the predisposition imparted by individual genes may act independently or interact with other genes to result in an additive effect or a

Table 4 Haplotype frequencies and genotype combinations of both *F5: Leiden* 1691G > A with *F5: R2* 4070A > G, and *MTHFR* 667C > T with 1298A > C polymorphisms in CAD patients and controls

Haplotypes[a]	Overall frequency	Controls ($n = 34$)	Patients ($n = 23$)	*P* values	OR (95% CI)
Genotype combination: *MTHFR* 667C > T/1298A > C					
CC-AA	11 (19.3)	8 (23.5)	3 (13.0)	0.150	*Reference*
CT-AA	3 (5.3)	2 (5.9)	1 (4.3)		1.3 (0.08–20.7)
TT-AA	4 (7.0)	0 (0.0)	4 (17.4)		21.8 (0.9–523)
CC-AC	9 (15.8)	6 (17.6)	3 (13)		1.3 (0.19–9.08)
CT-AC	14 (24.6)	10 (29.4)	4 (17.4)		1.06 (0.18–6.2)
TT–AC	1 (1.8)	0 (0.0)	1 (4.3)		7.2 (0.23–225)
CC-CC	14 (24.6)	8 (23.5)	6 (26.1)		2.0 (0.3–10.9)
CT-CC	1 (1.8)	0 (0.0)	1 (4.3)		7.2 (0.23–225)
Genotype combination: *FVL* 1691G > A/*FVR* 4070A > G					
GG-AA	41 (71.9)	28 (82.4)	13 (56.5)	0.080	*Reference*
GG-AG	11 (19.3)	4 (11.8)	7 (30.4)		3.7 (0.9–15.18)
GA–AA	3 (5.3)	2 (5.9)	1 (4.3)		1.07 (0.08–12.9)
GA-AG	2 (3.5)	0 (0.0)	2 (8.7)		10.5 (0.47–235)
Block 1: *MTHFR* 667C > T/1298A > C					
CC	0.446	45.9	42.8	0.7437	
CA	0.308	36.5	22.4	0.1114	
TA	0.218	16.5	29.8	0.0926	
TC	0.027	1.1	5	0.2134	
Block 2: *FVL* 1691G > A/*FVR* 4070A > G					
GA	0.856	91.2	77.4	**0.0397**	
GG	0.1	5.9	16.1	0.075	
AA	0.03	2.9	3	0.9767	
AG	0.014	0	3.5	0.121	

MTHFR, Methylenetetrahydrofolate reductase; *FV*, coagulation factor 5
[a]Haploview version 4.1 was used for data analysis. Bold values indicate statistically significant at $p < 0.05$

synergistic coeffect. The *FV:R2* A4070G variant causes amino acid replacement of histidine for arginine at the codon 1299 in the FV B domain. This polymorphism, which marked by the HR2 haplotype was reported to affect the plasma level of FV and contribute to the APC resistance [49]. Although the homo mutant genotype was absent in CAD patients and controls in the current work, this variant confers high susceptibility to CAD risk under the heterozygous and allelic models. Segers et al. [50] suggested that the reduced level of expression of *FV: R2* is the most likely explanation for the enhanced thrombophilic phenotype in *R2* carriers. Although there are no conclusive data available that associate the *R2* haplotype *per se* with a relevant increased risk of thrombosis (i.e. taken in consideration that *FV: Leiden* frequency was comparable between CAD patient and control groups in the current study), it was observed previously that male carriers of the *FV: R2* polymorphism, have increased circulating levels of FVIII [51]. Although there was no biochemical explanation has been given for this observation, it has been speculated that altered FV anticoagulant activity of *FV: R2* results in diminished the proteolytic control of FVIII levels by the protein C pathway [50]. Since increased levels of FVIII are an independent risk factor for the occurrence of venous thrombosis, this may explain the potential association between *FV: R2* and thrombosis. Nevertheless, we found that patients carrying the G allele unexpectedly displayed a mild phenotype (i.e. lower Genseni score and lower number of MVD) than wild-type genotype carriers. It seems therefore that the HR2 haplotype in our population preferentially increases the CAD susceptibility but correlates with mild disease severity. It should be kept in mind, however, that thrombosis is a multifactorial disease in which genetic and acquired risk factors interact dynamically. Therefore, the role that FV plays in the etiology of thrombosis is largely dependent on other factors that influence the impact of any altered FV phenotype [50] and the disease outcome depends on

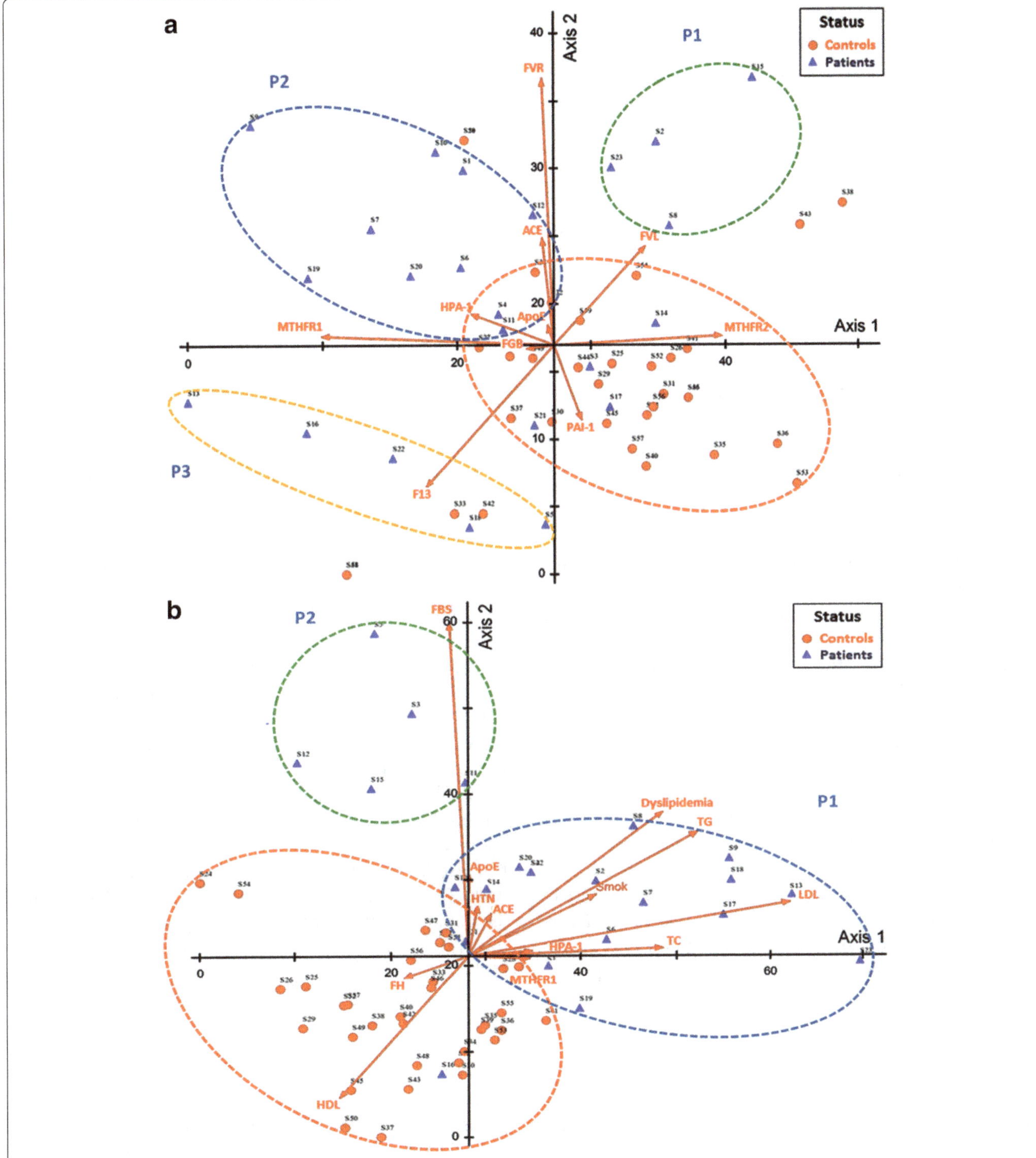

Fig. 3 Detrended correspondence analysis ordination plots showing the distribution of patient and control samples. DCA was done to show the relations among subject groups and genes (**a**) along with other environmental risk factors (**b**). DCA was done after rescaling axes. Red circle surrounds a control group while other colored circles for patient groups. Results were plotted on Axes 1 and 2

the sum of other multiple interacting factors determine the severity of the disease. This finding should be validated in future larger scale studies to be conclusive.

The mutant homozygote TT genotype of *MTHFR* 667C > T (rs1801133) was found to be more frequent among the studied CAD Egyptian patients (21.7%) and was not found in the controls. This variant showed

Table 5 Association between traditional risk factors and clinical characteristics of CAD patients

Risk factor	Gensini score		*P* value	Occlusion		*P* value	No of BVs		*P* value
	Low	High		<50%	≥50%		SVD	MVD	
Number	14	9		8	15		8	10	
Gender									
Females	6 (42.9)	0 (0.0)	**0.048**	2 (25.0)	4 (26.7)	1.00	5 (62.5)	1 (10)	**0.043**
Males	8 (57.1)	9 (100)		6 (75.0)	11 (73.3)		3 (37.5)	9 (90)	
Obesity	2 (14.3)	3 (33.3)	0.343	0 (0.0)	5 (33.3)	0.122	2 (25)	3 (30)	1.00
Smoking	6 (42.9)	7 (77.8)	0.197	4 (509	9 (60.0)	0.685	2 (25)	8 (80)	**0.020**
FH CAD	2 (14.3)	4 (44.4)	0.162	2 (25.0)	4 (26.7)	1.00	1 (12.5)	4 (40)	0.314
Hypertension	7 (50.0)	3 (33.3)	0.669	3 (37.5)	7 (46.7)	1.00	5 (62.5)	4 (40)	0.637
Diabetes	4 (28.6)	3 (33.3)	1.00	2 (25.0)	5 (33.3)	1.00	3 (37.5)	3 (30)	1.00
Dyslipidemia	11 (79)	8 (88.9)	1.00	6 (75.0)	13 (86.7)	0.589	5 (62.5)	9 (90)	0.275
Premature CAD	5 (35.7)	4 (44.4)	1.00	3 (37.5)	6 (40)	1.00	3 (37.5)	4 (40)	1.00
Previous events	9 (64.3)	9 (100)	0.116	4 (50.0)	14 (93.3)	**0.033**	7 (87.5)	9 (90)	1.00

Data are presented as number (percentage). *CAD* coronary artery disease, *FH* family history; premature coronary artery disease, <55 years in males and <65 years in females; previous events, previous acute coronary ischemic events, *No of BVs* number of blood vessels, *SVD* single vessel disease, *MVD* multivessel disease. Fisher's exact test was used. Bold values indicate statistically significant at $p < 0.05$

significantly higher susceptibility for CAD under homozygote and allelic models and it was one of the most effective associated gene variants in combination with other variants for clustering our CAD patients by multivariate analysis (i.e. the combined occurrence of the *MTHFR* 677TT, *ACE* DD and *FVR* 4070AG genotypes seems to magnify the CAD risk in our population). *MTHFR* gene is located on chromosome 1p36.3 and contains more than hundred SNPs, the most studied variants are rs1801133 and rs1801131 that included in the current study. The 667C > T transition in exon 5 of the first SNP is resulting in a change of alanine to valine (A222V) near the FAD (flavin-adenine-dinucleotide) cofactor binding region, and the other variant caused by the point mutation of A to C at nucleotide 1298 of coding sequence leads to substitution of glutamine by alanine at the amino acid number 470 in the protein structure [52]. In silico tools predicted the former variant (i.e. 667C > T) in exon 5 to be deleterious in contrast to the later neutral one. This could explain why *MTHFR 667C > T*; was associated with CAD risk in our population as the enzyme with valine was shown previously to be associated with increased thermoliability and reduced enzymatic activity to about 30% if mutant homozygous and 65% if heterozygous [53]. This reduced activity resulting in hyperhomocysteinemia when folate status is low that has been linked to thrombosis and considered as a major independent risk factor for cardiovascular diseases [54]. Similar to our results, when Almawi et al. [55] studied *FV* 1691 G > A, *PT* 20210 G > A, and *MTHFR* 677 C > T gene variants in angiographically documented CAD, they found a strong association of hyperhomocysteinemia and homozygosity of the *MTHFR* 677 C > T, but not *FV: Leiden* or *PT* 20210 G > A mutations with CAD. The results of the present study are also in agreement with Neto et al. [56] who found the *MTHFR* 677 T/T genotype to predispose to premature atherosclerotic coronary artery disease, and with Yamada et al. [57] and Schürks et al. [58] who reported increased risk for MI and ischemic stroke, respectively. Otherwise, our findings were in contrast to Hsu et al. [59], Yilmaz et al. [60] and Caner et al. [61] who reported that the *MTHFR* C677T mutation was not associated with the risk of CAD or venous thrombosis among Chinese in Taiwan nor among Turkish patients, respectively. These contradictory results between different studies could be attributed to relatively small sample size, low frequency of gene variants and ethnic heterogeneity [50].

The plasminogen activator inhibitor-1 (PAI-1) is a 52 kDa glycoprotein encoded by the serine protease inhibitor (*SERPINE1*) gene [62]. It is secreted by endothelial cells and is stored and released from the platelets during activation to downregulate the fibrinolysis process by inhibiting plasminogen to plasmin conversion induced by either tissue-plasminogen activator or urokinase [63]. The current study functional insertion/deletion promoter variant at -675 position (rs1799889), has been associated with increased risk of atherosclerosis and thrombosis previously with inconsistent results [20, 64–67]. As both the -675 4G and 5G alleles have a binding site for a common transcription activator and the 5G allele has an additional binding site for a repressor, this leads to 5G allele is slightly less transcriptionally active

Table 6 Association between SNP genotypes and clinical characteristics of CAD patients

Gene SNP	G	Gensini score		*P* value	Occlusion		*P* value	No of BVs		*P* value
		Low	High		<50%	≥50%		SVD	MVD	
Number		14	9		8	15		8	10	
FVL	N	11 (78.6)	9 (100)	0.253	7 (87.5)	13 (86.7)	1.00	7 (87.5)	9 (90)	1.00
	H	3 (21.4)	0 (0.0)		1 (12.5)	2 (13.3)		1 (12.5)	1 (10)	
FVR	N	6 (42.9)	8 (88.9)	**0.040**	2 (25)	12 (80)	**0.023**	4 (50)	9 (90)	0.118
	H	8 (57.1)	1 (11.1)		6 (75)	3 (20)		4 (50)	1 (10)	
F13A1	N	12 (85.7)	5 (55.6)	0.162	6 (75)	11 (73.3)	1.00	7 (87.5)	6 (60)	0.314
	H	2 (14.3)	4 (44.4)		2 (25)	4 (26.7)		1 (12.5)	4 (40)	
MTHFR 1	N	8 (57.1)	4 (44.4)	0.558	4 (50)	8 (53.3)	0.962	6 (75)	5 (50)	0.234
	H	4 (28.6)	2 (22.2)		2 (25)	4 (26.7)		2 (25)	2 (20)	
	M	2 (14.3)	3 (33.3)		2 (25)	3 (20)		0 (0.0)	3 (30)	
MTHFR 2	N	4 (28.6)	4 (44.4)	**0.035**	4 (50)	4 (26.7)	0.250	2 (25)	4 (40)	0.167
	H	3 (21.5)	5 (55.6)		1 (12.5)	7 (46.7)		2 (25)	5 (50)	
	M	7 (50)	0 (0.0)		3 (37.5)	4 (26.7)		4 (50)	1 (10)	
PAI-1	N	5 (35.7)	2 (22.2)	0.730	2 (25)	5 (33.3)	0.660	3 (37.5)	3 (30)	0.869
	H	6 (42.9)	4 (44.4)		3 (37.5)	7 (46.7)		3 (37.5)	5 (50)	
	M	3 (21.4)	3 (33.3)		3 (37.5)	3 (20)		2 (25)	2 (20)	
FGB	N	7 (50)	5 (55.6)	0.490	3 (37.5)	9 (60)	0.583	5 (62.5)	5 (50)	0.799
	H	5 (35.7)	4 (44.4)		4 (50)	5 (33.3)		2 (25)	4 (40)	
	M	2 (14.3)	0 (0.0)		1 (12.5)	1 (6.7)		1 (12.5)	1 (10)	
HPA-1	N	7 (50)	6 (66.7)	0.595	4 (50)	9 (60)	0.851	6 (75)	6 (60)	0.610
	H	6 (42.9)	2 (66.7)		3 (37.5)	5 (33.3)		2 (25)	3 (30)	
	M	1 (7.1)	1 (22.2)		1 (12.5)	1 (6.7)		0 (0.0)	1 (10)	
ACE	N	1 (7.1)	1 (11.1)	0.829	1 (12.5)	1 (6.7)	0.894	0 (0.0)	1 (10)	0.287
	H	5 (35.7)	4 (44.4)		3 (37.5)	6 (40)		2 (25)	5 (50)	
	N	8	4 (44.4)		4 (50)	8 (53.3)		6 (75)	4 (40)	
ApoE	2/2	0 (0.0)	1 (11.1)	0.492	0 (0.0)	1 (6.7)	0.658	0 (0.0)	1 (10)	0.834
	2/3	2 (14.3)	1 (11.1)		1 (12.5)	2 (13.3)		1 (12.5)	1 (10)	
	2/4	1	0 (0.0)		1 (12.5)	0 (0.0)		0 (0.0)	0 (0.0)	
	3/3	10	5 (55.6)		5 (62.5)	10 (66.6)		6 (75)	7 (70)	
	3/4	1	2 (66.7)		1 (12.5)	2 (13.3)		1 (12.5)	1 (10)	

Data are presented as number (percentage). *CAD* coronary artery disease, *SNP* single nucleotide polymorphism, *G* genotype, *N* normal, *H* heterozygote, *M* mutant, *No of BVs* number of blood vessels, *SVD* single vessel disease, *MVD* multivessel disease, *FV* coagulation factor 5, *MTHFR* 1 and 2 Methylenetetrahydrofolate reductase (rs1801133) and (rs1801131), respectively, *PAI-1* plasminogen activator inhibitor-1, *FGB* fibrinogen beta polypeptide chain, *HPA-1* human platelet antigen 1, *ACE* angiotensin converting enzyme, *ApoE* apolipotprotein E. Fisher's exact test was used. Bold values indicate statistically significant at $p < 0.05$. *PTH* (Prothrombin) and *ApoB* (Apolipoprotein B-100) gene variants were excluded from analysis as all patients were normal

than the 4G and subsequently is associated with lower PAI-1 plasma levels and lower risk of thrombus stabilization [68]. Our results showed no association between *PA1* 4G/5G and the studied sample of CAD patients. This is in line with a previous study on Egyptian population [69] and others [20, 65, 70, 71] that also showed lack of association of this risk variant with MI or CAD. A number of evidences could elucidate our findings; first, the pathogenesis of CAD is complex and multifactorial with multiple interacting environmental and genetic determinants; hence PAI-1 is influenced not only by the gene SNP, but also by environmental factors, such as blood sugar, insulin and triglyceride concentrations among others [66]. Considering this fact, in subgroup stratified analysis, the 4G/4G genotype has been shown to be associated with obesity under the dominant genetic model to be in concordance with Mertens et al. [72], who found increased PAI-1 levels are associated with increased visceral obesity due to its production by ectopic fat depots [73]. In addition, Fernandes and Sandrim [74], found that obese women with 4G/4G genotypes were at increased risk of thrombotic diseases. The

5G/5G genotype in our cases has shown to be protective in patients with positive family history for CAD, to be in line with Margaglione et al. [75]. Second, variability in plasma concentrations of PAI-1 has been reported in different ethnic groups worldwide. The 4G/5G variant has been shown to be the predominant effector in some cases [76–78], while in others environmental factors such as smoking are involved [79].

Human platelet antigens (HPA), platelet surface receptors, play a key role in the adhesion, activation, and aggregation of platelets. They are formed of two glycoprotein (GP) subunits (GPIIb/IIIa) [80]. The GPIIIa subunit is polymorphic [81]. One of the most studied GPIIIa variant, *HPA-1* a/b (c.176 T > C; Lys59Pro), also known as PIA1/A2, has been suggested as an important genetic key player in the CAD pathogenesis [82]. In the current study, our data demonstrated an association between *HPA-1* a/b polymorphism and the occurrence of CAD. We found a significant higher prevalence of *HPA-1* a/b and HPA b/b genotypes among CAD patients compared to controls. This was consistent with the studies of Weiss et al. [83] and Abboud et al. [84] which reported a strong association between the *HPA-1* b allele and genotypes and the risk of CAD. The mutant allele encodes proline instead of lysine at an amino acid position located near the ligand binding site [81]. Bennet et al. [85] showed no impact on ligand binding using static model system. Similarly, our *in silico* analysis demonstrated L59P mutation to be benign and tolerated. However, *in vitro* cell culture showed enhanced binding of both fibrinogen and von Willebrand factor (vWF) to the receptor. In the normal population, the *HPA-1*b phenotype results in increased platelet aggregation and increased fibrinogen binding, thus conferred an increased risk of MI [23, 86], especially in early onset heart disease [83], ischemic stroke [87] and resistance to aspirin [88]. In contrast, other studies reported the absence of any association between the *HPA-1*a/b missense mutation and the occurrence of coronary diseases [89–92]. This discrepancy could be explained by the finding of Zotz et al. [93] who reported that *HPA-1* a/b is a risk determinant in patients with already existing atheromatous burden, but not for the development of atheromata.

One of the most popular genetic risk factors in CAD is the *ACE* insertion/deletion (rs1799752) polymorphism [94]. The *ACE* gene is located on chromosome 17q23.3 with 26 exons and 25 introns spreading over about 2 Kb [95]. The presence (insertion) or absence (deletion) of an Alu repetitive element (287-bp repeat sequence) in intron 16 results in I and D alleles, respectively [92]. This common polymorphism accounts for 47% of variations within *ACE* gene [94]. The results of the current study showed that DD genotype could be a considerable risk factor for CAD susceptibility, particularly in females. There was an increased frequency of D allele in CAD patients (0.72) compared to controls (0.44). No association of the gene was observed with other cardiovascular risk factors highlighting more strong effect of *ACE* with CAD. In 1992, Cambien and his colleagues reported the earliest significant relationship between the DD homozygosity and the risk of CAD [96], and that was followed by the study of Morris et al. [97] who suggested that the DD genotype represents a robust risk factor for MI and sudden death compared to II genotype. In addition, DD genotype was associated with coronary artery spasm that is considered one of the mechanisms of MI [98] and increased risk of restenosis with atherosclerotic lesions after percutaneous transluminal angioplasty [99]. Similar findings were further reported in two meta-analysis studies conducted by Samani et al. [100] and Zhou et al. [101]. Furthermore, numerous studies implicated the DD homozygosity as a key risk factor in other cardiovascular diseases, including hypertension [102], coronary and carotid atherosclerosis [103], cardiomyopathy [104], peripheral arterial disease [105], ischemic stroke [106], and recurrent venous thromboembolism [107]. In contrast, Lindpaintner et al. [108] did not confirm the association between D variant and increased risk of CAD in a large population of American males, and this finding was consistent with that of ours as stratification analysis by gender revealed significant association among females only. ACE, the key regulator in the renin angiotensin system (RAS), has two main physiological functions; converts angiotensin I into a physiologically active peptide angiotensin II (Ang II) and degrades bradykinin, a potent vasodilator [105]. Ang II is the atherogenic component of RAS that increases vascular permeability, stimulates proliferation and migration of vascular smooth muscle cells, induces the expression of inflammatory mediators, and enhances the deposition of extracellular matrix [109]. Reduced bradykinin by ACE decreased endothelium-dependent vasodilators nitric oxide and prostacyclin thus controls blood pressure [103]. The circulatory ACE level is genetically determined by the I/D variant [105]. Individuals with DD genotype have a twofold increase in the serum ACE concentration in the normal population, with ID subjects having intermediate levels [110], leading to higher levels of circulating Ang II and vasoconstriction which are common in MI and hypertensive patients [95]. The results of these studies correlate with those of Suehiro et al. [111] which showed an association between D allele and higher expression of the *ACE* mRNA that may affect the renin-angiotensin system in local regions. The mechanisms underlying this variation in levels of circulating enzymes by the absence of the Alu repeat sequence within the intron in DD genotype still need to be elucidated.

Two apolipoprotein variants were examined in our study; *ApoB-100* R3500Q mutation and *ApoE* (rs7412 and rs429358). ApoB is the primary apolipoprotein of chyomicrons, VLDL and LDL, which is responsible for carrying fat molecules throughout the body to all tissue cells. The ApoB on the LDL particle acts as a ligand for LDL receptors. High levels of ApoB are the primary drivers of atheroma formation [112]. It is well established that ApoB100 levels are associated with coronary heart disease [113, 114]. Mutations in ApoB gene can cause familial hypercholesterolemia [115]. The R3500Q (rs5742904) mutation in *ApoB* was found to be a major determinant of LDL levels and coronary artery calcification in the Amish population [112]. Substitution of Arginine with Glutamine is believed to prevent proper folding of ApoB and thereby reducing the ability of LDL particle to bind to the LDL receptor [116]. R3500Q mutation was absent in our study population, possible due to low sample size or ethnic variations. This was consistent with population-based surveys which reported low frequency of R3500Q mutation in non-Amish population [117]. The *ApoB* gene mutations were not detected in Lebanon [118], Russia [119], Iran [26], and Turkey [120].

The other studied apolipoprotein *ApoE* is found in chylomicrons and intermediate density lipoprotein (IDL) that is essential for the normal catabolism of triglyceride-rich lipoprotein constituents and cholesterol metabolism [121]. The *ApoE* gene, mapped on chromosome 19q13.32 in a cluster with *ApoC1* and *ApoC2*, is highly polymorphic [122], with 3 major alleles according to the amino acids at positions 130 (rs429358; c.388 T > C) and 176 (rs7412; c.526C > T) in exon 4: *ApoE2* (cys130/cys176), *ApoE3* (cys130/arg176), and *ApoE4* (arg130/arg176) (ensemble.org). The *ApoE* polymorphisms were found to affect mRNA transcription and result in increased plasma cholesterol and triglyceride with impaired clearance of lipids from the bloodstream [121]. Moreover, knockout mice lacking *ApoE* developed extreme hypercholesterolemia after a high-fat diet [123]. In the present study, E3 (rs429358*T, rs7412*C) was the predominant form of gene in both patients and controls followed by E2 variant (rs429358*T, rs7412*T) among the study population, E2 carriers showed protection against developing CAD compared to E3 and E4. Both E3/E3 and E3/E4 genotypes had higher disease risk more than three times when compared to E2 genotypes. *ApoE* variants were also significantly associated with abnormal triglyceride and LDL-c among our CAD patients. Similar to our findings, E3 isoform was the most frequent *ApoE* variant in several populations, including Americans [124], Indians [125], Turkish [126], and Saudians [127], thus is considered the wild type *ApoE* genotype. The presence of E4 isoform (rs429358*C, rs7412*C) was previously associated with increased risk of CAD and mortality [128], atherosclerosis [129], and ischemic cerebrovascular disease [130]. Further meta-analyses studies showed *ApoE2* allele to be protective while E4 allele rendered higher susceptibility to heart diseases [119, 131–133]. Although these allelic forms differ from each other by only one or two amino acids at 2 sites, these differences alter the ApoE protein structure and function, and thereby have significant physiological consequences [134]. E2 variant with 2 cystienes binds poorly to LDL cell surface receptor compared to E3 and E4, thus can increase the LDLR number, and lowering cholesterol level [122]. On the other hand, E4 isoform with two arginine amino acids exhibits enhanced transfer from HDL to TG-rich lipoproteins, promoting hepatic remnant clearance by ApoE receptors and decreasing LDLR, thereby increasing circulating cholesterol levels [122]. The same variant has also been associated with increased calcium ion levels and apoptosis following mechanical injury [135].

Conclusions

With the caveat that our sample size for this analysis was low, and the current analyses are likely to have been underpowered, our study confirms that CAD development requires more complex interactions among several risk factors [89], including genetic and environmental one. More specifically, it has been found that five variants; rs1800595 (*FVR*), rs1801133 (*MTHFR*), rs5918 (*HPA-1*), rs1799752 (*ACE*), and rs7412 and rs429358 (*ApoE*) were significantly associated with CAD susceptibility under different genetic models in the current sample of Egyptian CAD patients. These variants interacted with different traditional risk factors to cluster the current study population into the patient and control subgroups by multivariate analysis application. However, there are some limitations in our study should be considered. First, the study is cross-sectional for the point of the coronary disease investigation and all the study participants were stable CAD patients. Thus, the clinical phenotype was determined up to the time that the study was performed thereby allowing us to detect an association, but not to predict the outcome. Hence, follow-up studies are highly recommended to estimate the effect of the study risk factors on the disease outcome. In addition, including CAD patients with different clinical presentations are recommended to be useful to differentiate the distribution of the genetic pattern analyzed. Second, it is possible that some of our control subjects could have subclinical atherosclerosis that might result in an underestimation of the true risk associated with certain alleles. Additional studies examining coronary angiography free controls, will be of even greater value to more clearly establish the magnitude of risk imparted by the presence of these genetic risk factors. Third, the lack of an association between some variants and CAD may be due to the relatively small sample size that warrant a larger cohort in the same population and in different ethnicity populations to validate the current results.

Additional files

Additional file 1: Table S1. Structural characteristics and functional impact of the studied single nucleotide polymorphisms. **Table S2** Odds ratio (95% confidence intervals) for the association between genotypes of thrombotic gene polymorphisms and CAD risk within strata of cardiovascular risk factors. **Table S3** Odds ratio (95% confidence intervals) for the association between genotypes of atherosclerotic gene polymorphisms and CAD risk within strata of cardiovascular risk factors. **Table S4** Correlation analysis matrix between genotypes and cardiovascular risk factors. (DOCX 41 kb)

Additional file 2: Figure S1. Genotyping results of the study CAD patients. (DOCX 174 kb)

Abbreviations

ACE: Angiotensin-converting enzyme; APC: Activated protein C; Apo B: Apolipoprotein B; BMI: Body mass index; CAD: Coronary artery disease; CVD: Cardiovascular disease; Cx: Circumflex coronary artery; DCA: Detrended correspondence analysis; FBG: Fasting blood glucose; FGB: Beta-fibrinogen; FV (L): Factor V Leiden; FXIII: Factor 13; HDL: High density lipoprotein; HPA-1: Human platelet antigen 1; LAD: Left anterior descending; LDL: Low density lipoprotein; LMCA: Left main coronary artery; MTHFR: 5,10-Methylenetetrahydrofolate Reductase; MVD: Multivessel disease; PAI-1: Plasminogen activator inhibitor 1; PTH: Prothrombin; RCA: Right coronary artery; SDS: Sodium dodecyl sulfate; TC: Total cholesterol; TG: Triglycerides

Acknowledgements

The authors thank the Oncology Diagnostic Unit and the Center of Excellence, Suez Canal University, Ismailia, Egypt for providing the facilities for performing the research work and thank the patients who agree to participate in the current study.

Funding

No sources of funding were used for this work.

Authors' contributions

MSF, EAT, NMA, AF-E and DIB conceived and designed the experiments, MHH recruited the study samples and clinical patient data, EAT, MSF, NMA, AF-E and DIB contributed parts of the experiments, EAT contributed to the statistical analysis. All authors contributed the reagents and materials needed for the current work, and all authors contributed in writing, reading and approval of the final manuscript.

Competing interest

The authors declare that they have no competing interests.

Author details

[1]Department of Medical Biochemistry, Faculty of Medicine, Suez Canal University, Ismailia, Egypt. [2]Department of Histology and Cell Biology (Genetics Unit), Faculty of Medicine, Suez Canal University, Ismailia, Egypt. [3]Clinical Pathology Department, Faculty of Medicine, Sohag University, Sohag, Egypt. [4]Pulmonologist, Ministry of Health, Cairo, Egypt.

References

1. Go AS, Mozaffarian D, Roger VL, Benjamin EJ, Berry JD, Borden WB, et al. Executive summary: heart disease and stroke statistics-2014 update: a report from the American heart association. Circulation. 2014;129:399–410.
2. Seef S, Jeppsson A, Stafström M. What is killing? People's knowledge about coronary heart disease, attitude towards prevention and main risk reduction barriers in Ismailia, Egypt (descriptive cross-sectional study). Pan Afr Med J. 2013;15:137.
3. Almahmeed W, Arnaout MS, Chettaoui R, Ibrahim M, Kurdi MI, Taher MA, et al. Coronary artery disease in Africa and the Middle East. Ther Clin Risk Manag. 2012;8:65–72.
4. Liu L, Li Y, Tollefsbol TO. Gene-environment interactions and epigenetic basis of human diseases. Curr Issues Mol Biol. 2008;10:25–36.
5. Raposo M, Sousa P, Nemeth S, Couto A, Santos M, Pinheiro J, et al. Polymorphism in cardiovascular diseases (CVD) susceptibility loci in the azores islands (Portugal). Open J Genet. 2011;1:48–53.
6. Roy H, Bhardwaj S, Yla-Herttuala S. Molecular genetics of atherosclerosis. Hum Genet. 2009;125:467–91.
7. Bustamante CD, Burchard EG, De la Vega FM. Genomics for the world. Nature. 2011;475:163–5.
8. Himabindu G, Rajasekhar D, Latheef K, Sarma PVGK, Vanajakshamma V, Chaudhury A, et al. Factor V Leiden mutation is not a predisposing factor for acute coronary syndromes. Indian Heart J. 2012;64:570–5.
9. Campo G, Pavasini R, Pollina A, Tebaldi M, Ferrari R. Coagulation factors and recurrence of ischemic and bleeding adverse events in patients with acute coronary syndromes. Thromb Res. 2013;132:151–7.
10. Kujovich JL. Factor V Leiden thrombophilia. Genet Med. 2011;13:1–16.
11. Burzotta F, Leone AM, Paciaroni K, De Stefano V, Rossi E, Testa L, et al. G20210A prothrombin gene variant and clinical outcome in patients with a first acute coronary syndrome. Haematologica. 2004;89:1134–8.
12. Ye Z, Liu EH, Higgins JP, Keavney BD, Lowe GD, Collins R, et al. Seven haemostatic gene polymorphisms in coronary disease: meta-analysis of 66,155 cases and controls. Lancet. 2006;367:651–8.
13. Poort SR, Rosendaal FR, Reitsma PH, Bertina RM. A common genetic variation in the 3'-untranslated region of the prothrombin gene is associated with elevated plasma prothrombin levels and an increase in venous thrombosis. Blood. 1996;88:3698–703.
14. Kobbervig C, Williams E. FXIII polymorphisms, fibrin clot structure and thrombotic risk. Biophys Chem. 2004;112:223–8.
15. Gemmati D, Serino ML, Ongaro A, Tognazzo S, Moratelli S, Resca R, et al. A common mutation in the gene for coagulation factor XIII-A (VAL34Leu): a risk factor for primary intracerebral hemorrhage is protective against atherothrombotic diseases. Am J Hematol. 2001;67:183–8.
16. Isotalo PA, Wells GA, Donnelly JG. Neonatal and fetal methylenetetrahydrofolate reductase genetic polymorphisms: an examination of C677T and A1298C mutations. Am J Hum Genet. 2000;67:986–90.
17. Zetterberg H, Regland B, Palmer M, Ricksten A, Palmqvist L, Rymo L, et al. Increased frequency of combined methylenetetrahydrofolate reductase C677T and A1298C mutated alleles in spontaneously aborted embryos. Eur J Hum Genet. 2002;10:113–8.
18. Hoekstra T, Geleijnse JM, Schouten EG, Kluft C. Plasminogen activator inhibitor-type 1: its plasma determinants and relation with cardiovascular risk. Thromb Haemost. 2004;91:861–72.
19. Ndrepepa G, Braun S, King L, Fusaro M, Keta D, Cassese S, et al. Relation of fibrinogen level with cardiovascular events in patients with coronary artery disease. Am J Cardiol. 2013;111:804–10.
20. Boekholdt SM, Bijsterveld NR, Moons AH, Levi M, Buller HR, Peters RJ. Genetic variation in coagulation and fibrinolytic proteins and their relation with acute myocardial infarction: a systematic review. Circulation. 2001;104:3063–8.
21. Jood K, Ladenvall P, Tjarnlund-Wolf A, Ladenvall C, Andersson M, Nilsson S, et al. Fibrinolytic gene polymorphism and ischemic stroke. Stroke. 2005;36:2077–81.
22. Rallidis LS, Gialeraki A, Fountoulaki K, Politou M, Sourides V, Travlou A, et al. G-455A polymorphism of beta-fibrinogen gene and the risk of premature myocardial infarction in Greece. Thromb Res. 2010;125:34–7.
23. Ghosh K, Kulkarni B, Nair S, Shetty S, Mohanty D. Human platelet alloantigen polymorphism in Glanzmann'sthrombasthenia and its impact on the severity of the disease. Br J Haematol. 2002;119:348–53.
24. Loncar R, Stoldt V, Hellmig S, Zotz RB, Mihalj M, Scharf RE. HPA-1 polymorphism of αIIbβ3 modulates platelet adhesion onto immobilized fibrinogen in an in-vitro flow system. Thromb J. 2007;5:2.

25. Kutluturk I, Karagöz A, Bezgin T, Oduncu V, Elveran A, Doğan C, et al. Relationship between angiotensin I-converting enzyme insertion/deletion gene polymorphism and retinal vein occlusion. Thromb J. 2014;12:17.
26. Farrokhi E, Shayesteh F, Asadi Mobarakeh S, Roghani Dehkordi F, Ghatreh Samani K, Hashemzadeh CM. Molecular characterization of Iranian patients with possible familial hypercholesterolemia. Indian J Clin Biochem. 2011;26:244–8.
27. Zhang M-d G, Gu W, Qiao S-b, Zhu E-j, Zhao Q-m, Lv SZ. Apolipoprotein E gene polymorphism and risk for coronary heart disease in the Chinese population: a meta-analysis of 61 studies including 6634 cases and 6393 controls. PLoS One. 2014;9:e95463.
28. Kamal HM, Ahmed AS, Fawzy MS, Mohamed FA, Elbaz AA. Plasma thrombin-activatable fibrinolysis inhibitor levels and Thr325Ile polymorphism as a risk marker of myocardial infarction in Egyptian patients. Acta Cardiol. 2011;66:483–8.
29. Saghafi H, Mahmoodi MJ, Fakhrzadeh H, Heshmat R, Shafaee A, Larijani B. Cardiovascular risk factors in first-degree relatives of patients with premature coronary artery disease. Acta Cardiol. 2006; 61(6):607–13.
30. Wilson PW, D'Agostino RB, Levy D, Belanger AM, Silbershatz H, Kannel WB. Prediction of coronary heart disease using risk factor categories. Circulation. 1998;97:1837–47.
31. Sheridan SL, Viera AJ, Krantz MJ, Ice CL, Steinman LE, Peters KE, et al. The effect of giving global coronary risk information to adults: a systematic review. Arch Intern Med. 2010;170:230–9.
32. Janssens ACJ, Ioannidis JP, van Duijn CM, Little J, Khoury MJ. Strengthening the reporting of genetic risk prediction studies: the GRIPS statement. Genome Med. 2011;3:16.
33. Schussler JM. Effectiveness and safety of transradial artery access for cardiac catheterization. Proc (Bayl Univ Med Cent). 2011;24:205–9.
34. Saha T, Khalequzzaman M, Akanda A-k, Saha S, Tushar AZ, Ahmed R, et al. Association of GRACE risk score with angiographic severity of coronary artery disease in patients with ST elevation myocardial infarction. Cardiovasc J. 2015;8:30–4.
35. Scognamiglio R, Negut C, Ramondo A, Tiengo A, Avogaro A. Detection of coronary artery disease in asymptomatic patients with type 2 diabetes mellitus. J Am Coll Cardiol. 2006;47:65–71.
36. Gökdeniz T, Kalaycıoğlu E, Aykan AÇ, Boyacı F, Turan T, Gü İ, et al. Value of coronary artery calcium score to predict severity or complexity of coronary artery disease. Arq Bras Cardiol. 2014;102:120–7.
37. Khandelwal G, Jain A, Rathore M. Prediction of angiographic extent of coronary artery disease on the basis of clinical risk scores in patients of unstable angina. J Clin Diagn Res. 2015;9:OC13–6.
38. Özdemir B, Emül A, Özdemir L, Sağ S, Biçer M, Aydınlar A. Association of aortic diameters with coronary artery disease severity and albumin excretion. Biomed Res Int. 2015;2015:857628.
39. Onaka L. Lipids. In: Anderson SC, Cockayne S, editors. Clinical chemistry: concepts and applications. London: WB Saunders; 1993. p. 166–83.
40. Kotze MJ, Kriegshäuser G, Thiart R, de Villiers NJ, Scholtz CL, Kury F, et al. Simultaneous detection of multiple familial hypercholesterolemia mutations facilitates an improved diagnostic service in South African patients at high risk of cardiovascular disease. Mol Diagn. 2003;7:169–74.
41. Strip assay evaluator Web-edition, Release 2 (version 2.10). http://viennalab.sci-design.at/webevaluator/. Accessed 14 Oct 2016.
42. Online Encyclopedia for Genetic Epidemiology studies (OEGE). Hardy-Weinberg equilibrium calculator including analysis for ascertainment bias. http://www.oege.org/software/hardy-weinberg.html. Accessed 14 Oct 2016.
43. Fawzy MS, Hussein MH, Abdelaziz EZ, Yamany HA, Ismail HM, Toraih EA. Association of MicroRNA-196a2 variant with response to short-acting β2-agonist in COPD: an Egyptian pilot study. PLoS One. 2016;11:e0152834.
44. McCune B, Mefford MJPC-ORD. Multivariate analysis of ecological data, version 5.0 for windows. 2006.
45. Roberts R, Stewart AF, Wells GA, Williams KA, Kavaslar N, McPherson R. Identifying genes for coronary artery disease: an idea whose time has come. Can J Cardiol. 2007;23:7A–15A.
46. Shaker O, Fayez S, Zarouk W, Shehata M. Fibrinogen b-455 G/A and prothrombin 20210 G/A polymorphisms and coronary heart disease: an Egyptian case–control study. Med Rese J. 2011;10:102–9.
47. Dai X, Wiernek S, Evans JP, Runge MS. Genetics of coronary artery disease and myocardial infarction. World J Cardiol. 2016;8:1–23.
48. Butt C, Zheng H, Randell E, Robb D, Parfrey P. Combined carrier status of prothrombin 20210A and factor XIII-A Leu34 alleles as a strong risk factor for myocardial infarction: evidence of a gene-gene interaction. Blood. 2003;101:3037–41.
49. Zaatari GS, Otrock ZK, Sabbagh AS, Mahfouz RA. Prevalence of factor V R2 (H1299R) polymorphism in the Lebanese population. Pathology. 2006;38:442–4.
50. Segers K, Dahlbäck B, Nicolaes GA. Coagulation factor V and thrombophilia: background and mechanisms. Thromb Haemost. 2007;98:530–42.
51. Martinelli I. Risk factors in venous thromboembolism. Thromb Haemost. 2001;86:395–403.
52. Trifonova EA, Spiridonova MG, Stepanov VA. Genetic diversity and the structure of linkage disequilibrium in the methylenetetrahydrofolate reductase locus. Genetika. 2008;44:1410–9.
53. Tajouri L, Martin V, Gasparini C, Ovcaric M, Curtain R, Lea RA, et al. Genetic investigation of methylenetetrahydrofolate reductase (MTHFR) and catechol-O-methyl transferase (COMT) in multiple sclerosis. Brain Res Bull. 2006;69:327–31.
54. Heidari MM, Khatami M, Hadadzadeh M, Kazemi M, Mahamed S, Malekzadeh P, et al. Polymorphisms in NOS3, MTHFR APOB and TNF-α Genes and Risk of Coronary Atherosclerotic Lesions in Iranian Patients. Res Cardiovasc Med. 2015;5:e29134.
55. Almawi WY, Ameen G, Tamim H, Finan RR, Irani-Hakime N. Factor V G1691A, prothrombin G20210A, and methylenetetrahydrofolate reductase (MTHFR]) C677T gene polymorphism in angiographically documented coronary artery disease. J Thromb Thrombolysis. 2004;17:199–205.
56. Neto AI, Moura Jr JR, Persuhn DC. Frequency of MTHFR G1793A polymorphism in individuals with early coronary artery disease: cross-sectional study. Sao Paulo Med J. 2013;131:296–300.
57. Yamada Y, Matsuo H, Segawa T, Watanabe S, Kato K, Hibino T, et al. Assessment of genetic risk for myocardial infarction. Thromb Haemost. 2006;96:220–7.
58. Schürks M, Zee RY, Buring JE, Kurth T. Interrelationships among the MTHFR 677C > T polymorphism, migraine, and cardiovascular disease. Neurology. 2008;71:505–13.
59. Hsu LA, Ko YL, Wang SM, Chang CJ, Hsu TS, Chiang CW, et al. The C677T mutation of the methylene tetrahydrofolate reductase gene is not associated with the risk of coronary artery disease or venous thrombosis among Chinese in Taiwan. Hum Hered. 2001;51:41–5.
60. Yilmaz H, Agachan B, Ergen A, Karaalib ZE, Isbir T. Methylene tetrahydrofolate reductase C677T mutation and left ventricular hypertrophy in Turkish patients with type II diabetes mellitus. J Biochem Mol Biol. 2004;37:234–8.
61. Caner M, Bircan R, Sevinç D, Benli F, Güney AI, Kurtoglu N. *MTHFR*, prothrombin and Factor V gene variants in Turkish patients with coronary artery stenosis. Genet Mol Biol. 2008;31:836–8.
62. Pepper MS. Role of the matrix metalloproteinase and plasminogen activator plasmin systems in angiogenesis. Arterioscler Thromb Va-sc Biol. 2001;21:1104–17.
63. Mehta R, Shapiro A. Plasminogen activator inhibitor type 1 deficiency. Haemophilia. 2008;14:1255–60.
64. Collet JP, Montalescot G, Vicaut E, Ankri A, Walylo F, Lesty C, et al. Acute release of plasminogen activator inhibitor-1 in ST segment elevation myocardial infarction predicts mortality. Circulation. 2003;108:391–4.
65. Ding J, Nicklas BJ, Fallin MD, de Rekeneire N, Kritchevsky SB, Pahor M, et al. Plasminogen activator inhibitor type 1 gene polymorphisms and haplotypes are associated with plasma plasminogen activator inhibitor type 1 levels but not with myocardial infarction or stroke. Am Heart J. 2006;152:1109–15.
66. Li Y, Di C, Li W, Cai W, Tan X, Xu L, et al. Oncomirs miRNA-221/222 and tumor suppressors miRNA-199a/195 Are crucial miRNAs in liver cancer: a systematic analysis. Dig Dis Sci. 2016;61:2315–27.
67. Zhang H, Dong P, Yang X, Liu Z. Plasminogen activator inhibitor-1 4G/5G polymorphism is associated with coronary artery disease risk: a meta-analysis. Int J Clin Exp Med. 2014;7:3777–88.
68. Tsantes AE, Nikolopoulos GK, Bagos PG, Bonovas S, Kopterides P, Vaiopoulos G. The effect of the plasminogen activator inhibitor-1 4G/5G gene polymorphism on the thrombotic risk. Thromb Res. 2008;122:736–42.
69. Ismail S, Abdel Azeem AA, Abdel Hamid MA, Nowier SR, Morad H. The role of 4G/5G genetic polymorphism of plasminogen activator inhibitor-1 gene in myocardial infarction among Egyptians. Life Sci J. 2011;8:32–9.
70. Anderson JL, Muhlestein JB, Habashi J, Carlquist JF, Bair TL, Elmer SP, et al. Lack of association of a common polymorphism of the plasminogen

activator inhibitor-1 gene with coronary artery disease and myocardial infarction. J Am Coll Cardiol. 1999;34:1778–83.
71. Crainich P, Jenny NS, Tang Z, Arnold AM, Kuller LH, Manolio T, et al. Lack of association of the plasminogen activator inhibitor-1 4G/5G promoter polymorphism with cardiovascular disease in the elderly. J Thromb Haemost. 2003;1:1799–804.
72. Mertens I, Verrijken A, Michiels JJ, Van der Planken M, Ruige JB, Van Gaal LF. Among inflammation and coagulation markers, PAI-1 is a true component of the metabolic syndrome. Int J Obes (Lond). 2006;30:1308–14.
73. Alessi M-C, Poggi M, Juhan-Vague I. Plasminogen activator inhibitor-1, adipose tissue and insulin resistance. Curr Opin Lipidol. 2007;18:240–5.
74. Fernandes KS, Sandrim VC. 4G/5G polymorphism modulates PAI-1 circulating levels in obese women. Mol Cell Biochem. 2012;364:299–301.
75. Margaglione M, Cappucci G, Colaizzo D, Giuliani N, Vecchione G, Grandone E, et al. The PAI-1 gene locus 4G/5G polymorphism is associated with a family history of coronary artery disease. Arterioscler Thromb Vasc Biol. 1998;18:152–6.
76. Dawson S, Hamsten A, Wiman B, Henney A, Humphries S. Genetic variation at the plasminogen activator inhibitor-1 locus is associated with altered levels of plasma plasminogen activator inhibitor-1 activity. Arterioscler Thromb. 1991;11:183–90.
77. Ye S, Green FR, Scarabin PY, Nicaud V, Bara L, Dawson SJ, et al. The 4G/5G genetic polymorphism in the promoter of the plasminogen activator inhibitor-1 gene is associated with differences in plasma PAI-1 activity but not with risk of myocardial infarction in the ECTIM study. Thromb Haemost. 1995;74:837–41.
78. Nordt TK, Lohrmann J, Bode C. Regulation of PAI-1 expression by genetic polymorphism. Impact on atherogenesis. Thromb Res. 2001;103:S1–5.
79. Eliasson M, Asplund K, Ervin PE, Lundblad D. Relationship of cigarette smoking and snuff dipping to plasma fibrinogen, fibrinolytic variables and serum insulin: the Northern Sweden MONICA study. Atherosclerosis. 1995;113:41–53.
80. Floyd CN, Ferro A, Warner TD. Expression of the PIA2 allele of glycoprotein IIIa and its impact on platelet function. JRSM Cardiovasc Dis. 2015;4: 2048004015610252.
81. Newman PJ, Derbes RS, Aster RH. The human platelet alloantigens, PIA1 and PIA2, are associated with a leucine33/proline33 amino acid polymorphism in membrane glycoprotein IIIa, and are distinguishable by DNA typing. J Clin Invest. 1989;83:1778–81.
82. Corral J, González-Conejero R, Rivera J, Iniesta JA, Lozano ML, Vicente V. HPA-1 genotype in arterial thrombosis-role of HPA-1b polymorphism in platelet function. Blood Coagul Fibrinolysis. 1997;8:284–90.
83. Weiss EJ, Bray PF, Tayback M, Schulman SP, Kickler TS, Becker LC, et al. A polymorphism of a platelet glycoprotein receptor as an inherited risk factor for coronary thrombosis. N Engl J Med. 1996;334:1090–4.
84. Abboud N, Amin H, Ghazouani L, Ben Haj Khalifa S, Ben Khalafallah A, Aded F, Almawi WY, Mahjoub T. Polymorphisms of human platelet alloantigens HPA-1 and HPA-2 associated with severe coronary artery disease. Cardiovasc Pathol. 2010;19:302–7.
85. Bennett JS, Catella-Lawson F, Rut AR, Vilaire G, Qi W, Kapoor SC, et al. Effect of the PI (A2) alloantigen on the function of beta (3)-integrins in platelets. Blood. 2001;97:3093–9.
86. Floyd CN, Mustafa A, Ferro A. The PIA1/A2 polymorphism of glycoprotein IIIa as a risk factor for myocardial infarction: a meta-analysis. PLoS One. 2014;9:e101518.
87. Floyd CN, Ellis BH, Ferro A. The PIA1/A2 polymorphism of glycoprotein IIIa as a risk factor for stroke: a systematic review and meta-analysis. PLoS One. 2014;9:e100239.
88. Krasopoulos G, Brister SJ, Beattie WS, Buchanan MR. Aspirin "resistance" and risk of cardiovascular morbidity: systematic review and meta-analysis. BMJ. 2008;336:195–8.
89. Ridker PM, Hennekens CH, Miletich JP. G20210A mutation in prothrombin gene and risk of myocardial infarction, stroke and venous thrombosis in a large cohort of US men. Circulation. 1999;99:999–1004.
90. Samani NJ, Lodwick D. Glycoprotein IIIa polymorphism and risk of myocardial infarction. Cardiovasc Res. 1997;33:693–7.
91. Scaglione L, Bergerone S, Gaschino G, Imazio M, Maccagnani A, Gambino R, et al. Lack of relationship between the P1A1/P1A2 polymorphism of platelet glycoprotein IIIa and premature myocardial infarction. Eur J Clin Invest. 1998;28:385–8.
92. Di Castelnuovo A, de Gaetano G, Donati MB, Iacoviello L. Platelet glycoprotein receptor IIIa polymorphism PLA1/PLA2 and coronary risk: a meta-analysis. Thromb Haemost. 2001;85:626–33.
93. Zotz RB, Winkelmann BR, Mu¨ller C, Boehm BO, Ma¨rz W, Scharf RE. Association of polymorphisms of platelet membrane integrins $\alpha_{IIb}\beta_3$ (HPA-1b/Pl^{A2}) and $\alpha_2\beta_1$ ($\alpha_2$807TT) with premature myocardial infarction. J Thromb Haemost. 2005;3:1522–9.
94. Zeinali N, Hashemi M, Mirmohammadsadeghi M, Mirmohammadsadeghi H, Eskandari N, Sabzghabaee AM. Association of angiotensin-converting enzyme genotype, insertion/deletion polymorphism and saphenous vein graft atherosclerosis in Iranian patients. Braz J Cardiovasc Surg. 2015;30:557–61.
95. Demurtas P, Orrù G, Coni P, Minerba L, Corrias M, Sirigu P, et al. Association between the *ACE* insertion/deletion polymorphism and pterygium in Sardinian patients: a population based case–control study. BMJ Open. 2014;4:e005627.
96. Cambien F, Poirer O, Lecerf L, Evans A, Cambou J-P, Arveiler D, et al. Deletion polymorphism in the gene for angiotensin-converting enzyme is a potent risk factor for myocardial infarction. Nature. 1992;359:641–4.
97. Morris BJ. Hypothesis: an angiotensin converting enzyme genotype present in one in three Caucasians, is associated with increased mortality rate. Clin Exp Pharmacol Physiol. 1996;23:1–10.
98. Oike Y, Hata A, Ogata Y, Numata Y, Shido K, Kondo K. Angiotensin converting enzyme as a genetic risk factor for coronary artery spasm: implication in the pathogenesis of myocardial infarction. J Clin Invest. 1995;96:2975–9.
99. Ohishi M, Fujii K, Minamino T, Hagaki J, Kamitani A, Rakugi H, et al. A potent genetic risk factor for restenosis. (Letter). Nature Genet. 1993;5:324–5.
100. Samani NJ, Thompson JR, O'Toole L, Channer K, Woods KL. A meta-analysis of the association of the deletion allele of the angiotensin-converting enzyme gene with myocardial infarction. Circulation. 1996;94:708–12.
101. Zhou L, Xi B, Wei Y, Shen W, Li Y. Meta-analysis of the association between the insertion/deletion polymorphism in ACE gene and coronary heart disease among the Chinese population. J Renin Angiotensin Aldosterone Syst. 2012;13:296–304.
102. Higaki J, Baba S, Katsuya T, Sato N, Ishikawa K, Mannami T, et al. Deletion allele of angiotensin-converting enzyme gene increases risk of essential hypertension in Japanese men: the Suita Study. Circulation. 2000;101:2060–5.
103. Butler R, Morris AD, Struthers AD. Angiotensin-converting enzyme gene polymorphism and cardiovascular disease. Clin Sci. 1997;93:391–400.
104. Bashyam MD, Savithri GR, Kumar MS, Narasimhan C, Nallari P. Molecular genetics of familial hypertrophic cardiomyopathy (FHC). J Hum Genet. 2003;48:55–64.
105. Tseng CH, Tseng FH, Chong CK, Tseng CP, Cheng JC. Angiotensin-converting enzyme genotype and peripheral arterial disease in diabetic patients. Exp Diabetes Res. 2012;2012:698695.
106. Zhang Z, Xu G, Liu D, Fan X, Zhu W, Liu X. Angiotensin-converting enzyme insertion/deletion polymorphism contributes to ischemic stroke risk: a meta-analysis of 50 case-control studies. PLoS One. 2012;7:e46495.
107. Fatini C, Gensini F, Sticchi E, Battaglini B, Prisco D, Fedi S, et al. ACE DD genotype: an independent predisposition factor to venous thromboembolism. Eur J Clin Invest. 2003;33:642–7.
108. Lindpaintner K, Pfeffer MA, Kreutz R, Stampfer MJ, Grodstein F, LaMotte F, et al. A prospective evaluation of an angiotensin-converting-enzyme gene polymorphism and the risk of ischemic heart disease. New Eng J Med. 1995;332:706–11.
109. Sprague AH, Khalil RA. Inflammatory cytokines in vascular dysfunction and vascular disease. Biochem Pharmacol. 2009;78:539–52.
110. Rigat B, Hubert C, Alhenc-Gelas F, Cambien F, Corvol P, Soubrier F. An insertion/deletion polymorphism in the angiotensin I-converting enzyme gene accounting for half the variance of serum enzyme levels. J Clin Invest. 1990;86:1343–6.
111. Suehiro T, Morita T, Inoue M, Kumon Y, Ikeda Y, Hashimoto K. Increased amount of the angiotensin-converting enzyme (ACE) mRNA originating from the ACE allele with deletion. Hum Genet. 2004;115:91–6.
112. Shen H, Damcott CM, Rampersaud E, Pollin TI, Horenstein RB, McArdle PF, et al. Familial defective apolipoprotein B-100 and increased low-density lipoprotein cholesterol and coronary artery calcification in the old order amish. Arch Intern Med. 2010;170:1850–5.
113. Tybjaerg-Hansen A, Humphries SE. Familial defective apolipoprotein B-100: A single mutation that causes hypercholesterolemia and premature coronary artery disease. Atherosclerosis. 1992;96:91–107.
114. Tybjaerg-Hansen A, Steffensen R, Meinertz H, Schnohr P, Nordestgaard BG. Association of mutations in the apolipoprotein B gene with hypercholesterolemia and the risk of ischemic heart disease. N Engl J Med. 1998;338:1577–84.

115. Ludwig EH, Hopkins PN, Allen A, Wu LL, Williams RR, Anderson JL, et al. Association of genetic variations in apolipoprotein B with hypercholesterolemia, coronary artery disease, and receptor binding of low density lipoproteins. J Lipid Res. 1997;38:1361–73.
116. Borén J, Lee I, Zhu W, Arnold K, Taylor S, Innerarity TL. Identification of the low density lipoprotein receptor-binding site in apolipoprotein B100 and the modulation of its binding activity by the carboxyl terminus in familial defective apo-B100. J Clin Invest. 1998;101:1084–93.
117. Austin MA, Hutter CM, Zimmern RL, Humphries SE. Genetic causes of monogenic heterozygous familial hypercholesterolemia: a HuGE prevalence review. Am J Epidemiol. 2004;160:407–20.
118. Sabbagh AS, Daher RT, Otrock ZK, Khalek RN, Zaatari GS, Mahfouz RA. ApoB-100 R3500Q mutation in the Lebanese population: prevalence and historical review of the literature. Mol Biol Rep. 2007;34:267–70.
119. Zakharova FM, Damgaard D, Mandelshtam MY, Golubkov VI, Nissen PH, Nilsen GG, et al. Familial hypercholesterolemia in St-Petersburg: the known and novel mutations found in the low density lipoprotein receptor gene in Russia. BMC Med Genet. 2005;6:6.
120. Sözen MM, Whittall R, Oner C, Tokatli A, Kalkanoğlu HS, Dursun A, et al. The molecular basis of familial hypercholesterolaemia in Turkish patients. Atherosclerosis. 2005;180:63–71.
121. Wang YL, Sun LM, Zhang L, Xu HT, Dong Z, Wang LQ, et al. Association between apolipoprotein E polymorphism and myocardial infarction risk: a systematic review and meta-analysis. FEBS Open Bio. 2015;5:852–8.
122. Ghebranious N, Ivacic L, Mallum J, Dokken C. Detection of ApoE E2, E3 and E4 alleles using MALDI-TOF mass spectrometry and the homogeneous mass-extend technology. Nucleic Acids Res. 2005;33:e149.
123. McNeill E, Channon KM, Greaves DR. Inflammatory cell recruitment in cardiovascular disease: murine models and potential clinical applications. Clin Sci. 2010;118:641–55.
124. Eichner JE, Kuller LH, Orchard TJ, Grandits GA, McCallum LM, Ferrell RE, et al. Relation of apolipoprotein E phenotype to myocardial infarction and mortality from coronary artery disease. Am J Cardiol. 1993;71:160–5.
125. Ventakaramana P, Reddy C, Ferrell RE. Apolipoprotein E polymorphism in two populations of Andhra Pradesh. Ind J Hum Genet. 1999;5:31–5.
126. Hergenc G, Taga Y, Emerk K, Cirakoglu B. Apolipoprotein E genotyping in Turkish myocardial infarction survivors and healthy controls. J Biomed Sci. 1995;2:46–9.
127. Dzimiri N, Meyer BF, Hussain SS, Basco C, Afrane B, Halees Z. Relevance of apolipoprotein E polymorphism for coronary artery disease in the Saudi population. Arch Pathol Lab Med. 1999;123:1241–5.
128. Lenzen HJ, Assmann G, Buchwalsky R, Schulte H. Association of apolipoprotein E polymorphism, low-density lipoprotein cholesterol, and coronary artery disease. Clin Chem. 1986;32:778–81.
129. Mahley RW. Apolipoprotein E: cholesterol transport protein with expanding role in cell biology. Science. 1988;240:622–30.
130. McCarron MO, Delong D, Alberts MJ. APOE genotype as a risk factor for ischemic cerebrovascular disease: a meta-analysis. Neurology. 1999;53:1308–11.
131. Liu S, Song Y, Hu FB, Niu T, Ma J, Gaziano M, Stampfer MJ. A prospective study of the APOA1 XmnI and APOC3 SstI polymorphisms in the APOA1/C3/A4 gene cluster and risk of incident myocardial infarction in men. Atherosclerosis. 2004;177:119–26.
132. Xu H, Li H, Liu J, Zhu D, Wang Z, Chen A, Zhao Q. Meta-analysis of apolipoprotein E gene polymorphism and susceptibility of myocardial infarction. PLoS One. 2014;9:e104608.
133. Zhang Y, Tang HQ, Peng WJ, Zhang BB, Liu M. Meta-analysis for the Association of Apolipoprotein E ε2/ε3/ε4 Polymorphism with Coronary Heart Disease. Chin Med J (Engl). 2015;128:1391–8.
134. Mahley RW, Rall Jr SC. Apolipoprotein E: far more than a lipid transport protein. Annu Rev Genomics Hum Genet. 2000;1:507–37.
135. Jiang L, Zhong J, Dou X, Cheng C, Huang Z, Sun X. Effects of ApoE on intracellular calcium levels and apoptosis of neurons after mechanical injury". Neuroscience. 2015;301:375–83.

8

Prevalence of coronary artery disease and its risk factors in Kerala, South India

M. N. Krishnan[1], G. Zachariah[2], K. Venugopal[3], P. P. Mohanan[4], S. Harikrishnan[5], G. Sanjay[5], L. Jeyaseelan[6] and K. R. Thankappan[7*]

Abstract

Background: There are no recent data on prevalence of coronary artery disease (CAD) in Indians. The last community based study from Kerala, the most advanced Indian state in epidemiological transition, was in 1993 that reported 1.4 % definite CAD prevalence. We studied the prevalence of CAD and its risk factors among adults in Kerala.

Methods: In a community-based cross sectional study, we selected 5167 adults (mean age 51 years, men 40.1 %) using a multistage cluster sampling method. Information on socio-demographics, smoking, alcohol use, physical activity, dietary habits and personal history of hypertension, diabetes, and CAD was collected using a structured interview schedule. Anthropometry, blood pressure, electrocardiogram, and biochemical investigations were done using standard protocols. CAD and its risk factors were defined using standard criteria. Comparisons of age adjusted prevalence were done using two tailed proportion tests.

Results: The overall age-adjusted prevalence of definite CAD was 3.5 %: men 4.8 %, women 2.6 % ($p < 0.001$). Prevalence of any CAD was 12.5 %: men 9.8 %, women 14.3 % ($p < 0.001$). There was no difference in definite CAD between urban and rural population. Physical inactivity was reported by 17.5 and 18 % reported family history of CAD. Other CAD risk factors detected in the study were: overweight or obese 59 %, abdominal obesity 57 %, hypertension 28 %, diabetes 15 %, high total cholesterol 52 % and low level of high density lipoprotein cholesterol 39 %. Current smoking was reported only be men (28 %).

Conclusion: The prevalence of definite CAD in Kerala increased nearly three times since 1993 without any difference in urban and rural areas. Most risk factors of CAD were highly prevalent in the state. Both population and individual level approaches are warranted to address the high level of CAD risk factors to reduce the increasing prevalence of CAD in this population.

Keywords: Coronary artery disease, Coronary risk factors, Prevalence, Kerala, India

Background

Coronary artery disease (CAD) is the foremost cause of disability and death the world over and is one of the top five causes of death in Indian population [1]. Mortality from CAD in Indians is predicted to increase rapidly and overtake that of the high-income countries. Among adults over 20 years of age, there has been a two-fold rise in CAD in rural areas and a 6-fold rise in urban areas during the period from 1960 to 2002 [2]. Previous studies have shown high prevalence of CAD in Asian Indians residing in the United States [3]. However there are no robust and contemporary data on CAD in native Indians. In a systematic review of CAD prevalence from India, Ahmed et al. commented that none of the studies conformed to the requirements of a high-quality epidemiologic study [4]. Kerala, with a population of over 33 million, is the most advanced state in epidemiological transition and has the highest prevalence of CAD risk factors in India [5]. The state has been reported to be

* Correspondence: kavumpurathu@yahoo.com; kr.thankappan@gmail.com
[7]Achutha Menon Centre for Health Science Studies, Sree Chitra Tirunal Institute for Medical Sciences and Technology, Trivandrum Medical College, P.O. 695011 Thiruvananthapuram, Kerala, India
Full list of author information is available at the end of the article

the harbinger of what the rest of India is going to face in the near future [5]. The INTERHEART study reported the importance of conventional risk factors associated with CAD [6]. Although the CAD risk factor prevalence is the highest in the state of Kerala, there are no recent studies on the prevalence of CAD in this state. The only one community based study in 1993 from the rural area of the southernmost district of the state reported a CAD prevalence of 7.4 % [7]. The environment in Kerala is conducive for increasing the CAD risk factors [8] which is likely to result in an increase in the CAD prevalence. Therefore we wanted to study the current prevalence of CAD and its major risk factors in Kerala.

Methods

A detailed description of the design, sample, and methods of the study has already been published [9]. Briefly, this was a cross-sectional community-based study during the period from January to June 2011. We estimated the sample size based on an anticipated prevalence of 7.4 % of CAD for rural Kerala based on the data by Kutty et al. [7] and 11 % for urban Kerala based on the study by Mohan et al. in Chennai [10]. The total sample size was estimated to be 3000 in rural and 2400 in urban areas. Sample selection procedure is given in Fig. 1. Subjects aged 20–79 years were selected using a multistage cluster sampling procedure. In the first stage three out of the 14 districts of Kerala state were selected. The 14 districts were grouped into five northern, five southern and four central districts. From the northern group of districts, Kozhikode district was selected which included the city corporation of Kozhikode. In the southern group of districts, Thiruvananthapuram and Kollam districts had city corporations. Of these Thiruvananthapuram was selected randomly. In the central group of districts there were two districts which included corporations; Ernakulam and Thrissur. Of these Thrissur district was selected randomly. In the second stage, one ward was randomly selected from each of the three city corporation wards in the urban area. Each of the selected wards was divided into six geographic regions. One of these geographic regions was selected randomly as the study area. All the households in this area were eligible to be included in this sample. One subject between 20 and 59 years was selected using KISH method [11] and all the subjects between 60 and 79 years were included.

In rural area, two of the Panchayats from the above three districts were randomly selected. From each of these Panchayats, one ward was randomly selected. All the households in the selected ward were eligible to be included on the sample. One subject between the age of 20 and 59 years was selected using KISH method and all subjects between 60 and 79 years were included.

Each selected individual was invited to visit an easily accessible facility with all past medical records after overnight fasting. Trained investigators collected all the relevant data.

Using a structured interview schedule, information on basic socio-economic and demographic details, smoking, physical activity, dietary habits, personal history of hypertension, dyslipidemia, diabetes mellitus and CAD were collected. The instrument also contained the Rose Angina Questionnaire (RAQ) [12, 13] and questions related to history of documented prior myocardial infarction, unstable angina, coronary artery bypass grafting (CABG) surgery, noninvasive investigations for CAD, coronary angiography, coronary angioplasty, documented use of drugs for CAD and hospital admission for CAD. Family history of ischemic heart disease, stroke and coronary risk factors was also recorded.

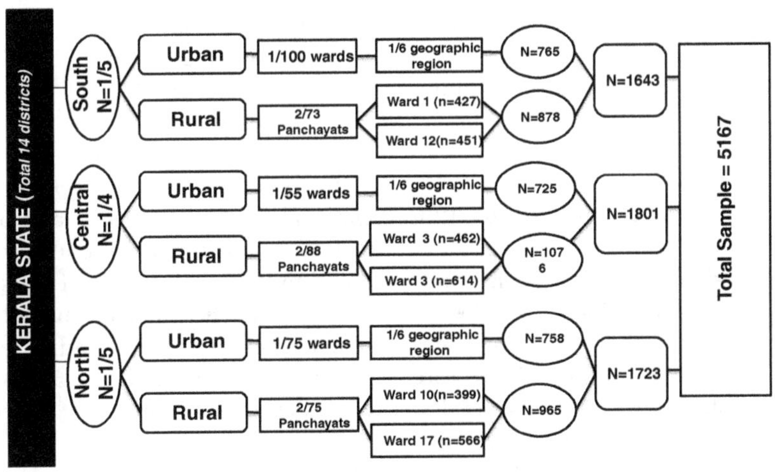

Fig. 1 Sample selection procedure

Anthropometric measurements

Height was measured by wall-mounted stadiometer (Model 206, Seca, Hamburg Germany) to the nearest centimeter. Subjects were asked to stand upright without shoes, with their back against the wall, heels together and eyes directed forward.

Weight was measured with a portable electronic weighing scale (Model HN 283, Omron Corporation, Shimogyo-ku, Kyoto, Japan) kept on a firm horizontal surface. The subjects were asked to wear light clothing and remove footwear. Weight was recorded in kilograms to the nearest 0.5Kg. Body mass index was calculated as weight in kg/(height in meter squared) [14].

Waist circumference was measured using a non-stretchable measuring tape. The subjects were asked to stand erect in a relaxed position with both feet together. Waist girth was measured at the midpoint between the iliac crest and the lower margin of the ribs at the end of expiration, to the nearest centimeter.

Blood pressure

Blood pressure was recorded with electronic apparatus (model 1A2, Omron Corporation, Shimogyo-ku, Kyoto, Japan) in sitting position, on the left arm resting on a table at heart level, after the subject having rested for at least 15 min. Three readings were taken 3 min apart and the mean of the last two readings was recorded as the BP. Heart rate was also recorded.

Electrocardiogram

Resting 12 lead electrocardiogram (ECG) was performed on all subjects by trained technicians with three-channel digital ECG recorders with facility for display and measured parameters. For each lead, five consecutive complexes were recorded. Minnesota coding [15] and application of CAD criteria were performed by an experienced cardiologist for the respective region; those subjects diagnosed to have CAD were re-evaluated by another cardiologist in a blinded manner. Disagreements were resolved by consensus. Similar procedure was followed for 10 % of randomly selected subjects without a diagnosis of CAD.

Biochemical investigations

Blood samples were drawn from individuals after 10–12 h of fasting. Plasma glucose was estimated immediately, onsite using the Glucose oxidase/ peroxidase- phenol-4-amenophenazone method (GOD-PAP). Blood samples for lipid profile measurement were transported on ice packs (4–6 °C) to an accredited core laboratory (Thyrocare Technologies Ltd, Navi Mumbai, India) on the same day. Estimation was carried out within 48 h in clinical chemistry instruments (Olympus AU2700) and Advia 1800 chemistry system (Siemens) using standard commercially available kits (Agappe Diagnostics). Photometry technology was used for lipid profile. Serum cholesterol was measured by cholesterol oxidase phenol 4- aminoantipyrine peroxidase (CHOD-PAP) method and serum triglycerides by glycerol-3 -phosphate oxidase -p - aminophenzone peroxidase (GPO-PAP) method. High density lipoprotein (HDL) cholesterol was estimated by enzyme selective protection method. The reaction between cholesterol assays is suppressed by the electrostatic interaction between polyanions & cationic substances. Low-density lipoprotein (LDL) cholesterol was calculated by using Friedwald's equation.

Ethical clearance

The present study was in compliance with the Helsinki Declaration. The study was approved by the Ethics Committee of Cardiological Society of India, Kerala Chapter. Informed written consent was obtained from all participants.

Definitions used

We defined coronary artery disease as: (a) Definite CAD based on any of: documented evidence of prior acute coronary syndrome (ACS) or treatment for CAD, documented history of undergoing coronary angioplasty or CABG, more than 50 % epicardial coronary stenosis by invasive coronary angiography, ECG showing pathological Q waves (any of Minnesota code 1-1-1 to 1-1-7 or 1-2-1 to 1-2-5 or 1-2-7), imaging evidence of a region of loss of viable myocardium that is thinned and has a motion abnormality, in the absence of a non-ischemic cause [16], RAQ angina plus ECG changes (any of Minnesota codes 4-1-1, 4-1-2, 4-2 or 5-l, 5-2), or RAQ angina plus positive treadmill ECG (exercise-induced horizontal or down-sloping ST depression of ≥ 1 mm at 80 ms from J point), or inducible ischemia on stress imaging;(b) Probable CAD based on any of (in the absence of any of the definite criteria): RAQ angina without significant ECG changes, ECG changes (any of Minnesota Code 4-1-1,4-1-2, 4-2 or 5-1, 5-2) without RAQ angina, or positive treadmill ECG without RAQ angina. Any CAD was defined as those who satisfied either definite or probable CAD criteria.

We defined diabetes mellitus as fasting blood glucose value of ≥ 7 mmol/L and/or if there was current use of medications for diabetes [17], hypertension as blood pressure $\geq$140 mm of Hg systolic and/or $\geq$90 mm of Hg diastolic and/or currently on drugs for high blood pressure [18], and dyslipidemia as any of: serum total cholesterol ≥ 5.18 mmol/L, serum LDL cholesterol ≥ 3.37 mmol/L, serum HDL cholesterol $<$1.04 mmol/L in men or $<$ 1.29 mmol/L in women, or serum triglycerides $\geq$1.69 mmol /L [19]. We categorized body mass index (BMI) as normal (18.0–22.9 kg/m^2), overweight (23.0–24.9 kg/m^2), or obesity (≥25 kg/m^2). Abdominal obesity was defined as a waist circumference of ≥90 cm in men or ≥80 cm in women [20]. Physical activity levels were classified into sedentary and non-sedentary. All subjects reporting physical activity for at least 30 min a day for a minimum of 5 days a week (household activities involving physical effort, walking to and from work involving at least 30 min., manual workers, those performing leisure-time physical activity) were considered non-sedentary. All others were classified as sedentary [21]. We determined the socioeconomic status of the participants using the validated standard of living Index tool developed by National Family Health Survey [22]. We divided our entire sample into tertiles, based upon the index score. Participants in the upper tertile were classified as high socioeconomic group, those in the middle tertile as intermediate socioeconomic group and lower tertile as low socioeconomic group.

Statistical analysis

We entered data into CS Pro software (the US Census Bureau) version 4·0 for Windows. Data cleaning and statistical analysis were performed using Stata (Stata Corp, Texas, USA) version 13·0 for Windows. All proportions were age-adjusted using WHO population data. Frequency distribution was done for categorical variables. Comparisons of age-adjusted prevalence between different categories were done using two-tailed proportion test. The difference in the age-adjusted prevalence and its 95 % confidence intervals are provided. *P* value <0·05 defined the level of statistical significance.

Results

Of the total 6477 individuals contacted, we could evaluate 5167 (men 40.1 %); overall response rate was 79.8 % (men 75.0 %, women 83.3 %). There were no missing data in the interview schedule, ECG or anthropometrics. Data on blood sugar and serum cholesterol were missing in 32 and 47 subjects respectively; these were excluded from analysis.

Table 1 depicts the demographic and behavioural characteristics of the participants by area. There were greater proportion of participants without formal education in rural area as compared to urban; those with >10 years of education were more in urban as compared to rural area. The proportion of subjects that reported current smoking was similar in rural and urban men. There was larger proportion of vegetarianism, obesity and abdominal obesity among urban participants.

Prevalence of coronary artery disease

The crude and age-adjusted prevalence of definite CAD in Kerala was 5.8 and 3.5 % respectively. The figures for men were 8.0 % and 4.8 % and for women 4.2 and 2.6 % respectively; the differences were significant across gender ($p < 0.001$). The overall crude and age-adjusted prevalence of any CAD in Kerala was 16.6 and 12.5 % respectively. The crude and age-adjusted prevalence of any CAD in men were 14.6 and 9.8 % and in women were 17.9 and 14.3 % respectively; the prevalence was significantly higher in women as compared to men ($p < 0.001$). Table 2 outlines the prevalence of CAD (any & definite) among different age groups and gender. As age increased, the prevalence of CAD increased in both gender.

The prevalence of definite CAD was similar irrespective of region or religion. The prevalence of any CAD was lowest among Christians and highest among Muslims (10 vs.15.8 % $p = 0\cdot002$). Of the three geographical regions of Kerala, Thirvananthapuram had lower prevalence of any CAD compared to Thrissur and Kozhikode (8.3 vs. 14.4 and 14.7 % $p < 0.001$).

Table 3 depicts the age-adjusted prevalence of CAD (any and definite) by gender, age group (age ≤ 45 and >45 years), and by area. Age-adjusted prevalence of any CAD in participants ≤45 years and >45 years was 7.8 and 18.7 % respectively. Similarly the age-adjusted prevalence of definite CAD was 0.9 % in participants ≤45 years and 6.8 % in >45 years. Age-adjusted prevalence of CAD (any and definite) was significantly higher in participants >45 years ($p < 0.001$). The prevalence of any CAD was significantly higher in rural women (15.6 %) as compared to urban women (11.7 %) ($p < 0.01$). The overall prevalence of any CAD was higher in rural (13.2 %) than urban (11·3 %) area ($p = 0.038$). However, there was no difference between urban and rural areas in the overall prevalence of definite CAD (3.4 vs. 3.6 %) ($p = 0.72$).

Table 4 shows the age-adjusted prevalence of various criteria for diagnosis of CAD. ST code, T code, and RAQ angina were significantly higher in women; all other criteria were higher in men ($p < 0.01$). Table 5 represents the age-adjusted prevalence of various criteria for diagnosis of CAD among participants with any CAD. Again, most of the definite criteria for CAD were higher in men. Except ST code, T code, and RAQ angina, there was higher prevalence of various coronary artery criteria among men as compared to women ($p < 0.001$); ST code was higher in women, while T code and RAQ angina showed no significant difference. Among participants diagnosed to have any CAD, the prevalence of known CAD was 7.8 and 2.7 % in men and women respectively. Symptomatic CAD (sum of those with known CAD and RAQ angina) was prevalent in 54 % with any CAD.

Coronary risk factors

Age-adjusted prevalence of major risk factors of CAD by gender and area is presented in Table 6. Conventional

Table 1 Baseline demographic and behavioural characteristics of the participants by area

Variable		Urban (*N* = 2248)		Rural (*N* = 2919)		Total (*N* = 5167)		
		n	(%)	n	(%)	n	(%)	*P* value
Age								
	20–29	111	4.94	225	7.71	336	6.50	<0.001
	30–39	345	15.35	543	18.60	888	17.19	
	40–49	507	22.55	692	23.71	1199	23.20	
	50–59	493	21.93	531	18.19	1024	19.82	
	60–69	566	25.18	650	22.27	1216	23.53	
	70–79	226	10.05	278	9.52	504	9.75	
Sex								
	Men	971	43.19	1101	37.72	2072	40.10	<0.001
	Women	1277	56.81	1818	62.28	3095	59.90	
Socio-economic status								
	Low	630	28.02	1303	44.64	1933	37.41	<0.001
	Middle	792	35.23	743	25.45	1535	29.71	
	High	826	36.74	873	29.91	1699	32.88	
Educational status								
	No formal education	87	3.87	203	6.95	290	5.61	<0.001
	1–4 years	208	9.25	437	14.97	645	12.48	
	5–10 years	1294	57.56	1729	59.23	3023	58.51	
	>10 years	659	29.31	550	18.84	1209	23.40	
Smoking[a]								
	Never	523	55.52	443	44.04	966	49.59	<0.001
	Past	111	11.78	220	21.87	331	16.99	
	Current	308	32.70	343	34.10	651	33.42	
Physical activity								
	Sedentary	1770	78.74	2328	79.75	4098	79.31	0.371
	Non-sedentary	478	21.26	591	20.25	1069	20.69	
Dietary habits								
	Vegetarian	161	7.16	110	3.77	271	5.24	<0.001
	Non-vegetarian	2087	92.84	2809	96.23	4896	94.76	
BMI								
	Low	111	4.95	244	8.37	355	6.88	<0.001
	Normal	685	30.53	1042	35.76	1727	33.48	
	Overweight	450	20.05	527	18.09	977	18.94	
	Obese	998	44.47	1101	37.78	2099	40.69	
Abdominal Obesity								
	Yes	1394	62.20	1709	58.67	3103	60.21	<0.001
	No	847	37.80	1204	41.33	2051	39.79	

[a] Smoking in men only

risk factors like diabetes mellitus, hypertension, high serum cholesterol, low serum HDL cholesterol, smoking, physical inactivity, and family history of CAD were highly prevalent in the state. Except low HDL cholesterol (23.9 % in urban men vs. 27.6 % in rural men), all other major risk factors were higher in urban men as compared to rural men. This pattern was also observed in urban women as compared to

Table 2 Crude and age-adjusted prevalence of CAD by age group and gender

Age group (yrs.)	Men			Women			Difference (%)	95 % CI	*p* value
Any CAD	n	P (%)	SE	n	P (%)	SE			
20–29	144	2.78	1.37	192	7.29	1.88	−4.51	(−9.07,0.04)	0.069
30–39	306	6.54	1.42	582	8.93	1.18	−2.40	(−6.01,1.21)	0.213
40–49	465	7.10	1.19	734	14.44	1.30	−7.34	(−10.80,−3.89)	<0.001
50–59	386	12.44	1.68	638	19.91	1.58	−7.47	(−11.99,−2.95)	0.002
60–69	537	22.72	1.81	679	25.77	1.68	−3.05	(−7.89,1.78)	0.218
70–79	234	32.05	3.06	270	29.26	2.77	2.79	(−5.28,10.87)	0.497
All	2072	14.58	0.78	3095	17.87	0.69	−3.29	(−5.32,−1.26)	0.002
Age adjusted	2072	9.80	0.65	3095	14.26	0.69	−4.46	(−6.24,−2.69)	<0.001
Definite CAD									
20–29	144	0.00	0.00	192	0.00	0.00	-	-	-
30–39	306	2.29	0.86	582	0.52	0.30	1.77	(0.00,3.55)	0.017
40–49	465	3.87	0.90	734	1.77	0.49	2.10	(0.10,4.10)	0.026
50–59	386	6.48	1.25	638	3.13	0.69	3.34	(0.54,6.14)	0.012
60–69	537	13.41	1.47	679	8.98	1.10	4.42	(0.83,8.02)	0.014
70–79	234	18.80	2.56	270	12.59	2.02	6.21	(−0.17,12.59)	0.055
All	2072	8.01	0.60	3095	4.23	0.36	3.78	(2.41,5.15)	<0.001
Age adjusted	2072	4.80	0.39	3095	2.63	0.23	2.17	(1.09,3.25)	<0.001

CAD coronary artery disease, *P* prevalence, *SE* standard error

rural women except high serum cholesterol (49.2 vs. 52.4 %; $p = 0.089$) and low HDL cholesterol (43.4 vs. 48.7 %; $p = 0.004$).

Risk factor analysis of any and definite CAD is presented in Table 7. The age adjusted prevalence of risk factors such as hypertension, low HDL and family history were significantly higher in any CAD group (p value <0.01). However, higher cholesterol and smoking were higher in no CAD group. In definite CAD, all risk factors except low HDL were statistically significant (p value <0.01). In addition, excluding higher cholesterol all age adjusted prevalence of these conventional risk factors was higher in definite CAD as compared to no CAD.

Table 3 Age-adjusted prevalence of CAD by gender, age, and area

	Gender	=/<45 years			>45 years			Difference (%)	95 % CI	*p* value
		n	P (%)	SE	n	P (%)	SE			
Any CAD	Men	728	5.12	0.82	1344	15.05	1.04	−9.92	(−12.42,−7.43)	<0.001
	Women	1239	9.48	0.92	1856	21.08	1.10	−11.60	(−14.07,−9.13)	<0.001
	All	1967	7.78	0.64	3200	18.68	0.78	−10.90	(−12.69,−9.10)	<0.001
Definite CAD	Men	728	1.82	0.43	1344	8.43	0.80	−6.61	(−8.39,−4.84)	<0.001
	Women	1239	0.36	0.15	1856	5.61	0.58	−5.25	(−6.35,−4.15)	<0.001
	All	1967	0.89	0.18	3200	6.80	0.47	−5.91	(−6.88,−4.95)	<0.001
		Urban			Rural					
Any CAD	Men	971	10.82	1.06	1101	8.94	0.81	1.88	(−0.70,4.46)	0.151
	Women	1277	11.66	0.88	1818	15.63	0.94	−3.97	(−6.40,−1.55)	0.002
	All	2248	11.31	0.68	2919	13.23	0.66	−1.92	(−3.72,−0.12)	0.038
Definite CAD	Men	971	4.92	0.57	1101	4.69	0.54	0.23	(−1.62,2.08)	0.806
	Women	1277	2.24	0.29	1818	2.84	0.33	−0.60	(−1.72,0.51)	0.299
	All	2248	3.38	0.29	2919	3.57	0.28	−0.18	(−1.19,0.82)	0.722

CAD coronary artery disease, *P* prevalence, *SE* standard error

Table 4 Age-adjusted prevalence of various CAD parameters among the total participant population

	Total		Men		Women		Difference (%)	95 % CI	*p* value
	n = 5167		*n* = 2072		*n* = 3095				
	P (%)	SE	P (%)	SE	P (%)	SE			
Q codes	0.87	0.11	1.65	0.24	0.32	0.08	1.33	(0.74,1.91)	<0.001
ST Code	1.87	0.19	1.00	0.18	2.46	0.29	−1.47	(−2.16,−0.77)	<0.001
T code	5.46	0.35	3.86	0.46	6.44	0.49	−2.59	(−3.79,−1.39)	<0.001
Documented ACS	1.59	0.14	2.70	0.30	0.84	0.13	1.86	(1.09,2.63)	<0.001
Documented treatment for CAD	2.26	0.16	3.55	0.34	1.39	0.16	2.17	(1.27,3.07)	<0.001
Angioplasty/CABG or Fibrinolysis	0.44	0.07	0.96	0.17	0.05	0.03	0.91	(0.48,1.34)	<0.001
Angiographic Coronary stenosis	0.63	0.09	1.15	0.19	0.27	0.07	0.88	(0.39,1.37)	<0.001
Imaging evidence of RWMA	0.06	0.09	1.34	0.20	0.10	0.05	1.24	(0.73,1.74)	<0.001
RAQ angina	6.38	0.35	4.71	0.44	7.47	0.51	−2.76	(−4.06,−1.46)	<0.001
Positive treadmill ECG	0.54	0.08	0.98	0.17	0.22	0.07	0.76	(0.30,1.21)	<0.001

Discussion

Prevalence of coronary artery disease

Coronary artery disease has been gaining importance as a major public health problem in India. In 2003, the prevalence of CAD was estimated to be 3–4 % in rural areas and 8–10 % in urban areas according to a population-based cross sectional survey [23]. Our study also showed high prevalence of CAD in Kerala. The age-adjusted overall prevalence of definite CAD was 3.5 % and any CAD was 12.5 %. We chose criteria for any CAD to detect all possible cases of CAD; for definite CAD we have avoided less specific criteria like RAQ angina, positive treadmill electrocardiogram or minor electrocardiographic changes in isolation and used combined criteria when these less specific components were incorporated.

Age-adjusted prevalence of definite CAD was higher in men. However, any CAD prevalence in women was significantly higher than in men. It is well known that women commonly have ECG with nonspecific ST −T changes and angina with normal coronary arteries; this may have resulted in overestimation of any CAD prevalence in women. In our study the prevalence of RAQ angina and ST-T changes were significantly higher among women whose proportion in rural area (62 %) was higher than that of urban area (57 %). Earlier population studies also consistently recorded much higher prevalence of CAD in women using RAQ angina and ST-T criteria for diagnosis of CAD [24–27]. It has also been noted that RAQ angina is less reliable in women [28] and non-white population [29]. Moreover, Patel et al. in a study from migrant South Asians observed that the

Table 5 Age-adjusted prevalence of various CAD parameters among any CAD

	Total		Men		Women		Difference (%)	95 % CI	*p* value
	n = 855		*n* = 302		*n* = 553				
	P (%)	SE	P (%)	SE	P (%)	SE			
Q codes	4.88	0.79	12.22	2.48	1.49	0.40	10.74	(6.91,14.57)	<0.001
ST Code	12.94	2.16	7.08	1.51	15.14	2.74	−8.07	(−12.23,−3.91)	<0.001
T code	43.06	3.44	45.84	6.35	42.61	3.92	3.23	(−3.74,10.20)	0.3625
Documented ACS	8.68	0.98	20.36	2.85	3.80	0.71	16.56	(11.75,21.37)	<0.001
Documented treatment for CAD	11.88	1.05	26.56	2.95	5.98	0.79	20.59	(15.23,25.94)	<0.001
Angioplasty/CABG or Fibrinolysis	2.18	0.41	6.63	1.44	0.19	0.11	6.43	(3.60,9.26)	<0.001
Angiographic Coronary stenosis	3.21	0.55	8.07	1.81	1.10	0.31	6.98	(3.78,10.17)	<0.001
Imaging evidence of RWMA	3.03	0.46	8.75	1.56	0.40	0.19	8.34	(5.11,11.57)	<0.001
RAQ angina	49.69	3.44	43.98	6.43	51.60	3.96	−7.62	(−14.60,−0.64)	0.033
Positive treadmill ECG	2.74	0.52	6.26	1.33	1.12	0.51	5.14	(2.27,8.01)	<0.001

Q code-any of the Minnesota Q code 1-1-1 to 1-1-7 or 1-2-1 to 1-2-5 or 1-2-7; ST code-any of the Minnesota ST code 4-1-1,4-1-2 or 4–2; T code -any of the Minnesota T code 5-1 or 5-2; *ACS* acute coronary syndrome, *CABG* coronary artery bypass graft surgery, *RWMA* regional wall motion abnormality, *ECG* electrocardiogram, *P* prevalence, *SE* standard error

Table 6 Age adjusted prevalence of major risk factors of CAD by gender and area

Risk factor	All			Men							Women							*p* value**
				Urban			Rural			*p* value*	Urban			Rural			*p* value*	
	n	%	SE	n	%	SE	n	%	SE		n	%	SE	n	%	SE		
Diabetes	5135	15.23	0.50	962	19.14	1.40	1097	16.23	1.16	0.0831	1272	15.40	0.95	1804	12.47	0.73	0.020	<0.001
Hypertension	5153	28.44	0.63	967	39.99	2.04	1095	26.24	1.33	<0.001	1275	30.15	1.29	1816	23.42	0.85	<0.001	<0.001
High cholesterol	5121	52.31	0.88	960	56.54	2.22	1092	53.36	1.85	0.1487	1264	49.23	1.76	1805	52.35	1.35	0.089	0.023
Low HDL	5120	38.55	0.88	959	23.92	1.94	1092	27.56	1.69	0.0603	1264	43.41	2.02	1805	48.73	1.44	0.004	<0.001
Smoking	2072	28.05	1.19	971	30.45	2.00	1101	26.88	1.48	0.0721	-	-	-	-	-	-	-	-
Physical inactivity	5167	17.45	0.64	971	30.72	2.06	1101	28.77	1.64	0.3315	1277	11.19	1.19	1818	9.38	0.64	0.101	<0.001
Family history	5167	18.35	0.64	971	18.97	1.47	1101	17.37	1.39	0.3467	1277	20.37	1.39	1818	16.92	1.02	0.015	0.939

P prevalence, *SE* standard error, *p value between urban and rural; ***p* value between men and women

value of ST-T changes alone as indicator of CAD was questionable, especially in women [30].

This study showed no difference in the prevalence of definite CAD between urban and rural population of Kerala while any CAD was slightly more in the rural population. Previous studies from other parts of India have highlighted the marked urban preponderance of CAD [25, 31, 32]. Some of the risk factors such as general obesity and abdominal obesity were higher in urban areas, whereas smoking was higher in rural area. There was no difference in physical inactivity in rural and urban areas. In most other Indian states there are huge differences between urban and rural areas. However, in Kerala these differences are either minimal or some risk factors are higher in urban while others are higher in rural as noted above. This could be the reason for not having significant difference of definite CAD prevalence in urban and rural areas of Kerala.

The overall age-adjusted prevalence of any CAD in subjects at or below the age of 45 years was 7.8 %. Our study showed a higher prevalence of CAD among young subjects compared to a previous study [7]; in this 1993 study, there were no subjects with definite CAD below the age of 45 years where as we found definite CAD in 0.9 %. It is well known that coronary artery disease occurs in Indians 5–10 years earlier [33, 34]. The average age of first myocardial infarction in Asians is 53 years; among the three Asian populations, Chinese, Malay, and Indian, the highest age-adjusted incidence of coronary events in both sexes was in Indians [6]. The age-adjusted prevalence of CAD in young subjects in our study was similar to the US data on prevalence of CAD in the young (1.2 %).

Comparisons with previous Indian studies on CAD prevalence may be problematic due to heterogeneity in period of study, sample characteristics, and criteria for diagnosis of CAD. We did a systematic search for articles in PubMed and EMBASE published during the period from 1990 to 2014 in English language on the prevalence of CAD in India by community-based surveys. We chose only studies that had a minimum sample size of 1000, and that based the diagnosis on documented history of CAD and ECG criteria. We could collect 11original articles, one systematic review [4] and one meta-analysis [35]. The studies were heterogeneous in terms of sampling methods, subject groups, and criteria for diagnosis. Most of the studies were from northern India. Only one study mentioned the period of field survey [25]. Only one study analyzed the data for definite CAD and probable CAD separately [7]. Most studies were on either rural or urban population; only four covered both the groups [25, 31, 32, 36]. Sample size calculations were reported in three studies [7, 25, 31]. In a study from Delhi during the period from 1984 to 1987, Chadda et al. reported unadjusted prevalence of 9.7 % in urban and 2.7 % in rural inhabitants [25]. The sample consisted of men and women aged 24–64 years; they used clinical history of CAD and electrocardiographic criteria for diagnosis of CAD. Gupta et al. published an epidemiological survey of urban inhabitants over 20 years of age in Rajasthan, India [27]. The prevalence of CAD was 7.6 % (6 % in men and 10.4 % in women). The age distribution of the sample was consistent with that of the population. Singh et al. in 1997 surveyed an urban and rural sample of 3575 subjects between the ages 25 and 64 years from North India and reported CAD prevalence of 9 and 3.3 % respectively [31]. Mohan and colleagues reported 9 % age-adjusted prevalence of CAD in an urban sample of Chennai, South India [10]. More recently, another study from India noted 12.6 % crude CAD prevalence in an urban population [37]. All these studies had used less specific criteria for diagnosis of CAD; definite CAD as we had analyzed had not been computed in these studies. A study from Pakistan showed a crude prevalence of definite CAD in 6.1 men and 4 % women; they found ischemic ECG changes much more prevalent in women [38].

Table 7 Risk factors analysis of any and definite CAD

Risk factor	Any CAD									Definite CAD								
	Yes			No			Difference (%)	95 % CI	*p* value	Yes			No			Difference (%)	95 % CI	*p* value
	n	%	SE	n	%	SE				n	%	SE	n	%	SE			
Diabetes	851	17.07	1.97	4284	14.89	0.52	2.18	(−0.56,4.93)	0.106	296	33.30	5.24	4839	14.73	0.50	18.57	(13.11,24.03)	<0.001
Hypertension	852	32.19	2.04	4301	27.67	0.67	4.51	(1.10,7.92)	0.008	295	51.32	5.34	4858	28.04	0.64	23.29	(17.44,29.13)	<0.001
High cholesterol	849	47.63	3.24	4272	52.82	0.92	−5.19	(−8.86,−1.51)	0.006	293	41.01	5.68	4828	53.01	0.88	−12.00	(−17.81,−6.20)	<0.001
Low HDL	849	43.62	3.53	4271	37.59	0.92	6.04	(2.40,9.68)	0.001	293	42.76	5.90	4827	38.33	0.89	4.44	(−1.39,10.26)	0.13
Smoking	855	6.91	1.02	4312	11.80	0.56	−4.89	(−6.85,−2.94)	<0.001	297	15.69	4.42	4870	11.22	0.53	4.46	(0.23,8.69)	0.019
Physical inactivity	855	15.55	2.17	4312	17.49	0.68	−1.94	(−4.62,0.74)	0.170	297	31.02	5.32	4870	17.13	0.65	13.89	(8.52,19.25)	<0.001
Family history	855	27.06	3.09	4312	17.37	0.66	9.70	(6.51,12.88)	<0.001	297	25.29	4.06	4870	18.03	0.65	7.27	(2.21,12.33)	0.002

The US statistics reported 6 % age-adjusted CAD prevalence in respondents above 18 years by survey based on self-reported CAD by telephonic interview [39]. The prevalence between ages 18–44 years was 1.2 %. The update on heart disease and stroke in the US reported CAD prevalence of 6.4%in adults ≥ 20 years of age. The prevalence of CAD was 7.9 for men and 5.1 % for women [40]. The higher figure in the US data may be due to differences in age, sample, survey methods, and criteria for diagnosis. The reported prevalence of CAD in the United Kingdom was 3.5 % [41]; this figure was similar to our data on definite CAD.

As to the figures for definite CAD, only one study [7] reported the prevalence (1.4 %); they found no participant below the age of 45 years with definite CAD. However, it should be noted that the age range in this study was 25–64 years and the population was rural only. Compared to this, our data show an increase in the prevalence of definite CAD (0.9 %). Any CAD prevalence of 11.3 % in urban and 13.2 % in rural area respectively in our study was higher compared to some previous studies in the same age group and similar definition for CAD (8.1–9 % for urban and 3.5–5 % for rural) [10, 27, 42, 43]. These data indicate an increase in the prevalence of any CAD over the past two decades. The increase in prevalence of any CAD may partially be due to improvement of treatment of CAD thus allowing better survival.

The urban prevalence data in this study may be comparable to other cities of India; however, the rural figures for prevalence may not be comparable to most rural areas in rest of India since rural Kerala is different from rest of rural India in social and economic development.

Prevalence of coronary risk factors

We found high prevalence of major conventional risk factors for CAD in our survey. The prevalence of various risk factors in our study like diabetes (15.2 %), hypertension (28.4 %), high cholesterol (52.3 %) and smoking in men (28.1 %) was comparable to the figures in a recent large study from Kerala, by Thankappan et al. [5]. The figures were also similar in the US adult population [44]. Physical activity in our study seems to be an overestimate due to the problems of self reports as has been reported by a recent study from Kerala [45].

Limitations of the study

Our study was the largest and most comprehensive contemporary community-based survey on the prevalence of CAD and its risk factors from India. The geographic spread of the survey enabled us to derive meaningful inferences of prevalence from the state. We could capture all the necessary data from participants with very little missing variables. One of the limitations for our study was the sub-optimal response rate, which could reach only ~ 80 %; the response rate was lower in rural men. We could not capture the reasons for the poor response in men although we surmise that, being manual laborers many of them would be working on Sundays. As a result the sample consisted of higher proportion of women than in the general population. Sex disaggregated data will partly take care of this problem. There was significantly higher proportion of older individuals compared to the population of Kerala although age-adjustment in analysis would have removed this bias.

Conclusion

Our study revealed a high age-adjusted prevalence of CAD and coronary risk factors in Kerala, South India. Our study did not show any difference in the CAD prevalence in urban and rural population. Our data on prevalence of CAD are comparable to the figures from the US and the United Kingdom. Compared to previous Indian studies and the 1993 study of Kerala, this study showed higher prevalence of CAD in Kerala. The prevalence of definite CAD in Kerala increased nearly three times since 1993 without any difference in urban and rural areas. Most risk factors of CAD were highly prevalent in the state. Both population and individual level approaches are warranted to address the high level of CAD risk factors to reduce the increasing prevalence of CAD in this population.

Abbreviations

ACS: acute coronary syndrome; CHOD-PAP: cholesterol oxidase phenol 4-aminoantipyrine peroxidase; CABG: coronary artery bypass grafting; CAD: coronary artery disease; ECG: electrocardiogram; GOD-PAP: glucose oxidase/ peroxidase-phenol-4-amenophenazone method; HDL: high density lipoprotein; LDL): low-density lipoprotein; RAQ: rose angina questionnaire.

Competing interests

There has been no financial relationship with any company or any other funding source. The authors declare that they have no competing interest.

Authors' contributions

MNK, GZ, KV, PPM and SH conceptualized and designed the study. MNK lead the study in northern region, GZ in Central region, and SH in southern region. LJ did the statistical analysis. All authors contributed to the writing of the manuscript, read the final version and approved it for submission.

Acknowledgements

We thankfully acknowledge the Cardiological Society of India Kerala Chapter for the generous and exclusive funding of the study. We also appreciate the important intellectual input provided by Dr. Mark Huffman.

Funding

The study was funded exclusively by the Cardiological Society of India, Kerala Chapter; this is the professional organization of cardiologists in this region. The funding source had no role in the design, data collection, analysis or interpretation or writing up of the article.

Author details
[1]Govt. Medical College, Kozhikode, Kerala, India. [2]Mother Hospital, Thrissur, Kerala, India. [3]Pushpagiri Hospital, Tiruvalla, Kottayam, Kerala, India. [4]Westfort High-tech Hospital, Thrissur, Kerala, India. [5]Sree Chitra Tirunal Institute for Medical Sciences and Technology, Trivandrum, Kerala, India. [6]Department of Biostatistics, Christian Medical College, Vellore, Tamil Nadu, India. [7]Achutha Menon Centre for Health Science Studies, Sree Chitra Tirunal Institute for Medical Sciences and Technology, Trivandrum Medical College, P.O. 695011 Thiruvananthapuram, Kerala, India.

References

1. Gupta R, Guptha S, Sharma KK, Gupta A, Deedwania P. Regional variations in cardiovascular risk factors in India: India Heart Watch. World J Cardiol. 2012;4:112–20.
2. Gupta R, Joshi P, Mohan V, Reddy KS, Yusuf S. Epidemiology and causation of coronary heart disease and stroke in India. Heart. 2008;94:16–26.
3. Enas EA, Garg A, Davidson MA, Nair VM, Huet BA, Yusuf S. Coronary heart disease and its risk factors in first-generation immigrant Asian Indians to the United States of America. Indian Heart J. 1996;48:343–53.
4. Ahmed N, Bhopal R. Is coronary heart disease rising in India? A systematic review based on ECG defined coronary heart disease. Heart. 2005;91:719–25.
5. Thankappan KR, Shah B, Mathur P, Sarma PS, Srinivas G, Mini GK, et al. Risk factor profile for chronic non-communicable diseases: results of a community-based study in Kerala, India. Indian J Med Res. 2010;131:53–63.
6. Yusuf S, Hawken S, Ounpuu S, Dans T, Avezum A, Lanas F, et al. Effect of potentially modifiable risk factors associated with myocardial infarction in 52 countries (the INTERHEART study): case-control study. Lancet. 2004;364:937–52.
7. Kutty VR, Balakrishnan KG, Jayasree AK, Thomas J. Prevalence of coronary heart disease in the rural population of Thiruvananthapuram district, Kerala, India. Int J Cardiol. 1993;39:59–70.
8. Sivasankaran S, Thankappan KR. Prevention of non-communicable diseases requires a life course approach: a case study from Kerala. Indian J Med Res. 2013;137:874–7.
9. Zachariah G, Harikrishnan S, Krishnan MN, Mohanan PP, Sanjay G, Venugopal K, et al. Prevalence of coronary artery disease and coronary risk factors in Kerala, South India: a population survey-design and methods. Indian Heart J. 2013;65:243–9.
10. Mohan V, Deepa R, Rani SS, Premalatha G. Prevalence of coronary artery disease and its relationship to lipids in a selected population in South India: The Chennai Urban Population Study (CUPS No. 5). J Am Coll Cardiol. 2001;38:682–7.
11. World Health Organization. WHO STEPS Manual, WHO STEPS Surveillance, Part 2: Planning and Set Up; Section 2: Preparing the sample. 2008. p. 2-2-24–25.
12. Rose GA. The diagnosis of ischemic heart pain and intermittent claudication in field surveys. Bull World Health Organ. 1962;27:645–58.
13. Rose GA, Blackburn H. Cardiovascular survey methods. Monogr Ser World Health Organ. 1968;56:1–188.
14. World Health Organization. WHO STEPS Part 3, Training and practical Guides. Section 3: Guide to physical measurements (Step 2). 2008. p. 3-3-1–3-3-14.
15. Ronald JP, Richards SC, Zhu-Ming Z. The Minnesota Code manual of electrocardiographic findings. Second edition Springer. 2010.
16. Mendis S, Thygesen K, Kuulasmaa K, Giampaoli S, Mähönen M, Ngu Blackett K, et al. World Health Organization definition of myocardial infarction:2008–09 revision. Int J Epidemiol. 2011;40:139–46.
17. American Diabetes Association. Diagnosis and classification of diabetes mellitus. Diabetes Care. 2010;33(1):S62–9.
18. Chobanian AV, Bakris GL, Black HR, Cushman WC, Green LA, Izzo Jr JL, et al. The Seventh report of the Joint National Committee on prevention, detection, evaluation, and treatment of high blood pressure: The JNC 7 Report. JAMA. 2003;289:2560–72.
19. Expert Panel on Detection, Evaluation, and Treatment of High Blood Cholesterol in Adults, Expert Panel on Detection, Evaluation, and Treatment of High Blood Cholesterol in Adults. Executive Summary of The Third Report of The National Cholesterol Education Program (NCEP) Expert Panel on detection, evaluation, and treatment of high blood cholesterol in Adults (Adult Treatment Panel III). JAMA. 2001;285:2486–97.
20. Misra A, Chowbey P, Makkar BM, Vikram NK, Wasir JS, Chadha D, et al. Consensus Statement for diagnosis of obesity, abdominal obesity and the metabolic syndrome for Asian Indians and recommendations for physical activity, medical and surgical management. J Assoc Physicians India. 2009;57:163–70.
21. World Health Organization. Global recommendations on physical activity for health. Geneva: World Health Organization; 2010. http://www.whqlibdoc.who.int/ publications/2010/9789241599979_eng.pdf. Accessed 5 Dec 2015.
22. International Institute of Population Sciences (IIPS), ORC Macro. National family health survey (NFHS –2), India, 1998–99. Mumbai: International Institute of Population Sciences; 2000.
23. Gupta R. Burden of coronary heart disease in India. Indian Heart J. 2005;57:632–8.
24. Sarvotham SG, Berry JN. Prevalence of coronary heart disease in an urban population in northern India. Circulation. 1968;37:939–53.
25. Chadha SL, Radhakrishnan S, Ramachandran K, Kaul U, Gopinath N. Epidemiological study of coronary heart disease in urban population of Delhi. Indian J Med Res. 1990;92:424–30.
26. Gupta R, Prakash H, Majumdar S, Sharma SC, Gupta VP. Prevalence of coronary heart disease and coronary risk factors in an urban population of Rajasthan. Indian Heart J. 1995;47:331–8.
27. Gupta R, Gupta VP, Sarna M, Bhatnagar S, Thanvi J, Sharma V, et al. Prevalence of coronary heart disease and risk factors in an urban Indian population: Jaipur Heart Watch-2. Indian Heart J. 2002;54:59–66.
28. Harris RB, Weissfeld LA. Gender differences in the reliability of reporting symptoms of angina pectoris. J Clin Epidemiol. 1991;44:1071–8.
29. Fischbacher CM, Bhopal R, Unwin N, White M, Alberti KG. The performance of the Rose angina questionnaire in South Asian and European origin populations: a comparative study in Newcastle. UK Int J Epidemiol. 2001;30:1009–16.
30. Patel DJ, Winterbotham M, Sutherland SE, Britt RG, Keil JE, Sutton GC. Comparison of methods to assess coronary heart disease prevalence in South Asians. Natl Med J India. 1997;10:210–3.
31. Singh RB, Sharma JP, Rastogi V, Raghuvanshi RS, Moshiri M, Verma SP, et al. Prevalence of coronary artery disease and coronary risk factors in rural and urban populations of north India. Eur Heart J. 1997;18:1728–35.
32. Kumar R, Singh MC, Singh MC, Ahlawat SK, Thakur JS, Srivastava A, et al. Urbanization and coronary heart disease: a study of urban–rural differences in northern India. Indian Heart J. 2006;58:126–30.
33. Hughes LO, Raval U, Raftery EB. First myocardial infarctions in Asian and white men. BMJ. 1989;298:1345–50.
34. Enas EA, Dhawan J, Petkar S. Coronary artery disease in Asian Indians: lessons learnt and the role of lipoprotein(a). Indian Heart J. 1997;49:25–34.
35. Gupta R, Gupta VP. Meta-analysis of coronary heart disease prevalence in India. Indian Heart J. 1996;48:241–5.
36. Kamili M, Dar I, Ali G, Wazir H, Hussain S. Prevalence of coronary heart disease in Kashmiris. Indian Heart J. 2007;59:44–9.
37. Latheef SA, Subramanyam G. Prevalence of coronary artery disease and coronary risk factors in an urban population of Tirupati. Indian Heart J. 2007;59:157–64.
38. Jafar TH, Qadri Z, Chaturvedi N. Coronary artery disease epidemic in Pakistan: more electrocardiographic evidence of ischemia in women than in men. Heart. 2008;94:408–13.
39. Centers for Disease Control and Prevention (CDC). Prevalence of coronary heart disease –United States, 2006–2010. MMWR Morb Mortal Wkly Rep. 2011;60:1377–81.
40. Go AS, Mozaffarian D, Roger VL, Benjamin EJ, Berry JD, Blaha MJ, et al. Executive summary: heart disease and stroke statistics–2014 update: a report from the American Heart Association. Circulation. 2014;129:399–410.
41. Townsend N, Wickramasinghe K, Bhatnagar P. Coronary heart disease statistics. London: British Heart Foundation; 2012. p. 82.
42. Gupta R, Gupta HP, Keswani P, Sharma S, Gupta VP, Gupta KD. Coronary heart disease and coronary risk factors in rural Rajasthan. J Assoc Physicians India. 1994;42:24–6.
43. Gupta AK, Bharadwaj A, Ashotra S, Gupta BP. Feasibility and training of multipurpose workers in detection, prevention and control of coronary artery disease in apple-belt of Shimla hills. South Asian J Prev Cardiol. 2002;6:17–22.

9

Percutaneous treatment of spontaneous left main coronary artery dissection using drug-eluting stent

Christos Graidis*, Dimokritos Dimitriadis, Vasileios Karasavvidis, Georgios Dimitriadis, Efstathia Argyropoulou, Fotios Economou, George Spiromitros, Antonios Antoniou and Georgios Karakostas

Abstract

Background: Spontaneous coronary artery dissection is a rare cause of ischemic heart disease and sudden death. Prompt diagnosis is of paramount importance, especially in cases when it manifests with ST elevation myocardial infarction (STEMI).

Case presentation: We report a case of a 42 year-old woman, who presented with an anterior STEMI in a hospital without on-site percutaneous coronary intervention (PCI) facilities. She was transferred to our hospital and coronary angiography revealed a spontaneous dissection of the left main stem coronary artery (LM). The dissection was successfully managed with PCI.

Conclusion: PCI appears to be a potential option, for the treatment of selected cases with spontaneous LM dissection, presenting with an acute coronary syndrome.

Keywords: Spontaneous coronary artery dissection, Left main, Percutaneous coronary intervention

Background

Spontaneous coronary artery dissection (SCAD) is a rare cause of ischemic heart disease and sudden death. The true incidence tends to be underestimated since most cases are diagnosed at autopsy, reflecting the significant mortality associated with this condition. The subtype of spontaneous LM coronary dissection is even less common (accounts for 6-12% of all primary coronary dissections), usually leading to sudden death or extensive infarction. Treatment options for SCAD include conservative treatment(medical), percutaneous coronary intervention(PCI) and coronary artery bypass graft surgery (CABG) still the optimal strategy for this disease process has not been clearly defined. We report here a case of spontaneous dissection of the LM coronary artery, with left anterior descending (LAD) and circumflex artery involvement (LCx), which occurred in a 42-year-old healthy woman and was unrelated with childbirth or other known risk factors. Rescue angioplasty with stenting was performed.

Case Presentation

A 42 years old Caucasian woman, without any previous medical history or any risk factors for coronary artery disease presented to a district general hospital, with no cardiac catheter laboratory facilities, complaining about a sudden-onset substernal chest pain lasting for the past 2 h. Her ECG findings on admission were ST elevation in leads I, aVL, aVF, V2-V6 (Figure 1). A thrombolytic agent was administered immediately, with regression of the angina and almost normalization of the ECG changes. The patient was not transferred to a hospital with PCI-capability for pharmaco-invasive strategy at that time, for unknown reasons. On the eighth in-hospital day, the patient complained of another episode of substernal chest pain, with hypotension and signs of left ventricular heart failure. The ECG showed extensive ST elevation in leads I, aVL, V1-V6 (Figure 2). Treatment with intravenous inotropic amines and re-thrombolysis (half-dose) was initiated and she was transferred to our hospital. On arrival to the coronary care unit, the patient was in cardiogenic shock. Echo on admission displayed anterior, apex and anteroseptum akinesia and severely impaired left ventricular function. The ejection

* Correspondence: dimitriadis1980@gmail.com
Department of Interventional Cardiology, Kyanous Stavros Hospital, Vizyis-Vyzantos 1 Street, Thessaloniki 54636, Greece

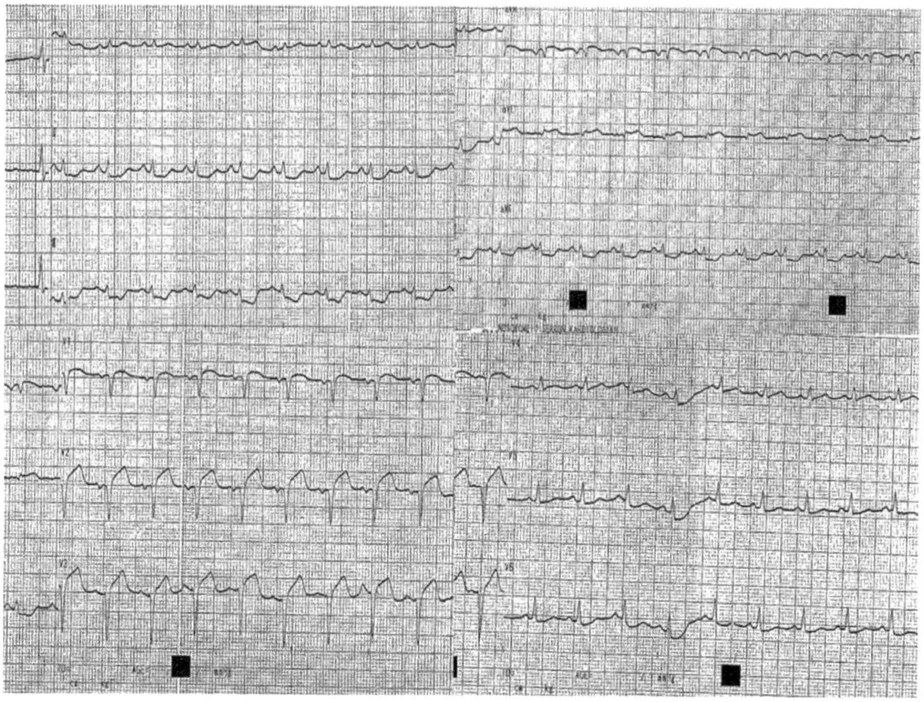

Figure 1 ECG findings on admission were ST elevation in leads I, aVL, aVF, V2-V6.

fraction of the patient was 25% with moderate mitral regurgitation. She was electively intubated, an intra-aortic balloon pump (IABP) was advanced and she was urgently transferred to the cardiac catheterization laboratory. Coronary angiography revealed the presence of a long dissection of the left coronary trunk (LCT) with a double distal extension: a. Towards the anterior left descending coronary artery (LAD), the proximal third of which was occluded (TIMI-1 flow) and b. towards the circumflex artery (Cx) with slowed distal flow (TIMI-2 flow), (Figure 3). The

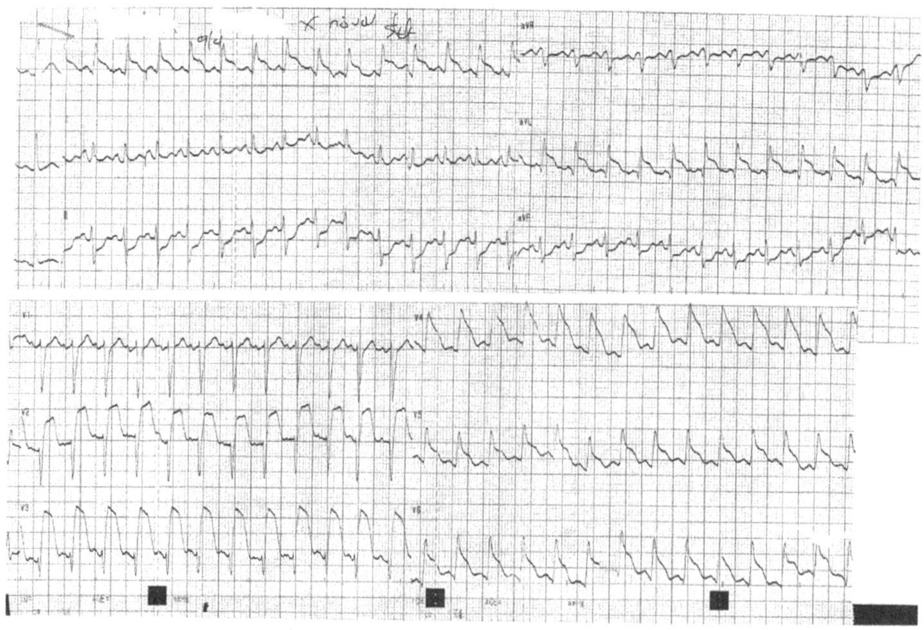

Figure 2 On the eighth in-hospital day, the patient suffered another episode of substernal chest pain. The ECG showed extensive ST elevation in leads I, aVL, V1-V6.

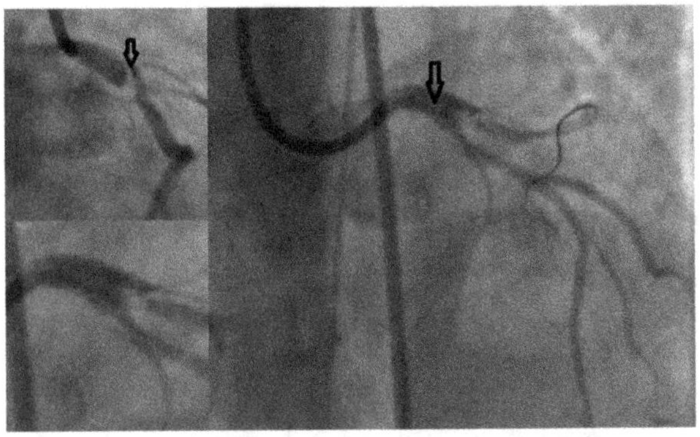

Figure 3 Coronary angiography revealed the presence of a long dissection with intimal flap (arrows) of the left coronary trunk (LCT) with a double distal extension to the left anterior descending and circumflex arteries.

right coronary artery (RCA) was normal. The diagnosis of a spontaneous coronary artery dissection was prompt, with these angiographic findings. The use of intravascular ultrasound (IVUS) or optical coherence tomography (OCT) was not plausible due to the emergency of the case. After a quick briefing with the heart team, immediate stenting was decided due to the hemodynamic compromise of the patient. Angioplasty and stenting with a drug eluting stent (DES) was therefore performed. After positioning a Q 3.5 SH 7Fr (Boston Scientific, Natick, MA, USA) guiding catheter using a Runthrough (Terumo Corporation, Tokyo, Japan) guide wire, the true lumen was crossed and the wire was placed in the distal Cx with free movement of the tip (Figure 4A). It was extremely difficult to place another guide wire to the distal LAD (despite multiple attempts and various J) and since there was a high risk of further extending the dissection, we decided to proceed with direct stenting of the left main. A 3.0 × 24 mm Taxus Element (Boston Scientific, Natick, MA, USA) stent was deployed at 14 atms into the left main and proximal Cx (Figure 5B). Due to the proximal sealing of the dissection, there was flow improvement in the LAD (Figure 4C). An Asahi Pro Water (Asahi Intecc, Japan) guide wire easily crossed the struts of the stent and was placed to the distal LAD, followed by inflations of two Sapphire (Orbus Neich Medical, B.V The Netherlands) 2.0 × 10 mm and a 2.5 × 15 mm balloons at the ostium and proximal of the LAD. A second Taxus Element 3.0X16mm was deployed, due to residual stenosis distally to the implanted stent of the Cx, overlapping it (Figure 4D). The procedure was concluded by placing a Taxus Element 3.0 × 16 mm stent, into the LAD, with TAP technique (T And Protrusion) (Figure 4E,F). The benefit of this combined technique is that the opportunity to first perform single-stenting is preserved, while side-branch stenting can be performed only if required. Final result was excellent, with no residual dissection and TIMI 3 flow in to the LAD and Cx. (Figure 5). She was discharged (day 8) on dual antiplatelet therapy, β-blocker, ACE inhibitor and statin. The patient remained asymptomatic at 3 months follow up and a MSCT coronary angiography showed the absence of restenosis in the segments treated with stents, followed by an improvement of left ventricular systolic function (Figure 6). A follow up cardiac catheterization angiography was recommended (class IIb) after 6 months according to European Society of Cardiology guidelines for high risk PCI (unprotected LM).

Discussion

Spontaneous coronary artery dissection (SCAD) is an unusual but increasingly recognised cause of acute coronary syndromes and sudden cardiac death. This entity was first described in 1931 by Pretty during a post-mortem study of a 42-year old woman with sudden cardiac death [1]. The overall incidence of SCAD in angiographic series ranges from 0.07% to 1.1% [2-6]. It is likely to be underestimated, since in a significant number of published cases, the diagnosis was only made at autopsy. The mean age at presentation is 35 to 45 years [3,6]. Seventy percent of the cases occur in women. One third of SCAD cases occur during the peripartum period, of which one third are in late pregnancy and two thirds in the early puerperal period. The LAD is the most common culprit vessel in women, whereas in men the RCA is more commonly affected [2-4]. Independently of gender, LAD is affected in 75% of the cases and RCA in 20% of the cases. Spontaneous dissection of the left main coronary artery (LMCA) accounts for 6-12% of all primary coronary dissections [3]. The circumflex artery was infrequently involved in men and women [7]. Multivessel involvement has also been described predominantly in women. The usage of modern techniques such as IVUS or OCT is of paramount importance in the diagnosis of SCAD. IVUS gained great importance in diagnosing SCAD especially of those that are angiographically unapparent. Typical IVUS features are the presence of intramural hematoma in the outer third of the media, visualization of the morphology of the vessel lumen, assessment of the intramural dissection and ensuring correct stent deployment. OCT being a new imaging modality provides extremely high resolution images of the coronary vessel. In cases of SCAD its exceptional spatial resolution provides a unique visualization of the intimal tear and the intramural hematoma. Although the pathophysiology remains unclear, it has been postulated that hemodynamic changes along with changes in the arterial wall architecture may predispose to intimal tears and intramural hematoma formation. The patients with SCAD have traditionally been divided into three groups: i) women in the peripartum period or in oral contraceptive therapy, ii) patients with concomitant atherosclerotic coronary artery disease

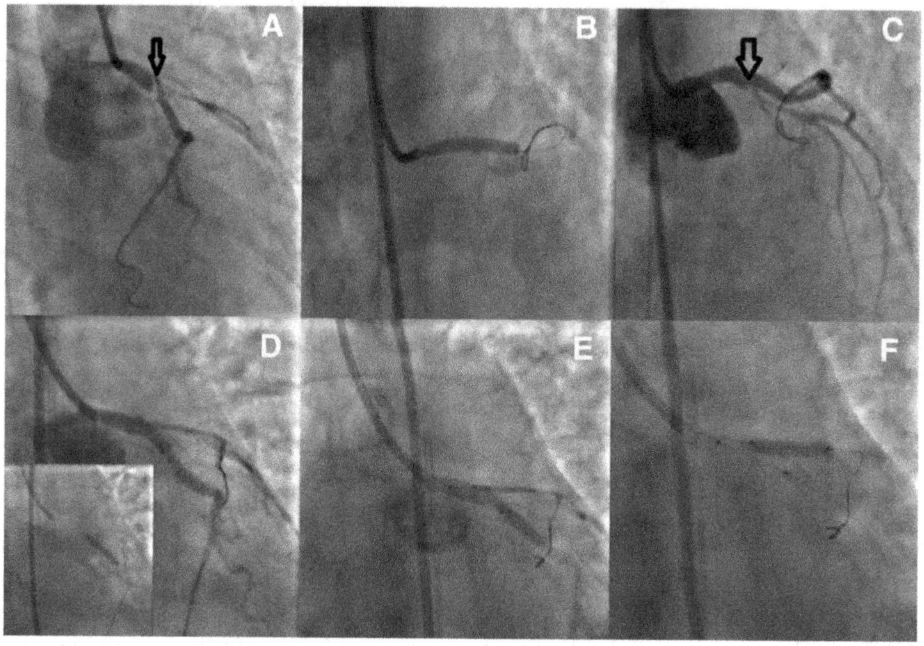

Figure 4 PCI with TAP technique (T And Protrusion), step by step analysis. A: The true lumen was crossed and the wire was placed in the distal Cx. **B**: A 3.0 × 24 mm Taxus Element stent was deployed at 14 atms into the left main and proximal LCx **C**: Due to the proximal sealing of the dissection (arrow), there was flow improvement in the LAD **D**: A second Taxus Element 3.0x16mm was deployed, due to residual stenosis distally to the implanted stent of the LCx, overlapping it **E**,**F**: The procedure was concluded by placing a Taxus Element 3.0 × 16 mm stent, into the LAD, with TAP technique (T And Protrusion).

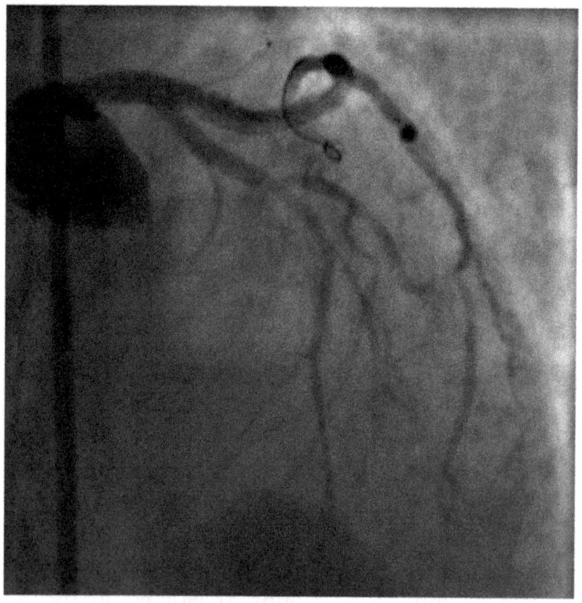

Figure 5 Final result was excellent, with no residual dissection and TIMI 3 flow in to the LAD and LCx.

and iii) idiopathic. SCAD has also been associated with cocaine use, blunt trauma, Marfan's syndrome, cystic medical necrosis, hypersensitivity vasculitis, coronary spasm, hypertension, fibromuscular dysplasia, after intense physical exercise and autoimmune thyroiditis [6].

There are no established guidelines available to guide treatment of patients with SCAD. Treatment options include medical therapy and revascularization with either CABG or PCI. The decision to pursue medical management or proceed to revascularisation with percutaneous intervention or coronary artery bypass grafting (CABG) should be individualized. Important factors to consider include location and extent of dissection, distal coronary blood flow, resolution or recurrence of symptoms following the initial event, hemodynamic stability and amount of myocardium at risk.

Conservative medical therapy is a reasonable approach in asymptomatic, stable patients with distal dissection or conserved coronary flow [7]. Medical therapy including aspirin, other antiplatelets, nitrates and beta-blockers has been successful in several cases with documentation of healing of the dissection on subsequent angiography. There are few data on the use of low molecular weight heparin or glycoprotein IIb/IIIa inhibitors [8]. Thrombolytic therapy is relatively contraindicated in SCAD due to the potential risk of worsening the dissection and

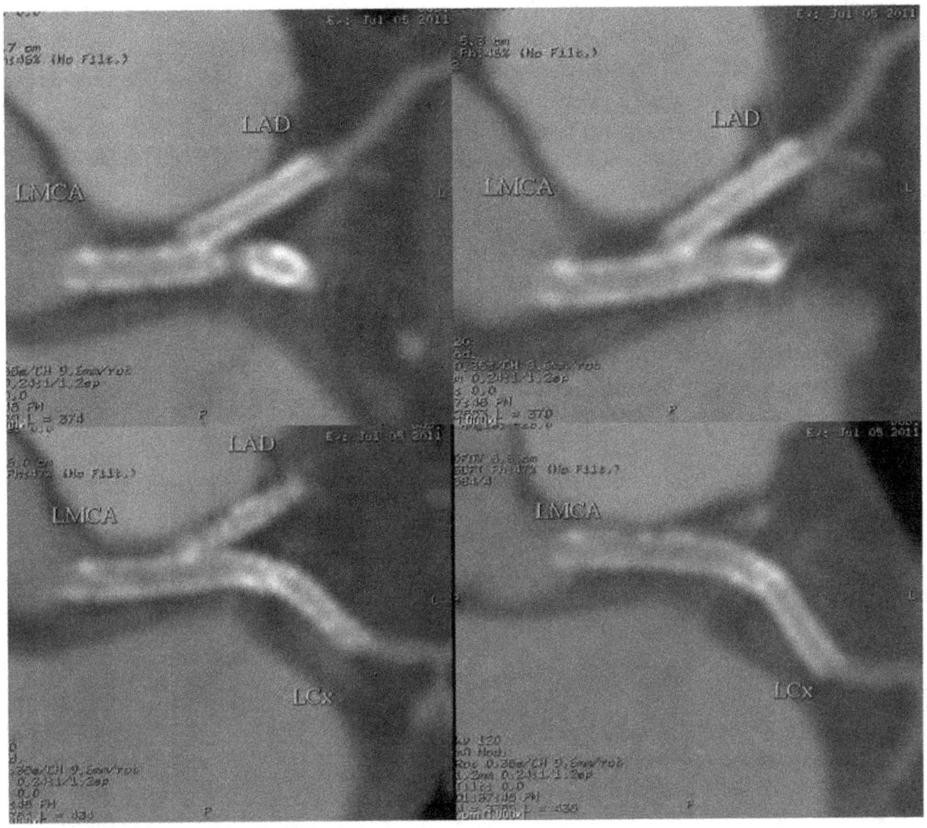

Figure 6 **A MSCT coronary angiography showed the absence of restenosis in the segments treated with stents at 3 months.**

contributing to expansion of the hematoma. Extension of dissection is possible [9], although successful use of thrombolysis has been described [10].

Revascularization for SCAD is warranted in those patients who present with ongoing ischemia refractory to medical treatment. Percutaneous coronary intervention [11] is the treatment of choice in patients with single-vessel involvement and signs of ongoing ischemia. Successful stenting for SCAD was first reported by Hong et al. [12] and since then percutaneous revascularisation has been increasingly performed resulting in very good long-term outcomes [13].

The interventionalist should be aware of the technical difficulties that may be encountered when dealing with such patients. It is essential to ensure that the guidewire is advancing in the true lumen. Passing the wire into the false lumen may occur more easily in these relatively non-fibrotic arteries were the use of OCT or IVUS would be a powerful weapon of the interventional cardiologist's arsenal. Predilation with balloons should be avoided because it may lead to expansion of the dissection; instead direct stent implantation should be performed. A potential complication of stenting includes the extrusion of intramural thrombus up- or downstream of the stent, due to lack of fibrous tissue in these non-atherosclerotic vessels. That seems to have occurred in our case after implantation of the first stent with distal propagation of the dissection.

Surgical management is advisable in patients with left main stem or multiple vessel dissection jeopardising a large area of myocardium and when percutaneous intervention has failed [4,14,15]. Surgical revascularisation is also technically challenging, especially in identifying the true lumen, since grafting of the false lumen can have catastrophic consequences. Especially off-pump coronary artery bypass surgery minimises the risk of aortic dissection [15] and it is also preferable in pregnant women. Reported cases of left main spontaneous dissection are mainly treated with CABG [16].

To the best of our knowledge, there have only been a few reported cases of spontaneous left main dissection treated with percutaneous coronary stenting [16-19]. In our case, given the rapidly progressive nature of the dissection presenting as acute myocardial infarction, the delay from the transfer to our hospital, the unstable and critical hemodynamics at the time of procedure and the severity of LV dysfunction, it was felt that percutaneous stenting of the left main coronary artery to seal the entry point of the dissection would be the most expeditious therapy.

The prognosis of patients with SCAD has improved in recent years, likely due to increased diagnosis by cardiac catheterization and advances in treatment. In earlier series, mortality from spontaneous dissection was approximately 50%. With contemporary medical therapy, the rate of recurrent dissection is much lower and most patients are asymptomatic at follow up, with a 95% survival and 5% recurrent dissection rate [2-6].

Conclusions

In summary PCI appears to be a potential option, for the treatment of selected cases with spontaneous left main coronary artery dissection, presenting with an acute coronary syndrome.

Consent

Written informed consent was obtained from the patient for publication of this Case Report and any accompanying images. A copy of the written consent is available for review by the Editor-in-Chief of this journal.

Abbreviations

STEMI: ST elevation myocardial infarction; SCAD: Spontaneous coronary artery dissection; PCI: Percutaneous coronary intervention; LCT: Left coronary trunk; LMCA: Left main coronary artery; LAD: Left anterior descending artery; RCA: Right coronary artery; LCx: Left circumflex artery; ECG: Electrocardiogram; CABG: Coronary artery bypass grafting.

Competing interests

The authors declare that they have no competing interests.

Authors' contributions

GrCh had a substantial contribution in drafting the manuscript, performing, analysis and interpretation of the coronary angiography data; DD made substantial contributions to the conception, design, drafting, and critical revision of the manuscript. He gave final approval for publication. KV analysed and interpreted the data regarding hospital admittance. He had substantial contribution to conception, in drafting the manuscript and revising it critically along with analysis and interpretation of MDCT data; DG had substantial contribution in drafting the manuscript, performing, analysis and interpretation of computed angiography data; AE and OF showed substantial contribution in collection and acquisition of data, drafting the manuscript. KG had contribution in drafting and revising the manuscript; GS and AA made substantial contributions to conception and design, acquisition of data, analysis and interpretation of data. He was involved in revising the manuscript critically and gave final approval for publication. All authors read and approved the final manuscript.

References

1. Pretty HC: **Dissecting aneurysm of coronary artery in a woman aged 42: rupture.** *BMJ* 1931, **1**:667.
2. Kamineni R, Sadhu A, Alpert JS: **Spontaneous coronary artery dissection: report of two cases and a 50-year review of the literature.** *Cardiol Rev* 2002, **10**:279–284.
3. Vrints CJM: **Acute coronary syndromes: spontaneous coronary artery dissection.** *Heart* 2010, **96**(10):801–808.
4. Shamloo BK, Chintala RS, Nasur A, Ghazvini M, Shariat P, Diggs JA, Singh SN: **Spontaneous coronary artery dissection, aggressive vs. conservative therapy.** *J Invasive Cardiol* 2010, **22**(5):222–228.
5. Vanzetto G, Berger-Coza E, Barone-Rochettea G, Chavanonb O, Bouvaista H, Hacinib R, Blinb D, Machecourta J: **Prevalence, therapeutic management and medium-term prognosis of spontaneous coronary artery dissection: results from a database of 11,605 patients.** *Eur J Cardiothorac Surg* 2009, **35**(2):250–254.
6. Thompson EA, Ferraris S, Gress T, Ferraris V: **Gender differences and predictors of mortality in spontaneous coronary artery dissection: a review of reported cases.** *J Invasive Cardiol* 2005, **17**:59–61.
7. Marijon E, Fressonnet R, Haggui A, Mousseaux E, Redheuil A: **Spontaneous coronary dissection of the left main stem after intense physical activity-regression under conservative strategy.** *Int J Cardiol* 2008, **128**:e16–e18.
8. Cheung S, Mithani V, Watson RM: **Healing of spontaneous coronary dissection in the context of glycoprotein IIB/IIIA inhibitor therapy: a case report.** *Catheter Cardiovasc Interv* 2000, **51**:95–100.
9. Zupan I, Noc M, Trinkaus D, Popovic M: **Double vessel extension of spontaneous left main coronary dissection in young women treated with thrombolytics.** *Catheter Cardiovasc Interv* 2001, **52**:226–230.
10. Leclercq F, Messner-Pellenc P, Carabasse D, Lucke N, Rivvaland FR, Grolleau R: **Successful thrombolysis treatment of a spontaneous left main coronary artery dissection without subsequent surgery.** *Eur Heart J* 1996, **17**:320–32123.
11. Naganuma T, Chieffo A, Meliga E, Capodanno D, Park SJ, Onuma Y, Valgimigli M, Jegere S, Makkar RR, Palacios IF, Costopoulos C, Kim YH, Buszman PP, Chakravarty T, Sheiban I, Mehran R, Naber C, Margey R, Agnihotri A, Marra S, Capranzano P, Leon MB, Moses JW, Fajadet J, Lefevre T, Morice MC, Erglis A, Tamburino C, Alfieri O, Serruys PW, *et al*: **Long-term clinical outcomes after percutaneous coronary intervention versus coronary artery bypass grafting for ostial/midshaft lesions in unprotected left main coronary artery from the DELTA registry: a multicenter registry evaluating percutaneous coronary intervention versus coronary artery bypass grafting for left main treatment.** *JACC Cardiovasc Interv* 2014, **7**(4):354–361.
12. Hong MK, Satler LF, Mintz GS, Wong SC, Kent KM, Pichard AD, Popma JJ, Leon MB: **Treatment of spontaneous coronary artery dissection with intracoronary stenting.** *Am Heart J* 1996, **132**:200–202.
13. Moukarbel GV, Alam SE: **Spontaneous coronary artery dissection: management options in the stent era.** *J Invasive Cardiol* 2004, **16**:333–335.
14. Thayer JO, Healy RW, Maggs PR: **Spontaneous coronary dissection.** *Ann Thorac Surg* 1987, **44**:97–102.
15. Carmi D, Touati G, Barry M, Dadez E: **Spontaneous coronary artery dissection: value of beating heart myocardial revascularisation.** *Interact CardioVasc Thorac Surg* 2003, **2**:694–696.
16. Adlam D, Cuculi F, Lim C, Banning A: **Management of spontaneous coronary artery dissection in the primary percutaneous coronary intervention era.** *J Invasive Cardiol* 2010, **22**:549–553.
17. Le MQ, D M, Ling FS: **Spontaneous dissection of the left main coronary artery treated with percutaneous coronary stenting.** *J Invasive Cardiol* 2007, **19**(8):59–61.
18. Jurado-Román A, Andreu J, Tejada JG, Velázquez M, Albarrán A, Hernández F, Unzué L, Tascón J: **A complicated spontaneous left main coronary artery dissection.is the initial conservative management safe in asymptomatic patients?** *Cardiovasc Revasc Med* 2012, **13**(6):362–364.
19. Lelasi A, Silvestro A, Personeni D, Saino A, Angeletti C, Costalunga A, Tespili M: **Outcomes following primary percutaneous coronary intervention for unprotected left main-related ST-segment elevation myocardial infarction.** *J Cardiovasc Med* Epub 2014 May 30.

10

The relation of location-specific epicardial adipose tissue thickness and obstructive coronary artery disease

Fu-Zong Wu[1,2,3], Kang-Ju Chou[2,3,4], Yi-Luan Huang[1] and Ming-Ting Wu[1,3*]

Abstract

Background: There is growing evidence about the importance of epicardial adiposity on cardiometabolic risk. However, the relation of location-specific epicardial adipose tissue (EAT) thickness to coronary atherosclerotic burden is still unclear.

Methods: This meta-analysis was used to study the relations between location-specific EAT thickness and obstructive coronary artery disease (CAD). A systemic literature search to identify eligible studies that met the inclusion criteria from the beginning until January 2014 was made. We conducted the meta-analysis of all included 10 published studies. Pre-specified subgroup analyses were performed according to ethnicity, body mass index, diagnostic tools for CAD, and measurement tool if presence of high heterogeneity between studies. Potential publication bias was also assessed.

Results: We identified ten observed studies with a total of 1625 subjects for planned comparison. With regard to the association between obstructive CAD and location-specific EAT thickness at the right ventricular free wall, caution is warranted. The pooled estimate showed that location-specific EAT thickness at the right ventricular free wall was significantly higher in the CAD group than non-CAD group (standardized mean difference (SMD): 0.70 mm, 95% CI: 0.26-1.13, P = 0.002), although heterogeneity was high ($I^2 = 93\%$). It should be clear that only the result of echocardiography-based studies showed a significant association (SMD: 0.98 mm, 95% CI: 0.43-1.53, P = 0.0005), and the result of all included CT-based studies showed a non-significant association (SMD: 0.06 mm, 95% CI: -0.12-0.25, P = 0.50). In the subgroup analysis, the "diagnostic tools for CAD" or "measurement tool of EAT thickness" are potential major sources of heterogeneity between studies. With regard to location-specific EAT thickness at the left atrioventricular (AV) groove, it was significantly higher in the CAD group than non-CAD group (SMD: 0.74 mm, 95% CI: 0.55-0.92, P <0.00001; $I^2 = 0\%$).

Conclusion: Our meta-analysis suggests that significantly elevated location-specific EAT thickness at the left AV groove is associated with obstructive CAD. Based on the current evidence, the location-specific EAT thickness at the left AV groove appears to be a good predictor in obstructive CAD, especially in Asian populations. Furthermore well-designed studies are warranted because of the current limited number of studies.

Keywords: Coronary artery disease, Location-specific epicardial adipose tissue thickness, Meta-analysis

* Correspondence: wu.mingting@gmail.com
[1]Department of Radiology, Section of Thoracic and Circulation Imaging, Kaohsiung Veterans General Hospital, Kaohsiung, Taiwan
[3]Faculty of Medicine, School of Medicine, National Yang Ming University, Taipei, Taiwan
Full list of author information is available at the end of the article

Background

Excessive epicardial adipose tissue (EAT) accumulation within the pericardial sac has been suggested to play an important role in the development of coronary artery atherosclerosis through potential paracrine or endocrine mechanism by exerting inflammatory mediators such as TNF-alpha, IL-6, adipocytokines, and leptin [1-5]. Several previous studies have found that CT-measured EAT volume played an important causal role in coronary atherosclerotic burden or coronary artery disease [6-8].

There is increasing attention on the location-specific EAT thickness as a potential predictor in cardiometabolic disease because of uneven regional distribution of EAT around the heart, especially mostly located in the atrioventricular (AV) groove and interventricular (IV) groove [9-11]. Echocardiographic EAT measurement is a non-invasive and simple way to measure location-specific EAT at the right ventricular free wall clinically [12-17]. Alternatively, CT (computed tomography) or MRI (magnetic resonance imaging) can also provide the simple but precise 2D measurement in the thickness of EAT in all cardiac segments [11,18,19]. Current evidence about the association between location-specific EAT thickness at the right ventricular free wall and coronary artery disease (CAD) is still controversial. Several studies using echocardiography have demonstrated a significant relationship between CAD and location-specific EAT thickness measured at right ventricular free wall [13,14,16,17], while some studies using echocardiography or CT failed to observe a significant association [11,12,19,20]. Recent evidence has suggested that there is increasing attention on location-specific EAT thickness at the left AV groove as a potentially new biomarker associated with cardiometabolic risks by using 2D CT or MR measurement [11,19,21,22]. In this study, we conducted a meta-analysis to study the relationship between location-specific EAT thickness and obstructive CAD, which may serve as a reliable predictor and improve CAD risk stratification in the future.

Methods

This meta-analysis was conducted according to the Meta-analysis Of Observational Studies in Epidemiology (MOOSE) statement [23].

Search strategy

We searched the Pubmed, Ovid Medline, Ovid Embase and Cochrane databases for relevant articles. Reviews were independently performed by two authors using the following search terms: "epicardial adipose tissue", "epicardial fat", "subepicardial adipose tissue", "subepicardial fat", "coronary artery disease [Mesh]", "atherosclerosis [Mesh]", and "cardiovascular disease [Mesh]", from the beginning of publication until January 2014. No language restrictions were applied. The pre-specified inclusion criteria were as follows: (a) observational studies to investigate the relationship between location-specific EAT thickness and CAD measured by echocardiography, CT or MRI-based quantitative measurements; (b) subjects with suspicion of CAD or at high risk of CAD clinically, and then subsequently divided into CAD and non-CAD groups assessed by coronary angiography, coronary CT angiography and coronary MR angiography. CAD group was defined as luminal stenosis ≥ 50% in one or more coronary arteries; and (c) for each study, the mean difference, standard deviation (SD) and sample size of subjects of CAD and non-CAD groups were reported in the literature. References within studies that met the inclusion criteria were reviewed for any possible missing relevant articles. Studies were excluded if any of the inclusion criteria were not met. All 10 published studies that met these inclusion criteria were considered eligible for further meta-analysis.

Data extraction and quality assessment

Data were abstracted and quality of studies was assessed independently by two reviewers (F.Z.W. and M.T.W.). Disagreement on specific studies between the two reviewers was resolved by consensus. Data were extracted from each study including the sample size and mean difference ± SD in location-specific EAT thickness in both CAD and non-CAD groups (regrouping and calculating the mean difference and mixed SD in the study of Eroglu et al. [14]). Methodological study quality was assessed using the Strengthening of Reporting of Observational Studies in Epidemiology (STROBE) checklist of 22 items [24].

Data analysis

All statistical analyses were performed using the Comprehensive Meta-Analysis version 2 (Biostat, Englewood, New Jersey) and the Review Manager 5.0 software, available through the Cochrane Collaboration. Both fixed- and random-effects models were used for analysis of the standardized mean difference (SMD) in the CAD and non-CAD group. Heterogeneity was assessed and quantified using Cochran's Q statistic and the I^2 statistic [25]. If I^2 was below 30%, fixed effects were chosen; if I^2 was equal to or greater than 30%, then random effects were applied [26]. Before the analysis, we formed a prior hypothesis that if heterogeneity existed in the studies, the source could be due to: (1) diagnostic tool for CAD (coronary angiography vs. coronary CT angiography); (2) ethnicity (Asian vs. non-Asian); (3) measurement tool of EAT (echocardiography vs. CT); and (4) body mass index (BMI). We also performed subgroup and univariate meta-regression analyses to investigate potential sources of variability. Publication bias was assessed if available by using Egger's test to examine the likely presence of publication bias.

Results

Study identification and selection

Overall, 312 articles were initially identified according to the broad criteria. After the initial screening of the title and abstract, 21 potentially relevant articles were retrieved for detailed review of their full text. Many studies that investigated the association between epicardial fat volume and CAD were excluded in this step.

In all these relevant studies, 11 studies were excluded after the detail review of their full text. Of these 11 studies, five studies were excluded because they did not report the detailed data for the meta-analysis [27-31]; two studies were excluded because of an investigation of the relationship between the EAT volume or area with CAD [32,33]; two studies were excluded because the study subjects were not well-defined or did not meet the criteria [15,34]; and the remaining two were letters and experimental studies [5,35]. The remaining 10 observational studies were eligible for the meta-analysis [11-14,16,17,19-21,36]. The flowchart of the search and selection of studies in this meta-analysis is illustrated in Figure 1. Overall, these studies included 1625 patients (924 subjects with CAD, and 701 subjects without CAD).

Table 1 summarize the characteristics of the nine observational studies investigating the association between location-specific EAT thickness at the right ventricular free wall and obstructive CAD. Table 2 summarizes the characteristics of the three observational studies investigating the association between location-specific EAT thickness at the left AV groove and obstructive CAD.

Location-specific EAT thickness at the right ventricular free wall and obstructive CAD

With regard to the association between the location-specific EAT thickness at the right ventricular free wall and obstructive CAD, there was a significant difference in the SMD between CAD and no-CAD groups (0.70 mm, 95% CI: 0.26-1.13, $p = 0.002$) in a random-effect pooled analysis of these studies (fixed-effect model in the Additional file 1: Figure S1). Statistically significant heterogeneity was observed in the study results ($p < 0.00001$, $I^2 = 93\%$). There was no indication of publication bias with Egger's test ($p = 0.229$, funnel plot shown in Additional file 2: Figure S2). A sensitivity analysis, in which one study was removed at a time, was performed to evaluate the stability of the results. Results were similar in all sensitivity analyses.

Subgroup analyses were performed in an attempt to explore the possible causes of heterogeneity, according to ethnicity, diagnostic tools for CAD, and measurement tool of EAT thickness. In subgroup analysis according to ethnicity shown in Table 3, the test for subgroup differences did not show a significant interaction. In contrast, the test for subgroup differences showed a significant interaction in the subgroup analysis according to diagnostic tools for CAD. In addition, the test for subgroup differences showed a significant interaction according to measurement tool of EAT thickness. In the subgroup of echocardiography-based studies, the random-effects model was used for the analysis, because the test for heterogeneity was statistically significant ($p < 0.00001$; $I^2 = 94\%$). There was a significant difference in the SMD between CAD and no-CAD groups (0.98 mm, 95% CI: 0.43-1.53, $p = 0.0005$).

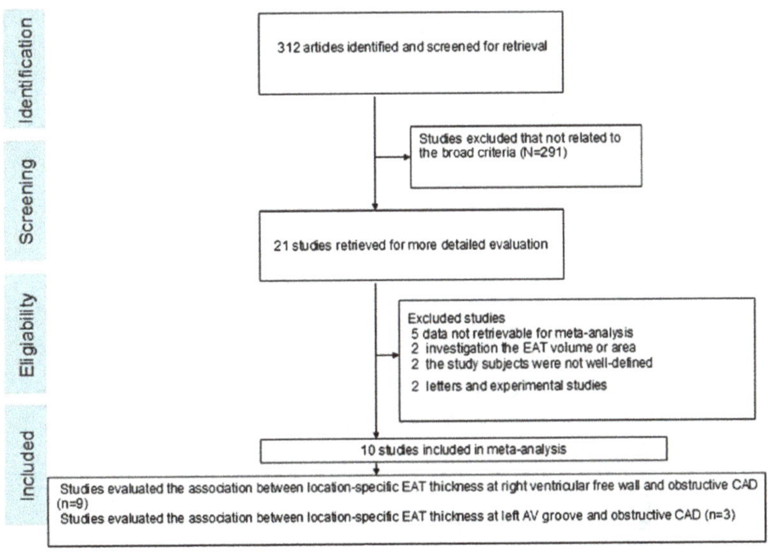

Figure 1 Flowchart of study selection process to determine the studies to be included in the meta-analysis. EAT, epicardial adipose tissue.

Table 1 Demographics of included studies in the association between location-specific EAT thickness at the right ventricular free wall and obstructive CAD

			CAD group EAT thickness (mm)			Non-CAD group EAT thickness (mm)							
References	Time	No. of patients	Mean	SD	Total	Mean	SD	Total	BMI (kg/m^2)	Diagnostic tool	Measurement tool	Ethnicity	Study quality
Chaowalit et al. [12]	2006	139	2.22	1.86	85	2.16	1.77	54	28.7 ± 5.5	Coronary angiography	Echocardiography	Non-Asian	20
Yun et al. [13]	2009	153	3.8	1.9	85	1.8	1.4	68	25.2 ± 3.1	Coronary angiography	Echocardiography	Asian	21
Eroglu et al. [14]	2009	150	7.3	1.2	80	4.68	1.13	70	28.9 ± 4.5	Coronary angiography	Echocardiography	Non-Asian	21
Wang et al. [11]	2010	224	4.3	1.8	140	4.1	2.0	84	26.1 ± 3.3	Coronary angiography	CT	Asian	21
Bastarrika et al. [20]	2010	45	8.57	2.08	23	7.69	2.68	22	29.1 ± 5.7	Coronary angiography	CT	Non-Asian	20
Mustelier et al. [16]	2011	250	6.6	2.8	185	4.7	2.3	65	27.4 ± 5.3	Coronary angiography	Echocardiography	Non-Asian	19
Shemirani et al. [17]	2012	292	5.4	1.9	171	4.4	1.8	121	NR	Coronary angiography	Echocardiography	Non-Asian	19
Wu et al. [19]	2013	208	5.8	2.3	97	5.9	2.3	111	24.8 ± 3.3	Coronary CT angiography	CT	Asian	21
Kaya et al. [36]	2013	64	6.43	0.9	34	5.35	0.75	30	26.0 ± 3.0	Coronary angiography	Echocardiography	Non-Asian	19

BMI, body mass index; EAT, epicardial adipose tissue; CAD, coronary artery disease; CT, computed tomography; NR, not reported.

Table 2 Demographics of included studies in the association between location-specific EAT thickness at left AV groove and obstructive CAD

			CAD group EAT thickness (mm)			Non-CAD group EAT thickness (mm)							
References	Time	No. of patients	Mean	SD	Total	Mean	SD	Total	BMI (kg/m^2)	Diagnostic tool	Measurement tool	Ethnicity	Study quality
Wang et al. [11]	2010	224	13.2	3.1	140	11.3	2.5	84	26.1 ± 3.3	Coronary angiography	CT	Asian	21
Kim et al. [21]	2012	100	13	2.6	24	11.5	2.1	76	25.3 ± 3.2	Coronary MR angiography	MRI	Asian	21
Wu et al. [19]	2013	208	17.8	3.9	97	14.3	4.3	111	24.8 ± 3.3	Coronary CT angiography	CT	Asian	21

BMI, body mass index; EAT, epicardial adipose tissue; CAD, coronary artery disease; CT, computed tomography; AV, atrioventricular.

Table 3 Subgroups analyses according to the ethnicity, diagnostic tool, and measurement tool comparing location-specific EAT thickness at the right ventricular free wall in subjects of CAD and non-CAD groups

Subgroups	Studies	Subjects	SMD (95% CI)	p Value
Ethnicity				
Asian	3	585	0.4 (-0.28 to 1.09)	0.36
Non-Asian	6	940	0.80 (0.30 to 1.29)	
Diagnostic tool				
Coronary angiography	8	1317	0.75 (0.34 to 1.16)	0.002
Coronary CT angiography	1	208	-0.04 (-0.23 to 0.32)	
Measurement tool				
Echocardiography	6	1048	0.98 (0.43 to 1.53)	0.002
CT	3	477	0.06 (0.17 to 1.09)	

p Value: test of interaction between subgroups. CAD, coronary artery disease; SMD, standardized mean difference; CT, computed tomography.

By contrast, there was no significant difference in the SMD between CAD and no-CAD groups (0.06 mm, 95% CI: -0.12-0.25, $p = 0.50$) in the subgroup of CT-based studies, and greater homogeneity was also observed within this subgroup shown in Figure 2 ($p = 0.43$; $I^2 = 0$). Therefore, diagnostic tools for CAD and measurement tool of EAT thickness were the potential sources of heterogeneity between studies. In univariate random effects meta-regression analysis, BMI was not significantly associated with effect size shown in Figure 3 (95% CI: -0.24 -0.17, $p = 0.59$).

Location-specific EAT thickness at the left AV groove and obstructive CAD

Figure 4 shows the forest plot of the pooled results of the SMD of the three studies in order to investigation the association between obstructive CAD and EAT thickness at the left AV groove. In a fixed-effect pooled analysis, there was a significant difference in the SMD between CAD and no-CAD groups (0.74 mm, 95% CI: 0.55-0.92, $p < 0.00001$), and low heterogeneity among the three studies shown in Figure 4 ($p = 0.61$, $I^2 = 0\%$). Overall, location-specific EAT thickness at the left AV groove was significantly thicker in the CAD group than the no-CAD group. Publication bias was not assessed because of limited studies.

Discussion

The role of location-specific EAT thickness at the right ventricular free wall in obstructive CAD

With regard to the association between the location-specific EAT thickness at the right ventricular free wall and obstructive CAD, the overall results of the meta-analysis in nine studies show a statistically significantly increase in EAT thickness at the right ventricular free wall in the CAD group than in the no-CAD group.

It should be clear that only the result of echocardiography-based studies (six studies) showed a significant association between CAD and the EAT thickness at right ventricular free wall, and the result of all included CT-based studies (three studies) showed a non-significant association. And low between-study heterogeneity was also observed in the CT-based studies (three studies) assessed at the right ventricular free wall. However, extreme between-study heterogeneity was also observed in the overall meta-analysis

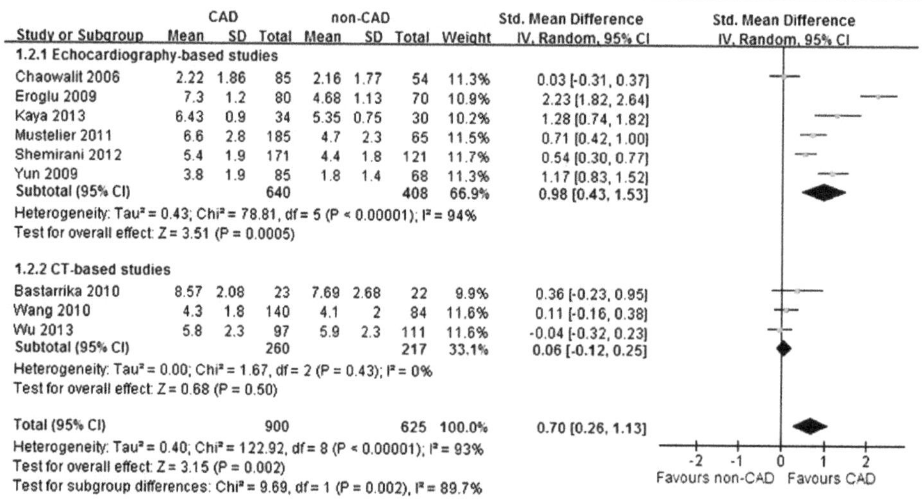

Figure 2 Forest plot for SMD (random-effect model) in location-specific EAT thickness at the right ventricular free wall between CAD and non-CAD group in the overall meta-analysis (including nine published studies). In addition, subgroup analyses were assessed by the measurement tool of EAT thickness (echocardiography or CT). SMD, standardized mean difference; CAD, coronary artery disease; EAT, epicardial adipose tissue.

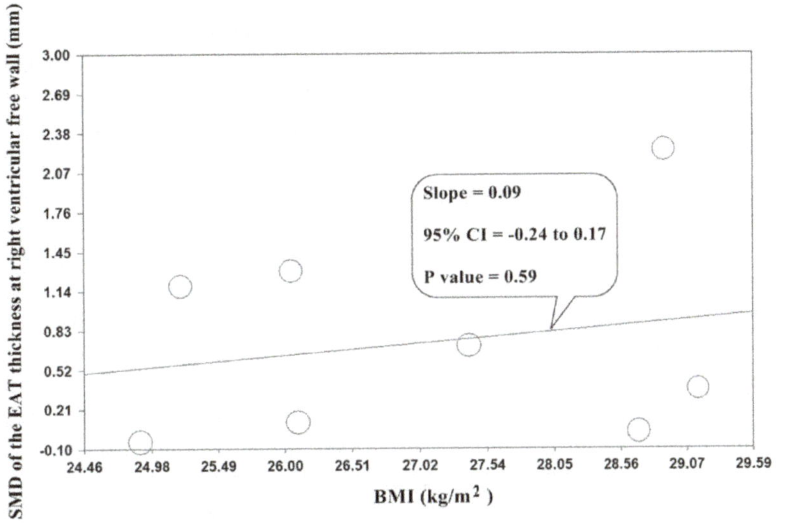

Figure 3 Meta-regression analysis between BMI and SMD of location-specific EAT thickness at right ventricular free wall. BMI, body mass index; SMD, standardized mean difference; EAT, epicardial adipose tissue.

(nine studies) and echocardiography-based studies (six studies). Therefore, all this evidence suggested that CT-based measurement may potentially be a more reliable tool than echocardiography-based measurement.

Regarding the association between location-specific EAT thickness at the right ventricular free wall and obstructive CAD, subgroup and meta-regression analyses for all covariates have been used to address the issues of heterogeneity between studies. A recent meta-analysis of worldwide study demonstrates a significant correlation between EAT and BMI, but shows a relationship between EAT and metabolic syndrome independent of BMI [37]. These findings support the meta-regression analysis in our study that revealed BMI was not considered a potential source of heterogeneity between eight studies.

We think a possible explanation for the high heterogeneity between studies was that the difference in reliability and reproducibility between the two tools (echocardiography vs. CT) should be seriously concerned. In comparison with CT-based measurement, echocardiography is a non-invasive imaging modality in EAT measurement that requires less cost and is less time-consuming. However, a recent study has shown the poor reproducibility of echocardiographic EAT measurements assessed by intraclass correlation coefficient, and low concordance observed between CT and echocardiographic measurement [38]. One the contrary, several studies have demonstrated high interobserver reliability and intraobserver reproducibility of EAT thickness measured by CT [11,39,40]. Potential measurement bias in the EAT measurement by echocardiography may contribute to the disparate results between echocardiography-based and CT-based studies. And recent longitudinal studies have also demonstrated non-association between EAT thickness assessed by echocardiography and cardiac events or major adverse cardiac events (MACE) [29,31], which also supports the negative result by CT-based studies in the subgroup analysis. Therefore, we suggest that the effect of location-specific EAT at the right ventricular free wall on CAD is still uncertain. However, future well-designed studies are warranted because of limited CT-based studies measuring location-specific EAT thickness at the right ventricular free wall.

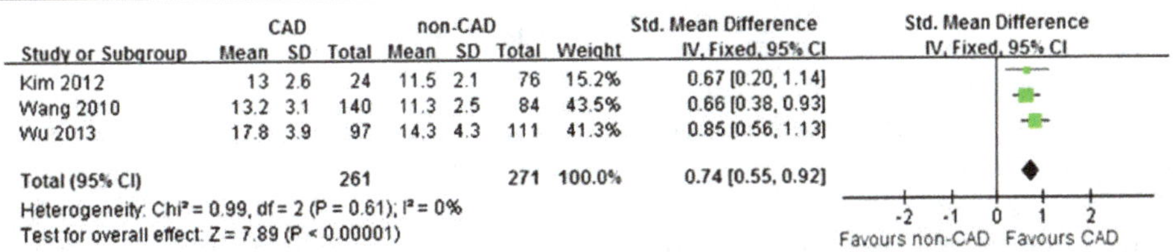

Figure 4 Forest plot for SMD in location-specific EAT thickness at the left AV groove between CAD and non-CAD groups in the meta-analysis (including three published studies). SMD, standardized mean difference; CAD, coronary artery disease; EAT, epicardial adipose tissue; AV, atrioventricular.

The role of location-specific EAT thickness at the left AV groove in obstructive CAD

With regard to the association between the location-specific EAT thickness at the left AV groove and obstructive CAD, the results from the current meta-analysis indicate increased location-specific EAT thickness at the left AV groove was associated with obstructive CAD assessed by CT or MRI.

And high homogeneity between studies was observed, despite diagnosis of CAD in different imaging modalities, including coronary angiography, coronary CT angiography and MR coronary angiography. Substantial evidence has also supported the diagnostic accuracy of coronary CT angiography and MR coronary angiography in the evaluation of coronary arteries stenosis [41-43].

While there is no obvious explanation for this observation, uneven regional distribution of EAT around the heart may provide clues. Recent studies also suggest that location-specific EAT thickness at the left AV groove may play a important causal role in cardiometabolic disease through a possible mechanism described by Wang et al. [11] whereby diffusion of EAT paracrine metabolites through thin-walled coronary venous networks into the coronary sinus is due to abundant coronary venous sinus drainage networks in the left AV groove. In addition, location-specific EAT thickness at the left AV groove can be easily and reliably assessed in 2D-based CT or MRI images available in routine clinical practice for cardiovascular risk assessment [11,19,21]. Taken together, these findings may indicate that combined measurement of EAT thickness in the left AV groove and coronary calcium score provides more in-depth information than conventional risk factor assessment in CAD prediction [44]. Because of the limited number of studies almost exclusively in Asian populations, future well-designed cohort studies are warranted to investigate the cause-effect relationship by CT or MRI.

Study strengths and limitations

It is our belief that the present study has demonstrated certain advantages over the previous meta-analysis [45]. First, in contrast to previous meta-analysis by Xu et al. [45] on this topic, we used explicit criteria to define inclusion criteria. To investigate the association between regional EAT thickness and CAD, we select the location-specific EAT thickness at the right ventricular free wall or left AV groove by echocardiography, CT or MRI rigorously. However, the previous meta-analysis has used these data of the "average" EAT thickness extracted from the study by Wang et al. [11]. Second, the aims of the previous meta-analysis and our study were both to investigate the relationship between EAT thickness and CAD. We found one included study in the previous meta-analysis that investigated the relationship between regional EAT thickness and descending thoracic aorta atherosclerosis [46], instead of all included nine studies rigorously assessing obstructive CAD in our study. Third, study quality was assessed using the STROBE statement to ensure that all studies reach a level of quality in this meta-analyses.

The current study had several potential limitations. First, all ten included studies in the present meta-analysis were case-control or cross-sectional studies despite assessing study quality using the STROBE statement, which has limitations in providing definite information about the cause-and-effect relationship. In addition, the best evidence comes primarily from meta-analyses of randomized controlled trials. Second, there are many confounding factors associated with CAD, such as the Framingham risk score and CAC score were not considered in this meta-analyses. However, we have investigated a number of factors to explore between-study heterogeneity. The included studies were different in diagnostic tools for CAD and measurement tools of EAT, which may contribute to the heterogeneity among the studies. Third, there are limited studies in assessing the association between left AVG EAT thickness and obstructive CAD despite recognition that homogeneity exists between studies, which may lead to insufficient evidence to support the result.

Conclusion

In summary, our meta-analysis suggests that significantly elevated location-specific EAT thickness at the left AV groove is associated with obstructive CAD, and homogeneity influenced agreement between studies. Based on the current evidence, the location-specific EAT thickness at the left AV groove appears to play an influential role in the prediction of obstructive CAD, especially in Asian populations. In addition, adding EAT thickness at the left AV groove on top of clinical CAD risk factors plus Agatston score may provide further evidence in predicting CAD in the population with suspicion of CAD [19,44]. Subsequent, large, more definitive studies are needed to confirm these findings and to establish if location-specific EAT thickness at the left AV groove be used in clinical context.

Additional files

Additional file 1: Figure S1. Forest plot for SMD (fixed-effect model) in location-specific EAT thickness at the right ventricular free wall between CAD and non-CAD groups in the overall meta-analysis (including nine published studies). Moreover, subgroup analyses were assessed by the measurement tool of EAT thickness (echocardiography or CT). SMD, standardized mean difference; CAD, coronary artery disease; EAT, epicardial adipose tissue.

Additional file 2: Figure S2. Funnel plot for potential publication bias in the overall meta-analysis of the association between location-specific EAT at the right ventricular free wall and obstructive CAD, including nine studies. EAT, epicardial adipose tissue; CAD, coronary artery disease.

Abbreviations

AV: Atrioventricular; BMI: Body mass index; CAC: Coronary arterial calcification; CAD: Coronary artery disease; CT: Computed tomography; EAT: Epicardial adipose tissue; MRI: Magnetic resonance imaging; MOOSE statement: Meta-analysis Of Observational Studies in Epidemiology statement; SD: Standard deviation; SMD: Standardized mean difference; STROBE checklist: Strengthening of Reporting of Observational Studies in Epidemiology checklist; MACE: Major adverse cardiac events.

Competing interests

The authors declare that they have no competing interests.

Authors' contributions

FZW and MTW participated in the conception, design of the study, collected the data, performed statistical analyses, and drafted the manuscript. YLH and KJC helped to collect data and draft the manuscript. All authors read and approved the final manuscript.

Acknowledgements

We are grateful to Dr. Carol C. Wu for reviewing the manuscript. This study was supported by Grants from National Science Council NSC97-2314-B-010-045-MY3 and Kaohsiung Veterans General Hospital, VGHKS101-020, VGHKS100-074, Taiwan, R.O.C.

Author details

[1]Department of Radiology, Section of Thoracic and Circulation Imaging, Kaohsiung Veterans General Hospital, Kaohsiung, Taiwan. [2]Centre for Evidence-Based Medicine, Kaohsiung Veterans General Hospital, Kaohsiung, Taiwan. [3]Faculty of Medicine, School of Medicine, National Yang Ming University, Taipei, Taiwan. [4]Department of Internal Medicine, Kaohsiung Veterans General Hospital, Kaohsiung, Taiwan.

References

1. Mazurek T, Zhang L, Zalewski A, Mannion JD, Diehl JT, Arafat H, Sarov-Blat L, O'Brien S, Keiper EA, Johnson AG, Martin J, Goldstein BJ, Shi Y: **Human epicardial adipose tissue is a source of inflammatory mediators.** *Circulation* 2003, **108**(20):2460–2466.
2. Baker A, da Silva N, Quinn D, Harte A, Pagano D, Bonser R, Kumar S, McTernan P: **Human epicardial adipose tissue expresses a pathogenic profile of adipocytokines in patients with cardiovascular disease.** *Cardiovasc Diabetol* 2006, **5**(1):1–7.
3. Sacks HS, Fain JN: **Human epicardial adipose tissue: a review.** *Am Heart J* 2007, **153**(6):907–917.
4. Iacobellis G, Corradi D, Sharma AM: **Epicardial adipose tissue: anatomic, biomolecular and clinical relationships with the heart.** *Nat Clin Pract Cardiovasc Med* 2005, **2**(10):536–543.
5. Iacobellis G, Pistilli D, Gucciardo M, Leonetti F, Miraldi F, Brancaccio G, Gallo P, di Gioia CR: **Adiponectin expression in human epicardial adipose tissue in vivo is lower in patients with coronary artery disease.** *Cytokine* 2005, **29**(6):251–255.
6. Iwasaki K, Matsumoto T, Aono H, Furukawa H, Samukawa M: **Relationship between epicardial fat measured by 64-multidetector computed tomography and coronary artery disease.** *Clin Cardiol* 2011, **34**(3):166–171.
7. Rosito GA, Massaro JM, Hoffmann U, Ruberg FL, Mahabadi AA, Vasan RS, O'Donnell CJ, Fox CS: **Pericardial fat, visceral abdominal fat, cardiovascular disease risk factors, and vascular calcification in a community-based sample: the Framingham Heart Study.** *Circulation* 2008, **117**(5):605–613.
8. Ahmadi N, Nabavi V, Yang E, Hajsadeghi F, Lakis M, Flores F, Zeb I, Bevinal M, Ebrahimi R, Budoff M: **Increased epicardial, pericardial, and subcutaneous adipose tissue is associated with the presence and severity of coronary artery calcium.** *Acad Radiol* 2010, **17**(12):1518–1524.
9. Gorter PM, de Vos AM, van der Graaf Y, Stella PR, Doevendans PA, Meijs MF, Prokop M, Visseren FL: **Relation of epicardial and pericoronary fat to coronary atherosclerosis and coronary artery calcium in patients undergoing coronary angiography.** *Am J Cardiol* 2008, **102**(4):380–385.
10. de Vos AM, Prokop M, Roos CJ, Meijs MF, van der Schouw YT, Rutten A, Gorter PM, Cramer MJ, Doevendans PA, Rensing BJ, Bartelink ML, Velthuis BK, Mosterd A, Bots ML: **Peri-coronary epicardial adipose tissue is related to cardiovascular risk factors and coronary artery calcification in post-menopausal women.** *Eur Heart J* 2008, **29**(6):777–783.
11. Wang TD, Lee WJ, Shih FY, Huang CH, Chen WJ, Lee YT, Shih TT, Chen MF: **Association of epicardial adipose tissue with coronary atherosclerosis is region-specific and independent of conventional risk factors and intra-abdominal adiposity.** *Atherosclerosis* 2010, **213**(1):279–287.
12. Chaowalit N, Somers VK, Pellikka PA, Rihal CS, Lopez-Jimenez F: **Subepicardial adipose tissue and the presence and severity of coronary artery disease.** *Atherosclerosis* 2006, **186**(2):354–359.
13. Yun KH, Rhee SJ, Yoo NJ, Oh SK, Kim NH, Jeong JW, Park DS, Park HY: **Relationship between the Echocardiographic Epicardial Adipose Tissue Thickness and Serum Adiponectin in Patients with Angina.** *J Cardiovasc Ultrasound* 2009, **17**(4):121–126.
14. Eroglu S, Sade LE, Yildirir A, Bal U, Ozbicer S, Ozgul AS, Bozbas H, Aydinalp A, Muderrisoglu H: **Epicardial adipose tissue thickness by echocardiography is a marker for the presence and severity of coronary artery disease.** *Nutr Metab Cardiovasc Dis* 2009, **19**(3):211–217.
15. Iacobellis G, Lonn E, Lamy A, Singh N, Sharma AM: **Epicardial fat thickness and coronary artery disease correlate independently of obesity.** *Int J Cardiol* 2011, **146**(3):452–454.
16. Mustelier JV, Rego JOC, González AG, Sarmiento JCG, Riverón BV: **Parâmetros ecocardiográficos de deposição de gordura epicárdica e sua relação com doença arterial coronariana.** *Arq Bras Cardiol* 2011, **97**:122–129.
17. Shemirani H, Khoshavi M: **Correlation of echocardiographic epicardial fat thickness with severity of coronary artery disease-an observational study.** *Anadolu Kardiyol Derg* 2012, **12**(3):200–205.
18. Liang KW, Tsai IC, Lee WJ, Lee IT, Lee WL, Lin SY, Wan CJ, Fu CP, Ting CT, Sheu WH: **MRI measured epicardial adipose tissue thickness at the right AV groove differentiates inflammatory status in obese men with metabolic syndrome.** *Obesity (Silver Spring)* 2012, **20**(3):525–532.
19. Wu FZ, Huang YL, Wang YC, Lin HS, Chen CS, Ju YJ, Chiou KR, Cheng CC, Wu MT: **Impact of location of epicardial adipose tissue, measured by coronary artery calcium-scoring computed tomography on obstructive coronary artery disease.** *Am J Cardiol* 2013, **112**(7):943–949.
20. Bastarrika G, Broncano J, Schoepf UJ, Schwarz F, Lee YS, Abro JA, Costello P, Zwerner PL: **Relationship between coronary artery disease and epicardial adipose tissue quantification at cardiac CT: comparison between automatic volumetric measurement and manual bidimensional estimation.** *Acad Radiol* 2010, **17**(6):727–734.
21. Kim HM, Kim KJ, Lee HJ, Yu HT, Moon JH, Kang ES, Cha BS, Lee HC, Lee BW, Kim YJ: **Epicardial adipose tissue thickness is an indicator for coronary artery stenosis in asymptomatic type 2 diabetic patients: its assessment by cardiac magnetic resonance.** *Cardiovasc Diabetol* 2012, **11**:83.
22. Wang TD, Lee WJ, Shih FY, Huang CH, Chang YC, Chen WJ, Lee YT, Chen MF: **Relations of epicardial adipose tissue measured by multidetector computed tomography to components of the metabolic syndrome are region-specific and independent of anthropometric indexes and intraabdominal visceral fat.** *J Clin Endocrinol Metab* 2009, **94**(2):662–669.
23. Stroup DF, Berlin JA, Morton SC, Olkin I, Williamson GD, Rennie D, Moher D, Becker BJ, Sipe TA, Thacker SB: **Meta-analysis of observational studies in epidemiology: a proposal for reporting. Meta-analysis Of Observational Studies in Epidemiology (MOOSE) group.** *JAMA* 2000, **283**(15):2008–2012.
24. von Elm E, Altman DG, Egger M, Pocock SJ, Gotzsche PC, Vandenbroucke JP: **The Strengthening the Reporting of Observational Studies in Epidemiology (STROBE) statement: guidelines for reporting observational studies.** *PLoS Med* 2007, **4**(10):e296.
25. Higgins JP, Thompson SG, Deeks JJ, Altman DG: **Measuring inconsistency in meta-analyses.** *BMJ* 2003, **327**(7414):557–560.
26. DerSimonian R, Kacker R: **Random-effects model for meta-analysis of clinical trials: an update.** *Contemp Clin Trials* 2007, **28**(2):105–114.
27. Ahn SG, Lim HS, Joe DY, Kang SJ, Choi BJ, Choi SY, Yoon MH, Hwang GS, Tahk SJ, Shin JH: **Relationship of epicardial adipose tissue by echocardiography to coronary artery disease.** *Heart* 2008, **94**(3):e7.
28. Jeong JW, Jeong MH, Yun KH, Oh SK, Park EM, Kim YK, Rhee SJ, Lee EM, Lee J, Yoo NJ, Kim NH, Park JC: **Echocardiographic epicardial fat thickness and coronary artery disease.** *Circ J* 2007, **71**(4):536–539.
29. Kaushik M, Saurav A, Smer A, Alla VM, Khan S, Madan R, Holmberg MJ, Mohiuddin S: **Epicardial adipose tissue as assessed by echocardiography and incident cardiac disease.** *J Am Coll Cardiol* 2012, **59**(13s1):E1159.
30. Nelson MR, Mookadam F, Thota V, Emani U, Al Harthi M, Lester SJ, Cha S, Stepanek J, Hurst RT: **Epicardial fat: an additional measurement for**

subclinical atherosclerosis and cardiovascular risk stratification? *J Am Soc Echocardiogr* 2011, **24**(3):339–345.

31. Albuquerque FN, Somers VK, Blume G, Miranda W, Korenfeld Y, Calvin AD, Qin R, Lopez-Jimenez F: **Usefulness of epicardial adipose tissue as predictor of cardiovascular events in patients with coronary artery disease.** *Am J Cardiol* 2012, **110**(8):1100–1105.
32. Bettencourt N, Toschke AM, Leite D, Rocha J, Carvalho M, Sampaio F, Xara S, Leite-Moreira A, Nagel E, Gama V: **Epicardial adipose tissue is an independent predictor of coronary atherosclerotic burden.** *Int J Cardiol* 2012, **158**(1):26–32.
33. Sironi AM, Petz R, De Marchi D, Buzzigoli E, Ciociaro D, Positano V, Lombardi M, Ferrannini E, Gastaldelli A: **Impact of increased visceral and cardiac fat on cardiometabolic risk and disease.** *Diabet Med* 2012, **29**(5):622–627.
34. Bachar GN, Dicker D, Kornowski R, Atar E: **Epicardial adipose tissue as a predictor of coronary artery disease in asymptomatic subjects.** *Am J Cardiol* 2012, **110**(4):534–538.
35. Cabrera-Rego JO: **Echocardiographic measurement of epicardial fat thickness: in search for a consensus/Correlation of echocardiographic epicardial fat thickness with severity of coronary artery disease-an observational study.** *Anadolu Kardiyol Derg* 2012, **12**(5):448–449. author reply 449.
36. Kaya H, Ertas F, Oylumlu M, Bilik MZ, Yildiz A, Yuksel M, Polat N, Acet H, Isik F, Ulgen MS: **Relation of epicardial fat thickness and brachial flow-mediated vasodilation with coronary artery disease.** *J Cardiol* 2013, **62**(6):343–347.
37. Rabkin SW: **The relationship between epicardial fat and indices of obesity and the metabolic syndrome: a systematic review and meta-analysis.** *Metab Syndr Relat Disord* 2014, **12**(1):31–42.
38. Saura D, Oliva MJ, Rodriguez D, Pascual-Figal DA, Hurtado JA, Pinar E, de la Morena G, Valdes M: **Reproducibility of echocardiographic measurements of epicardial fat thickness.** *Int J Cardiol* 2010, **141**(3):311–313.
39. Abbara S, Desai JC, Cury RC, Butler J, Nieman K, Reddy V: **Mapping epicardial fat with multi-detector computed tomography to facilitate percutaneous transepicardial arrhythmia ablation.** *Eur J Radiol* 2006, **57**(3):417–422.
40. Gorter PM, van Lindert AS, de Vos AM, Meijs MF, van der Graaf Y, Doevendans PA, Prokop M, Visseren FL: **Quantification of epicardial and peri-coronary fat using cardiac computed tomography; reproducibility and relation with obesity and metabolic syndrome in patients suspected of coronary artery disease.** *Atherosclerosis* 2008, **197**(2):896–903.
41. Yonezawa M, Nagata M, Kitagawa K, Kato S, Yoon Y, Nakajima H, Nakamori S, Sakuma H, Hatakenaka M, Honda H: **Quantitative analysis of 1.5-T whole-heart coronary MR angiograms obtained with 32-channel cardiac coils: a comparison with conventional quantitative coronary angiography.** *Radiology* 2014, **271**(2):356–364.
42. Meijboom WB, Meijs MF, Schuijf JD, Cramer MJ, Mollet NR, van Mieghem CA, Nieman K, van Werkhoven JM, Pundziute G, Weustink AC, de Vos AM, Pugliese F, Rensing B, Jukema JW, Bax JJ, Prokop M, Doevendans PA, Hunink MG, Krestin GP, de Feyter PJ: **Diagnostic accuracy of 64-slice computed tomography coronary angiography: a prospective, multicenter, multivendor study.** *J Am Coll Cardiol* 2008, **52**(25):2135–2144.
43. Budoff MJ, Dowe D, Jollis JG, Gitter M, Sutherland J, Halamert E, Scherer M, Bellinger R, Martin A, Benton R, Delago A, Min JK: **Diagnostic performance of 64-multidetector row coronary computed tomographic angiography for evaluation of coronary artery stenosis in individuals without known coronary artery disease: results from the prospective multicenter ACCURACY (Assessment by Coronary Computed Tomographic Angiography of Individuals Undergoing Invasive Coronary Angiography) trial.** *J Am Coll Cardiol* 2008, **52**(21):1724–1732.
44. Canpolat U, Ozcan F, Ozeke O, Turak O, Aydogdu S: **Usefulness of screening left atrioventricular groove epicardial adipose tissue thickness.** *Am J Cardiol* 2013, **112**(7):1054–1055.
45. Xu Y, Cheng X, Hong K, Huang C, Wan L: **How to interpret epicardial adipose tissue as a cause of coronary artery disease: a meta-analysis.** *Coron Artery Dis* 2012, **23**(4):227–233.
46. Yorgun H, Canpolat U, Hazirolan T, Sunman H, Ates AH, Gurses KM, Ertugrul O, Kaya EB, Aytemir K, Tokgozoglu L, Kabakci G, Oto A: **Epicardial adipose tissue thickness predicts descending thoracic aorta atherosclerosis shown by multidetector computed tomography.** *Int J Cardiovasc Imaging* 2012, **28**(4):911–919.

Effectiveness and safety of a home-based cardiac rehabilitation programme of mixed surveillance in patients with ischemic heart disease at moderate cardiovascular risk

Raquel Bravo-Escobar[1*], Alicia González-Represas[2*], Adela María Gómez-González[1], Angel Montiel-Trujillo[1,3], Rafael Aguilar-Jimenez[1], Rosa Carrasco-Ruíz[1] and Pablo Salinas-Sánchez[4]

Abstract

Background: Previous studies have documented the feasibility of home-based cardiac rehabilitation programmes in low-risk patients with ischemic heart disease, but a similar solution needs to be found for patients at moderate cardiovascular risk. The objective of this study was to analyse the effectiveness and safety of a home-based cardiac rehabilitation programme of mixed surveillance in patients with ischemic cardiopathology at moderate cardiovascular risk.

Methods: A randomised, controlled clinical trial was designed wherein 28 patients with stable coronary artery disease at moderate cardiovascular risk, who met the selection criteria for this study, participated. Of these, 14 were assigned to the group undergoing traditional cardiac rehabilitation in hospital (control group) and 14 were assigned to the home-based mixed surveillance programme (experimental group). The patients in the experimental group went to the cardiac rehabilitation unit once a week and exercised at home, which was monitored with a remote electrocardiographic monitoring device (NUUBO®). The in-home exercises comprised of walking at 70% of heart rate reserve during the first month, and 80% during the second month, for 1 h per day at a frequency of 5 to 7 days per week. A two-way repeated measures analysis of variance (ANOVA) was performed to evaluate the effects of time (before and after intervention) and time-group interaction regarding exercise capacity, risk profile, cardiovascular complications, and quality of life.

Results: No significant differences were observed between the traditional cardiac rehabilitation group and the home-based with mixed surveillance group for exercise time and METS achieved during the exertion test, and the recovery rate in the first minute (which increased in both groups after the intervention). The only difference between the two groups was for quality of life scores (10.93 [IC95%: 17.251, 3.334, $p = 0.007$] vs −4.314 [IC95%: −11.414, 2.787; $p = 0.206$]). No serious heart-related complications were recorded during the cardiac rehabilitation programme.

(Continued on next page)

* Correspondence: rbravoescobar@yahoo.es; alicia@uvigo.es
[1]Unidad de Rehabilitación Cardiaca, Hospital universitario Virgen de la Victoria de Málaga, Campus de Teatinos s/n, 29010 Málaga, España
[2]Facultad de Fisioterapia, Departamento de Biología Funcional y Ciencias de la Salud, Universidad de Vigo, Campus A Xunqueira s/n, 36005 Pontevedra, España
Full list of author information is available at the end of the article

(Continued from previous page)

Conclusions: The home-based cardiac rehabilitation programme with mixed surveillance appears to be as effective and safe as the traditional model in patients with ischemic heart disease who are at moderate cardiovascular risk. However, the cardiac rehabilitation programmes carried out in hospital seems to have better results in improving the quality of life.

Keywords: Telemedicine, Rehabilitation, Exercise therapy, Myocardial ischemia

Background

Cardiovascular diseases are the main causes of mortality in today's society and the primary cause of hospital admissions. They are responsible for up to 30% of all deaths worldwide and 48% of deaths in Europe, and it is expected that these figures will increase in the coming years [1].

Cardiac rehabilitation is not a new concept. Various studies have shown the effectiveness of these programmes in reducing cardiac mortality [2–4] by between 27 and 31% in patients with coronary heart disease; unfortunately, participation levels in these programmes continue to be low in some countries [1]. Sociodemographic factors, factors related to programme availability and accessibility, and the low referral rates of patients to this service are associated with lower rates of patient participation in cardiac rehabilitation programmes [5, 6].

All of these challenges have led to the recent development of alternative models of cardiac rehabilitation, with innovative approaches to improve the delivery and use of these programmes and to provide solutions to these barriers [7].

The effectiveness of home-base cardiac rehabilitation/secondary prevention programs is not new [8]. Studies carried out in the 1980's documented the feasibility of home-based cardiac rehabilitation programmes in low-risk patients with ischaemic cardiomyopathy [9]. While some authors maintained that such programmes provided a solution to the low patient participation in rehabilitation programmes [9], a solution also needs to be found for moderate-risk patients so that they can follow a safe and effective home-based cardiac rehabilitation programme.

Implementing telemedicine in cardiac rehabilitation through the use of technology could partially reduce the logistical problems described above. Telemonitoring devices can allow the patient to be monitored at home so that the patient does not have to travel, and they can improve the efficiency of health care processes by incorporating this information in a comprehensive management programme for cardiac patients [10, 11].

As with any other form of health technology, the effectiveness and safety of these devices must be assessed before their use is extended [10]. In this sense, some alternative home-based cardiac rehabilitation/secondary prevention program with remote monitoring has been previously described [12], but clinical trials evaluating the efficacy of these programs in patients with high risk, greater comorbidity, and also with stable angina are necessary [8].

If home-based cardiac rehabilitation programmes with telemonitoring offer the same safety and effectiveness in moderate-risk patients, it could herald a change in health insurance policies to extend the coverage of these programmes. This would allow a greater number of patients to access cardiac rehabilitation programmes without increasing the total costs [6].

Very few studies have evaluated a home-based cardiac rehabilitation programme model with mixed surveillance, and the studies to date have focused on patients with a low-risk profile. For this reason, it was necessary to develop an alternative home-based cardiac rehabilitation model aimed at higher-risk patients.

The objective of this study was to analyse the effectiveness and safety of a home-based cardiac rehabilitation programme with mixed surveillance in moderate-risk patients with ischaemic cardiomyopathy.

Methods

Study population

Patients with stable ischaemic cardiomyopathy who had undergone revascularisation by either stent-angioplasty or by-pass surgery, who were at moderate risk according to the Spanish Cardiology Society's clinical practice guidelines (Table 1) [8, 13–17], aged ≤ 75, with a good cognitive level, a capacity to perform aerobic exercise on a treadmill or stationary bike, and knowledge of how to use a smartphone or tablet were included in this study. Patients also had to meet at least one of the following inclusion criteria: ventricular dysfunction using ejection fraction (EF) 40–55%, functional capacity 5–7 METS, and/or raised blood pressure with exertion.

We excluded patients with malignant arrhythmias (ventricular fibrillation >24 h after the acute myocardial infarction, ventricular tachycardia, grade 2 or 3 AV block, atrial fibrillation in patients with Wolff-Parkinson-White syndrome, fibrillation or paroxysmal flutter with rapid ventricular response and haemodynamic deterioration, ventricular extrasystole which increases during exertion and uncontrolled supraventricular tachycardia), previous infarctions, ischemia induced by exercise, unstable angina, disease not amenable to revascularisation, poorly-controlled

Table 1 Classification criteria

Risk	Clinical Variables	Complementary Tests	Physical Capacity
Low	Age <50 years Clinical course with no complications. Killip I No previous infarct. Asymptomatic.	No signs of ischemia. Ejection fraction >50%. Normal BP response to exercise. No arrhythmias.	≥7 METS
Moderate	Age >50 years Killip I or II No previous infarct. Mild symptomology.	Effort angina or mild signs of ischemia. Ejection fraction between 35-49%. Mild BP elevation with effort. Low grade arrhythmias. Reversible thallium defect with effort.	>5 METS
High	Killip II or III Previous infarct. Symptoms with low load.	Severe ischemia. ST depression of >2 mm at a rate of less than 135 beats per minute. Hypertensive response to effort. Malignant arrhythmias.	<5 METS

high blood pressure, associated valvular heart disease, pacemaker or ICD-CRT and locomotor system, or a neurological or respiratory pathology that would make walking for prolonged periods difficult.

The study protocol complied with the Declaration of Helsinki and was reviewed and approved by the Comité de Ética Interprovincial de Málaga [Malaga Interprovincial Ethics Committee] belonging to the Consejería de Salud [Health Council] of the Junta de Andalucía [Regional Government of Andalusia] and registered in the clinical trials register (NCT02796404). The study met the requirements of the Andalusian Health System order SAS 3470/2009 and with Organic Law 15/1999 of 13 December for the Protection of Data of a personal nature.

The participants received information about the study methods and gave their written informed consent.

Study design

This is an ongoing randomised controlled multicentre clinical trial (NCT02796404). In this paper, we present preliminary data from one of the participating centres, the Hospital Virgen de la Victoria in Malaga (Spain).

The patients were assigned randomly by an independent investigator to either the control group, which participated in the usual cardiac rehabilitation programme at the hospital, or to the experimental group, which participated in the home-based mixed surveillance programme. The software program Epidat was used for the randomization, ensuring a balanced distribution in both groups. The algorithm generated by this program established that every time a new subject was assigned to a particular group, the probability that that subject was assigned to that group would be inversely proportional to the number of individuals included in it up to that point.

The cardiac rehabilitation programme in both cases had a duration of 2 months. There was only one patient who withdrew from the home-based mixed surveillance group due to personal reasons. The outline design is shown in Fig. 1.

Intervention

The two cardiac rehabilitation programs were started 4–6 months after the patients were discharged from the hospital. Both programs included physical exercise, health education, and physiotherapy, with a duration of 2 months in both cases.

The usual cardiac rehabilitation programme took place in the cardiac rehabilitation unit of the Hospital Virgen de la Victoria in Malaga (Spain). The patients in this group attended the hospital exercise programme 3 times a week (24 sessions) and were encouraged to do exercise at home according to the European Society of Cardiology guidelines [18].

The patients in the home-based cardiac rehabilitation with mixed surveillance group only went to the cardiac rehabilitation unit once a week. During this visit, they had a supervised physical exercise session that was identical to the usual cardiac rehabilitation session. Then they exercised at home following a walking program for 1 h in duration at 70% of the reserve heart rate following the Karvonen formula during the first month and 80% during the second, which was monitored with a remote electrocardiographic monitoring device NUUBO®, for at least two more days a week, although they were encouraged to exercise every day.

The NUUBO® system uses Bluetooth wireless technology and biometric vests using textile electrodes developed and patented by Nuubo, BlendFix Sensor Electrode Technology, which makes its use simple. On the first day, the patients were instructed on how to use this device's mobile application and they were all given a smartphone with Internet connection and the NUUBO® application pre-installed. Each patient

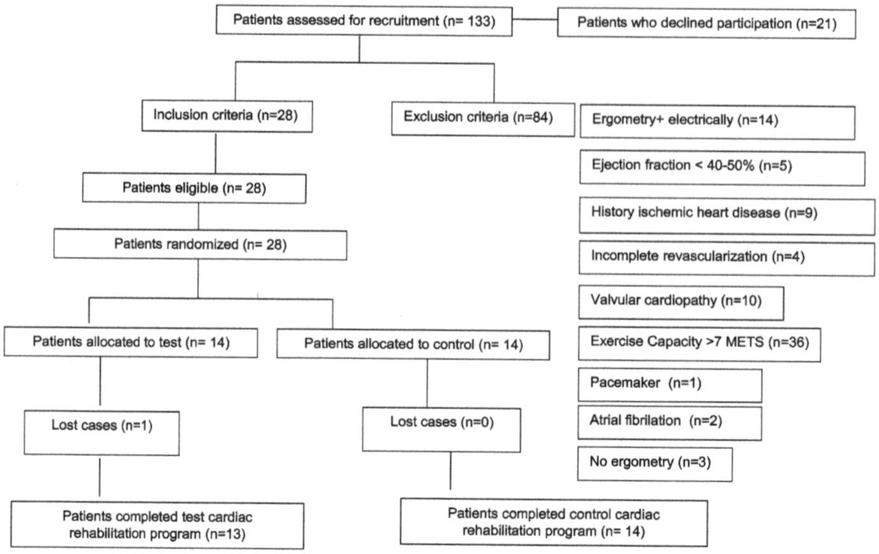

Fig. 1 Flowchart of the study design

was registered on the server; clinical details were entered along with the previously calculated and adjusted exercise heart rate and exercise time (60 min).

The exercise program prescribed for both groups consisted of 15 min of warm-up exercise (stretching and isotonic exercises), followed by 30 min of continuous aerobic exercise, alternating between treadmill training 1 day and stationary bike training the next day, at 70% of the reserve heart rate, following the Karvonen formula during the first month and 80% during the second. The intensity of the exercise was calculated using the heart rate value obtained during the stress test. The patients ended the exercise session with a 15-min cool-down period. Once a week the patients also did a prescribed strength-training session consisting of one or two series of 10 repetitions of exercise for the brachial biceps, brachial triceps, pectoris major, deltoids, and quadriceps at 20 MR (maximum resistance) that is equivalent to 50% of 1MR, with a recovery time of 2–3 min recovery time between each set of repetitions.

Both groups had a health education session at the hospital once a week to improve awareness and understanding about subjects related to the anatomy and function of the heart, cardiovascular risk factors, physical exercise, medication, diet, erectile dysfunction, and returning to work.

All of the patients also attended a group psychotherapy support and assessment session once a week to reduce the emotional impact of the disease, improve their state of health, reduce their chances of another infarction, help them accept their diagnosis, and improve their quality of life.

Measurements

The following measurements were taken at the start of the study and at the end of the 2-months cardiac rehabilitation programmes.

Anthropometric measurements

The body weight of the patients was recorded using a calibrated scale. The measurements were taken with patients wearing light clothes and no shoes. The body mass index (BMI) was calculated based on the formula weight (kg)/height^2 (m). The abdominal circumference was measured with a metric tape with the patient standing up with legs together, arms by the side, and abdomen relaxed after a deep breath. The circumference of the area located at mid-point between the costal edge and the upper edge of the iliac crest was then measured.

Blood pressure

Systolic and diastolic blood pressure readings were taken with an Omro M5-I ® electric sphygmomanometer. The measurements were taken after 10 min of rest with the arm on a table, and the average of three readings was recorded.

Exercise capacity

The participants took an exertion test before enrolling in the study to ensure that they could tolerate the exercise and to determine their METS and exercise time (minutes). The exertion test was done on a treadmill (General Electrics®, Marquette - CASE 8000 Exercise Testing System), following the clinical practice guidelines with continual monitoring with 12-derivation electrocardiogram, using the Bruce protocol. The test ended when the participants were exhausted or showed signs and/or symptoms of intolerance.

Maximum heart rate reached in the stress test was recorded. The heart rate recovery rate during the first minute and the perceived exertion level according to the Borg scale, RPE 6–20, were also recorded.

Laboratory parameters

The participant's total cholesterol, HDL cholesterol, LDL cholesterol, triglycerides, blood glucose and glycated haemoglobin (HbA1c) were analysed in the Clinical Analysis Laboratory of the Laboratory and Haematology Clinical Management Unit of the Hospital Virgen de la Victoria. The glucose, cholesterol and triglycerides levels were recorded using the "Dimension Vista" measuring equipment from Siemens of Grunelwald, Germany. The HbA1c levels were determined using the Adams A1c, HA-8180 V analyser. The glucose levels were measured using the glucose hexokinase method. The total cholesterol levels were analysed using the cholesterol oxidase method, the HDL cholesterol levels were analysed with the enzymatic magnesium dextransulphate method, and the LDL cholesterol levels were analysed using the selective detergent method. Finally, the triglycerides levels were determined using the lipase/glycerol kinase method.

Assessment of health-related quality of life

The Medical Outcome Survey Short Form (SF-36) questionnaire was used to measure the quality of life. The SF-36 consists of 36 items which assess 8 different dimensions, and the possible scores range from 0–100; the variables assessed include limitations due to physical problems, body pain, social function or role, mental health, limitation due to emotional problems, vitality, energy or fatigue, and general perception of health. Studies published on the metric characteristics of the Spanish version of the SF-36 have provided enough evidence in support of its reliability, validity, and sensitivity [19].

Cardiovascular complications

Complications that arose during the hospital and home-based cardiac rehabilitation programmes were recorded, and they included AMI, severe arrhythmias, cardiorespiratory arrest or death, arterial hypotension, arterial hypertension, hypoglycaemia, hyperglycaemia, or intermittent claudication due to peripheral arterial disease.

Statistical analysis

A two-way repeated measures analysis of variance (ANOVA) was carried out to evaluate the effect of the time (before and after intervention) and the effect of time-group interaction. The normality of distributions was verified using the Shapiro-Wilk test. Descriptive analyses were performed to characterise the sample and the study outcomes using the central tendency, confidence interval, and percentage measures. The level of significance was set at $p < 0.05$ for all tests.

Results

A total of 28 patients initially participated in the study, all men with an average age of 56.07 (±8.92); 14 of the participants were assigned to the usual cardiac rehabilitation group (control group) and 14 were assigned to the home-based mixed surveillance programme (experimental group). During the intervention phase, one patient from the experimental group withdrew from the study for personal reasons. The initial characteristics of the sample are shown in Table 2. No significant differences were seen between both groups except for the number of patients presenting with diabetes mellitus and the maximum heart rate achieved in the stress test. The differences in this latter parameter probably can be related to the response to the medication of some patients since there are no differences in METS achieved nor in the time of exercise.

The right coronary and anterior descending arteries were the most affected among patients with either single-vessel disease or double-vessel lesions in both groups; while in patients with triple-vessel disease the affected arteries were either the anterior descending, circumflex, and marginal obtuse arteries, or the anterior descending, right coronary, and circumflex arteries. In general, the majority of patients underwent PCI, and 78.6% of the patients received pharmacoactive stents.

The medication prescribed to patients is similar in both groups (Table 3). Therapeutic doses were adjusted in each case to maintain heart rate, blood pressure and blood glucose levels within the recommended levels according to clinical practice guidelines for the control of cardiovascular risk factors in patients with heart disease Ischemic.

The exercise time and METS achieved during the exertion test as well as the recovery rate in the first minute increased in both groups after the intervention, with no significant differences being found between the usual cardiac rehabilitation group and the home-based with mixed surveillance group (Table 4).

The maximum heart rate reached during the stress test, however, appeared to be significantly differences between both groups, although it is not possible to affirm that the heart rate in any individual significantly changed (usual cardiac rehabilitation group: −17.57 [IC95%: −35.348, .205, $p = 0.052$]; home-based with mixed surveillance group 9.46 [IC95%: −.133, 19.056, $p = 0.053$]).

The only differences found between the two groups were in quality of life. The results obtained in the SF-36 post-intervention were significantly higher in the usual

Table 2 Baseline characteristics of the study population

	Hospital ($n = 14$)	Home ($n = 13$)	p-value
Age (years)	55.64 (11.35)	56.50 (6.01)	ns
Sex Male n (%)	14 (100)	14 (100)	ns
Risk factors			
Hypertension n (%)	11 (78.57)	9 (64.28)	ns
Hyperlipidaemia n (%)	5 (35.71)	7 (50)	ns
Diabetes n (%)	1 (7.14)	6 (42.85)	0.029*
Overweight n (%)	8 (57.14)	5 (35.71)	ns
Obese n (%)	6 (42.85)	6 (42.85)	ns
BMI (kg/m^2)	29.29 (3.62)	28.64 (3.65)	ns
Waist-hip ratio (cm)	106.42 (8.84)	104.14 (10.21)	ns
Current smokers n (%)	2 (14.28)	2 (14.28)	ns
Coronary artery disease			
Monovessel n (%)	3 (21.42)	8 (57.14)	ns
Double vessel n (%)	5 (35.71)	4 (28.57)	ns
Triple vessel n (%)	5 (35.71)	1 (7.14)	ns
Revascularization technique			
CABG n (%)	2 (14.3)	1 (7.1)	ns
PCI n (%)	11 (78.6)	11 (78.6)	ns
PCI & CABG n (%)	1 (7.1)	2 (14.3)	ns
Blood pressure			
Systolic blood pressure (mmHg)	115.35 (23.73)	119.35 (24.05)	ns
Diastolic blood pressure (mmHg)	69.28 (11.41)	71.50 (9.48)	ns
Exercise stress test			
Exercise time (min)	5.47 (2.08)	5.84 (2.66)	ns
METS	7.10 (1.97)	7.55 (2.77)	ns
Heart rate maximal (bpm)	132.84 (16.11)	106.21 (32.58)	0.02*
% of predicted peak HR.	79.86 (12.27)	65.10 (20.09)	0.02*
Hypertension response n (%)	5 (41.7)	4 (28.6)	ns
Clinical positive response n (%)	1 (7.1)	0 (0)	ns
Electrical positive response n (%)	2 (14.3)	0 (0)	ns
Ejection Fraction (EF)	52.33 (3.51)	51.00 (7.9)	ns
Laboratory values			
Total cholesterol (mg/dL)	130.50 (32.16)	145.71 (29.35)	ns
HDL cholesterol (mg/dL)	37.85 (8.07)	39.84 (9.21)	ns
LDL cholesterol (mg/dL)	67.17 (23.19)	73.68 (25.62)	ns
Triglycerides (mg/dL)	161.21 (72.31)	148.35 (58.16)	ns
Glucose (mg/dL)	94.92 (13.56)	111.00 (28.03)	ns
HbA1c	5.62 (1.05)	5.72 (0.93)	ns
Health-related quality of life			
SF-36 (score)	53.33 (19.80)	48.44 (20.89)	ns

Values are presented as mean (SD) unless stated otherwise
* Significance level $p < 0.05$

Table 3 Prescribed medication to patients

Medication	Hospital ($n = 14$)	Home ($n = 13$)
Antiplatelet agents	-	-
Acetylsalicylic acid	14	14
Clopidrogrel	3	5
Tricagrelor	8	5
Rivaroxavan	-	-
Plasugrel	2	4
Stomach protectors	14	14
Antiarrhythmics		
Bisoprolol	13	13
Carvedilol	1	-
Ranazolina	-	1
Antihypertensives	-	-
IECA	10	9
ARA-II	3	4
Diuretic	4	4
Amlodipino	4	1
Oral antidiabetic agents	1	7
Insulin	1	3
Anxiolytic	8	7
Statins	14	14
Hipnotic	2	2
Antidepressant	1	2
Epleronona	1	1

cardiac rehabilitation group (10.93 [IC95%: 17.251, 3.334, $p = 0.007$]) with no changes compared to the initial status in the home-based with mixed surveillance group (−4.314 [IC95%: −11.414, 2.787; $p = 0.206$]).

During the training sessions, two patients from the control group presented with angina-type pain without electrical changes evident on telemonitoring which subsided with rest, one patient presented an arrhythmia (*de novo* atrial fibrillation), two patients had a hypertensive response to the exercise which subsided with rest, and one patient had a hypotensive response which required the administration of intravenous saline solution.

In the experimental group, one patient had a hypertensive response to exercise which subsided during the cool-down phase, and one patient had a hypotensive response which required the intravenous administration of saline solution; both events occurred during the supervised training sessions carried out at the hospital.

No patient required treatment at the hospital's Accident & Emergency (A&E) department.

The control group had 24 supervised training sessions in the hospital. Although it was recommended that the control group also exercise at home, we do not have a record of -home sessions. The experimental group's patients completed an average of 36 sessions at home. The home-based training sessions lasted over an hour in 83.3% of cases. During the home-based exercise sessions supervised using the NUUBO® device, 8 patients pressed the alarm button in 20 training sessions, of which 3 patients reported angina-type pain during the exercise which subsided with rest; no ECG changes were seen on the recording in any of the cases. None of the other patients presented with angina-type pain or ECG changes during the home-based training sessions.

No serious cardiovascular complications were recorded during the cardiac rehabilitation programme.

Discussion

The majority of patients who participate in cardiac rehabilitation programmes are middle-aged men. A number of studies have identified the patients who could benefit the most from cardiac rehabilitation and they include patients with significant functional deterioration, patients of advanced age, women, and ethnic groups, although these patients are the least likely to participate in cardiac rehabilitation programmes [1, 5]. Several studies have concluded that the effectiveness and safety of these home-based programmes could reduce inequality by improving access to this type of health service [20–23].

This study demonstrated that the cardiac rehabilitation with a mixed surveillance programme was as effective as the usual programme for improving functional capacity in moderate-risk patients.

Other studies have obtained similar results in low-risk patients after coronary revascularisation surgery and in patients of advanced age [8, 22, 24, 25]. While some of these studies analysed exercise capacity based on other parameters such as oxygen consumption, the shuttle walk test, or total cycle work capacity, the studies all found that home-based exercise programmes improved exercise capacity, and they found no differences when they compared them to hospital programmes [25].

When the training protocols for the different intervention models were compared, considerable variation was seen in the duration, frequency, and intensity of the exercise [25]. Despite these variations, all of the studies showed a beneficial short-term impact on exercise capacity after low-risk or moderate-risk patients completed a home-based cardiac rehabilitation programme. Furthermore, some of the studies demonstrated that long-term home-based programmes had better results than programmes carried out in hospitals.

The improved exercise time and recovery rate detected in the first minute also suggest an improved survival prognosis in patients with coronary heart disease [26]. All of these factors, together with the intensity of the exercise attained over the final weeks, could explain the increased subjective perception of the exertion measured

Table 4 Measures results obtained before and after the two different cardiac rehabilitation programs

	Hospital based cardiac rehabilitation program		Home based cardiac rehabilitation program		p-value[a]	p-value[b]
	Before	After	Before	After		
METS	7.10 (1.97)	8.45 (1.71)	7.55 (2.77)	8.28 (2.62)	**0.03***	0.49
Exercise time (min)	5.47 (2.08)	6.87 (1.67)	5.84 (2.66)	6.38 (1.80)	**0.03***	0.32
Heart rate maximal (bpm)	132.84 (16.11)	123.38 (17.38)	107.23 (32.58)	123.84 (22.61)	-	**0.009****
% of predicted peak HR.	79.86 (12.27)	75.16 (9.2)	65.10 (20.09)	75.81 (14.07)	.	**0.008****
Borg Scale	12.57 (1.15)	13.57 (1.22)	13.07 (1.49)	13.69 (1.18)	**0.015***	0.54
Recovery rate 1 min (bpm)	13.85 (5.02)	17.21 (6.29)	11.63 (7.41)	13.81 (4.46)	**0.008****	0.54
BMI (kg/m^2)	29.29 (3.62)	29.08 (37.6)	28.60 (3.80)	29.08 (4.33)	0.54	0.13
Waist-hip ratio (cm)	106.42 (8.84)	105.35 (9.96)	103.84 (10.56)	103.69 (10.59)	0.24	0.37
Total cholesterol (mg/dL)	130.50 (32.16)	138.21 (25.41)	142.66 (29.44)	135.91 (23.43)	0.91	0.10
HDL cholesterol (mg/dL)	37.85 (8.07)	20.57 (8.75)	39.45 (8.99)	40.45 (7.01)	0.24	0.58
LDL cholesterol (mg/dL)	62.17 (23.19)	68.62 (16.63)	70.30 (26.14)	61.13 (15.50)	0.74	0.06
Triglycerides (mg/dL)	161.21 (72.31)	161.07 (102.20)	149.83 (61.56)	160.08 (84.71)	0.77	0.76
Glucose (mg/dL)	94.92 (13.56)	104.07 (27.73)	109.83 (28.67)	106.75 (14.61)	0.57	0.26
HbA1c	5.62 (1.05)	5.75 (1.30)	6.05 (1.18)	6.15 (1.36)	0.35	0.90
Systolic blood pressure (mm Hg)	115.76 (24.65)	119.23 (19.45)	119.35 (24.05)	120.35 (16.69)	0.65	0.80
Diastolic blood pressure (mm Hg)	69.23 (11.87)	72.30 (11.65)	71.50 (9.48)	72.14 (11.21)	0.45	0.62
SF-36 (score)	53.33 (19.80)	63.63 (21.00)	47.93 (22.57)	43.62 (24.20)	-	**0.004****

Data are presented as mean values (SD)
[a]Significance level for the hypothesis of no time effect
[b]Significance level for the hypothesis of no time x group effect (difference in outcome improvement between the two programs)
*Significance level $p < 0.05$
**Significance level $p < 0.01$
Significant values are highlighted in bold

using the Borg scale in both groups, and the improved risk profile of these patients.

With respect to the maximum heart rate achieved in the stress test, although the sample is not large enough to affirm that the changes observed in each separate group are statistically significant, it is sufficient to affirm the different effects of exercise on both groups. The decrease in heart rate in the stress test of the control group together with the increase in exercise time and the METs that were achieved, translate into a better adaptation to exercise than that of the experimental group. This is probably due to the fact that it was not possible to control caloric consumption per training session, the amount of time they remained at goal intensity during the -home exercise session, and walking speed, which are aspects that are related to improvement in prognosis and reduction in mortality [3, 4] and hospitalizations of these patients [2]. In this sense, the results obtained from this pilot study allow for the introduction of improvements in the design of these devices, which allow not only the monitoring of these patients, offering an efficient and safe way to exercise, but they also provide the patient enough flexibility to exercise anywhere with a workload that is adequate and easily modifiable [12].

The beneficial effect of exercise on lipids and the metabolism of carbohydrates has been documented in several studies, but in this study we found no significant differences when we compared the readings in both groups. The patients who participated in the study from the start presented with blood glucose, cholesterol and triglycerides readings within the normal ranges; only the HDL levels were below optimal levels. Other authors have also not seen improvements in HDL levels in patients with coronary heart disease [27]. In general, there is a high variability in results when the effect of exercise on the metabolism of lipids are analysed due to the heterogeneity of the study methods, duration of studies, populations, exercise protocols, and other contributory factors such as diet or lipid-lowering pharmacological agents. It is also known that in adults aged 50 and over, prolonged periods of exercise are needed to achieve a change in lipid metabolism, so the intervention duration of two months may not have been long enough to achieve an effect comparable to the results seen in other studies [28–30] on the lipid profile, body mass index, and abdominal circumference.

In terms of the quality of life, other studies have shown a significant improvement in both groups [30–34], and sometimes the effect was even greater in the home-based group [30]. However, in this study we detected an improvement in the usual cardiac rehabilitation group. The differences in the risk profile of the patients as well as other associated psychosocial factors may partially explain the results we obtained [35].

The exercise sessions at the hospital likely promoted social support due to the nature of the programmes and this could have impacted on patients' perceived quality of life, as they feel like they were part of a group, with everything that entails [36]. It is be plausible that the exercise group in the traditional cardiac rehabilitation model achieved greater social cohesion and thus the programme had a greater impact on their quality of life.

The strategies which increased the frequency of exercise could in turn have contributed to a faster improvement in the perceived quality of life [30].

These and other factors, such as creating a home-based support network, will need to be taken into consideration when designing home-based cardiac rehabilitation programmes in order to achieve better results when it comes to the quality of life.

The safety of the exercise programme for moderate-risk patients was an important question, particularly when the programme was performed at home [37]. The safety of the exercise programme for patients with coronary heart disease has generally been related to the intensity and duration of the training and the patient selection. The individual risk assessment is a fundamental starting point here which serves as a guide for decision-making, among other things, when it comes to determining the right level of surveillance [11].

There are a wide variety of monitoring and surveillance strategies for home [9, 38, 39], but there are very few studies which use ECG monitoring systems through various devices [1, 12, 21, 22, 39–41]. Ades et al. [9] maintained that not all patients require transtelephonic monitoring in all sessions. Indeed, they suggested the selective use of this technology only in the initial sessions, and/or depending on the characteristics of each patient and their individual progress, probably because they did not differentiate between low and moderate-risk patients in their sample. However, Giallura et al. [21] maintained that telemonitoring improved compliance and the results of a home-based cardiac rehabilitation programme, particularly the functional capacity profile, compared with patients who participated in a home-based cardiac rehabilitation programme without ECG monitoring.

Bearing in mind the characteristics of the patients in this study, the mixed surveillance model described required, for the whole programme, the use of a telemetric monitoring system which allowed the information stored on the device during the exercise session to be sent from home so that it could be evaluated at the hospital without the patient needing to go to the centre. We have not found any other study which assessed a similar mixed surveillance model for the whole programme in moderate-risk patients.

Patients generally accepted this new exercise monitoring model away from the hospital, which made the telemonitoring system mixed surveillance exercise programme a viable option for moderate-risk patients.

However, this intervention model in higher-risk patients establishes a new scenario in which it is not only necessary to have a clear definition of the risks and responsibilities, but also the various clinical skills among the health professionals [10].

Other studies have demonstrated the safety of home-based cardiac rehabilitation programmes in lower-risk patients [23, 38, 39]. Bearing in mind that the complications recorded in the home-based group with mixed surveillance were minor, we believe that this model of intervention was safe in low-risk patients with coronary heart disease.

There are some limitations derived from the sample size. Although the sample size in the current study are small, this is a preliminary investigation regarding an alternative method for mixed-home supervision, which that could improve access to this type of program for cardiac patients with a risk-profile that is greater than has been previously reported. The study currently continues to recruit patients. Further, another limitation of the current study is that the sample only consists of men since none of the women who came in for an evaluation for the cardiac rehabilitation program met the inclusion criteria for taking part in this study. Additionally, with relation to heart disease, despite the randomization procedure described in the manuscript, the experimental group consisted of a majority of patients presenting with monovessel disease, while the majority of the control group had presented with two or three vessel disease. However, all the patients had stable ischemic heart disease and met the moderate risk criteria. Finally, although it was recommended that the control group exercise at home, we do not have a record of in-home sessions.

In spite of these limitations, the results of this study may help with the design of home-based programs that are adapted to different sociodemographic situations for moderate-risk coronary patients and also in the design of new technologies that are adapted to the profiles of these patients, which can improve access to Cardiac Rehabilitation services. However, the long-term effects need to be assessed for this patient population through multicentre studies to determine the effectiveness and acceptability of these mixed surveillance programmes based on telemedicine in different contexts. It is necessary to point out that the study is continuing with the added participation of different hospitals (multicentre study) and we will soon have the first results on long-term monitoring.

Conclusion

A home-based cardiac rehabilitation programme with mixed surveillance was as effective and safe as the usual model in moderate-risk patients with ischaemic cardiomyopathy. However, the cardiac rehabilitation programmes carried out at the hospital had a greater impact on the patients' quality of life. The results presented here suggest that the implementation of this programme would represent an improvement in the care quality of the public health services as it could offer benefits in the type and number of potential patients helped, the possibility of personalised treatment tailored to the different lifestyles or needs of patients, and thus enhance treatment adherence. Future lines of research should analyse how the design of home-based programmes could improve these results, bearing in mind the multidimensional nature of quality of life.

Abbreviations

AMI: Acute myocardial infarction; AV: Atrioventricular; BMI: Body mass index; BP: Blood pressure; CABG: Coronary artery bypass grafting; CRT: Cardiac resynchronization therapy; ECG: Electrocardiogram; EF: Ejection fraction; HR: Heart rate; ICD: Implantable cardioverter-defibrillator; PCI: Percutaneous coronary intervention; RPE: Rating of perceived exertion

Acknowledgements

The authors would like to thank the Fundación Pública Andaluza para la Investigación de Málaga en Biomedicina y Salud (FIMABIS), this study's sponsor, and Belén Pimentel (AME Unit_IBIMA-FIMABIS) for critically reviewing the manuscript.

Funding

The sponsor of this study was the Fundación Pública Andaluza para la Investigación de Málaga en Biomedicina y Salud [Andalusian Malaga Public Foundation for Research in Biomedicine and Health] (FIMABIS). The sponsor has provided the legal support to this independent clinical trial and in addition has provided with the resources to conduct the clinical trial, these are, the Clinical Trial Platform in Málaga that provides with monitoring and the clinical trials specialists for the assessment and support with the protocol design services and liason with the Institutional ethics committee and the AEMPS, the Spanish Agency for the regulation of medicines and health products. In addition, the sponsor provides with the Statistics Unit for the statistical analysis of data. The liason with patients community, the design of the study and interpretation of results have been performed and conducted by the IP in collaboration with all the authors of the manuscript. The collection of data has been performed by the clinicians with authorship in the manuscript. RBE and AGR have done the writing of the manuscript. The funding body for the work contracts of the authors is the Andalusian Health Public Service (SAS) for RBE, AMGG, RAJ and RCR; the University of Vigo for AGR; and University of Malaga for PSS.

Authors' contributions

RBE and AMGG conceived the idea for this study and designed the study in collaboration with PSS. The selection of patients was done by RBE, AMGG and AMT, and also participated in the collection of data with RAJ and RCR. RBE, AMGG, RAJ and RCR participated in the delivery and surveillance of the hospital and home-based cardiac rehabilitation programmes. RBE and AGR performed the statistical analysis, the interpretation of the results, and wrote the manuscript. All of the authors participated in the critical review of the content of the article and approved the final manuscript.

Competing interest

NUUBO provided, exclusively and without payment, the NUUBO® remote electrocardiographic monitoring biometric vests to carry out this independent trial. The authors have no conflicts of interest to declare.

Author details

[1]Unidad de Rehabilitación Cardiaca, Hospital universitario Virgen de la Victoria de Málaga, Campus de Teatinos s/n, 29010 Málaga, España. [2]Facultad de Fisioterapia, Departamento de Biología Funcional y Ciencias de la Salud, Universidad de Vigo, Campus A Xunqueira s/n, 36005 Pontevedra, España. [3]Servicio de Cardiología, Hospital universitario Virgen de la Victoria de Málaga, Campus de Teatinos s/n, 29010 Málaga, España. [4]Facultad de Medicina, Departamento de Anatomía Humana, Medicina legal e Historia de la Ciencia, University of Málaga, Campus de Teatinos s/n, 29010 Malaga, España.

References

1. Antypas K, Wangberg SC. E-Rehabilitation—an Internet and mobile phone based tailored intervention to enhance self-management of cardiovascular disease: study protocol for a randomized controlled trial. BMC Cardiovasc Disord. 2012. doi:10.1186/1471-2261-12-50.
2. Grazzi G, Mazzoni G, Myers J, Codecà L, Pasanisi G, Napoli N, Guerzoni F, Volpato S, Conconi F, Chiaranda G. Improved walking speed is associated with lower hospitalization rates in patients in an exercise-based secondary prevention program. Heart. 2016. doi:10.1136/heartjnl-2015-309126.
3. Chiaranda G, Bernardi E, Codecà L, Conconi F, Myers J, Terranova F, Volpato S, Mazzoni G, Grazzi G. Treadmill walking speed and survival prediction in men with cardiovascular disease: a 10-year follow-up study. BMJ Open. 2013. doi:10.1136/bmjopen-2013-003446.
4. Grazzi G, Myers J, Bernardi E, Terranova F, Grossi G, Codecà L, Volpato S, Conconi F, Mazzoni G, Chiaranda G. Association between VO_2 peak estimated by a 1-km treadmill walk and mortality. A 10-year follow-up study in patients with cardiovascular disease. Int J Cardiol. 2014;173(2):248–52. doi: 10.1016/j.ijcard.2014.02.039.
5. Walters DL, Sarela A, Fairfull A. A mobile phone-based care model for outpatient cardiac rehabilitation: the care assessment platform (CAP). BMC Cardiovasc Disord. 2010. doi:10.1186/1471-2261-10-5.
6. Kraal JJ, Peek N, Van den Akker-Van Marle ME, Kemps HM. Effects and costs of home-based training with telemonitoring guidance in low to moderate risk patients entering cardiac rehabilitation: The FIT@Home study. BMC Cardiovasc Disord. 2013. doi:10.1186/1471-2261-13-82.
7. Pfaeffli L, Maddison R, Whittaker R, Stewart R, Kerr A, Jiang Y, et al. A mHealth cardiac rehabilitation exercise intervention: findings from content development studies. BMC Cardiovasc Disord. 2012. doi:10.1186/1471-2261-12-36.
8. Anderson L, Oldridge N, Thompson DR, Zwisler AD, Rees K, Martin N, Taylor RS. Exercise-Based Cardiac Rehabilitation for Coronary Heart Disease: Cochrane Systematic Review and Meta-Analysis. J Am Coll Cardiol. 2016. doi:10.1016/j.jacc.2015.10.044.
9. Ades PA, Pashkow FJ, Fletcher G, Pina IL, Zohman LR, Nestor JR. A controlled trial of cardiac rehabilitation in the home setting using electrocardiographic and voice transtelephonic monitoring. Am Heart J. 2000;139:543–8.
10. Currell R, Urquhart C, Wainwright P, Lewis R. Telemedicine versus face to face patient care: effects on professional practice and health care outcomes. Cochrane Database Syst Rev. 2000;2:CD002098.
11. Clark RA, Conway A, Poulsen V, Keech W, Tirimacco R, Tideman P. Alternative models of cardiac rehabilitation: a systematic review. Eur J Prev Cardiol. 2015. doi:10.1177/2047487313501093.
12. Worringham C, Rojek Stewart. Development and feasibility of a smartphone, ECG and GPS based system for remotely monitoring exercise in cardiac rehabilitation. PLoS One. 2011. doi:10.1371/journal.pone.0014669.
13. Boraita Péreza A, Baño Rodrigo A, Berrazueta Fernándeza JR, Lamiel Alcainea R, Luengo Fernándeza E, Manonelles Marquetaa P, et al. Guías de práctica clínica de la sociedad Española de cardiología sobre la actividad física en el cardiópata. Rev Esp Cardiol. 2000;53:684–726.
14. Velasco JA, Cosín J, Maroto JM, Muñiz J, Casanovas JA, PLaza I, et al. Guidelines of the Spanish society of cardiology for cardiovascular disease prevention and cardiac rehabilitation. Rev Esp Cardiol. 2000;53:1095–120.

15. Gómez-González A, Miranda-Calderín G, Pleguezuelos-Cobos E, Bravo-Escobar R, López-Lozano A, Expósito-Tirado JA, Heredia-Torres A, Montiel-Trujillo A, Aguilera-Saborido A. Recomendaciones sobre rehabilitación cardiaca en la cardiopatía isquémica de la Sociedad de rehabilitación Cardio-respiratoria (SORECAR) *(Recommendations for cardiac rehabilitation in ischemic heart disease from the Cardio-respiratory Society)*. Rehabilitación (Rehabilitation) (Madr). 2015;49:1.
16. Castillo JI, Moreno-Atanasio E, Tinoco-González J, Pleguezuelos-Cobo E. Rehabilitación cardiaca en el Síndrome Coronario Agudo. *(Cardiac rehabilitation in Acute Coronary Syndrome)*. In: Pleguezuelos AA, Miranda E, Gómez G, Capellas A, editors. L. Principios de rehabilitación cardiaca. *(Principles of cardiac rehabilitation)*. Madrid: Editorial Médica Panamericana; 2011. p. 170–81.
17. Castillo Marín JI, Miranda Vivas T, Rozalén Pinedo M, Jiménez Esteso JM. Rehabilitación cardiaca en el síndrome coronario agudo. Reahbilitación *(Cardiac rehabilitation in acute coronary syndrome. Rehabilitation)*. Madr. 2006;40:318–32.
18. Task Force Members. 2013 ESC guidelines on the management of stable coronary artery disease: The Task Force on the management of stable coronary artery disease of the European Society of Cardiology. Eur Heart J. 2013. doi:10.1093/eurheartj/eht296.
19. Vilagut G, Ferrer M, Rajmil L, Rebollo P, Permanyer-Miralda G, Quintana JM, et al. El Cuestionario de Salud SF-36 español: una década de experiencia y nuevos desarrollos. Gac Sanit. 2005;19:135–50.
20. Taylor RS, Dalal H, Jolly K, Moxham T, Zawada A. Home-based versus center-based cardiac rehabilitation. Cochrane Database Syst Rev. 2010. doi:10.1002/14651858.CD007130.pub2.
21. Giallauria F, Lucci R, Pilerci F, De Lorenzo A, Manakos A, Psaroudaki M, et al. Efficacy of telecardiology in improving the results of cardiac rehabilitation after acute myocardial infarction. Arch Chest Dis. 2006;66:8–12.
22. Scalvini S, Zanelli E, Comini L, Dalla Tomba M, Troise G, Febo O, et al. Home-based versus in-hospital cardiac rehabilitation after cardiac surgery: a nonrandomized controlled study. Phys Ther. 2013. doi:10.2522/ptj.20120212.
23. Kraal JJ, Niels P, Van den Akker-Van Marle ME, Kemps HMC. Effects of home-based training with telemonitoring guidance in low to moderate risk patients entering cardiac rehabilitation: short-term results of FIT@home study. Eur J Prev Cardiol. 2014;21:26–31.
24. Dangenais JR, Rouleaus JR, Christen A, Fabia J. Survival of patient with strongly positive exercise electrocardiogram. Circulation. 1982;65:452–6.
25. Dalal HM, Zawada A, Jolly K, Moxham T, Taylor RS. Home based versus center based cardiac rehabilitation: Cochrane systematic review and meta-analysis. BMJ. 2010. doi:10.1136/bmj.b5631.
26. McNeer JF, Margolis JR, Lee KL, et al. The role of exercise test in the evaluation of patients for ischemic heart disease. Circulation. 1978;57:64–70.
27. Astengo M, Dahl A, Karlsson T, Mattsson-Hultén L, Wiklund O, Wennerblom B. Physical training after percutaneous coronary intervention in patients with stable angina: effects on working capacity, metabolism, and markers of inflammation. Eur J Cardiovasc Prev Rehabil. 2010;17:349–54.
28. Karapolat H, Demir E, Bozkaya YT, Eyigor S, Nalbantgil S, Durmaz B, et al. Comparison of hospital-based versus home-based exercise training inpatients with heart failure: effects on functional capacity, quality of life, psychological symptoms, and hemodynamic parameters. Clin Res Cardiol. 2009;98:635–42.
29. Coghill N, Cooper AR. The effect of a home-based walking program on risk factors for coronary heart disease in hypercholesteremic men. A randomized controlled trial. Prev Med. 2008. doi:10.1016/j.ypmed.2008.01.002.
30. Arthur HM, Smith KM, Kodis J, McKelvie R. A controlled trial of hospital versus home-based exercise in cardiac patients. Med Sci Sports Exerc. 2002;34:1544–50.
31. Dalal HM, Evans PH, Campbell JL, Taylor RS, Watt A, Read KLQ, et al. Home-based versus hospital based rehabilitation after myocardial infarction: a randomized trial with preference arms- Cornwall heart attack management study (CHARMS). Int J Cardiol. 2007;119:202–11.
32. Jolly K, Taylor R, Lip GYH, Greenfield SM, Raftery J, Mant JWF, et al. The Birmingham uptake maximisation study (BRUM). home-based compared with hospital based cardiac rehabilitation in a multiethnic population: cost effectiveness and patient adherence. Health Technol Assess. 2007;11:1–118.
33. Smith KM, Arthur HM, McKelvie RS, Kodis J. Differences in sustainability of exercise and health-related quality of life outcomes following home or hospital-based cardiac rehabilitation. Eur J Cardiovasc Prev Rehabil. 2004;11:313–9.
34. Marchionni N, Fattirolli F, Fumagalli S, Oldridge N, Del Lungo F, Morosi L, et al. Improved exercise tolerance and quality of life with cardiac rehabilitation of older patients after myocardial infarction: results of a randomized controlled trial. Circulation. 2003;107:2201–6.
35. Salvetti XM, Filho JAO, Servantes DM, Vicenzo de Paola AA. How much do the benefits cost? Effects of a home based training program cardiovascular fitness, quality of life, program cost and adherence for patients with coronary disease. Clin Rehabil. 2008. doi:10.1177/0269215508093331.
36. Estabrooks P. Sustaining exercise participation through group cohesion. Exerc Sport Sci Rev. 2000;28:63–7.
37. Frederix I, Driessche NV, Hansen D, Berger J, Bonne K, Alders T, Densale P. Increasing the medium-term clinical benefits of hospital-based cardiac rehabilitation by physical activity telemonitoring in coronary artery disease patients. Eur J Prev Cardiol. 2015. doi:10.1177/2047487313514018.
38. Piotrowicz E, Baranowski R, Bilinska M, Stepnowska M, Piotrowska M, Wójcik A, et al. A new model of home-based telemonitored cardiac rehabilitation in patients with heart failure: effectiveness, quality of life, and adherence. Eur J Heart Fail. 2010;12:164–71.
39. Korzaniowska-kubacka I, Dobraszkoewicz-Wasilewska B, Bilinska M, Rydzewska E, Piotrowicz R. Two models of early cardiac rehabilitation in male patients after myocardial infarction with preserved left ventricular function: comparison of estándar out-patient versus hybrid training programs. Kardiol Pol. 2011;69:220–6.
40. Fletcher GF, Balady GJ, Amsterdam EA, Chaitman B, Eckel R, Fleg J, et al. Exercise standards for testing and training: a statement for healthcare professionals from the American heart association. Circulation. 2001;104:1694–740.
41. Lee YH, Hur SH, Sohn J, Lee HM, Park NH, Cho YK, et al. Impact of home-based exercise training with wireless monitoring n patients with acute coronary syndrome undergoing percutaneous coronary intervention. J Korean Med Sci. 2013;28:564–8.

12

Genetic association study of coronary collateral circulation in patients with coronary artery disease using 22 single nucleotide polymorphisms corresponding to 10 genes involved in postischemic neovascularization

Joan Duran[1], Pilar Sánchez Olavarría[1,2], Marina Mola[1,3], Víctor Götzens[1], Julio Carballo[4], Eva Martín Pelegrina[4], Màrius Petit[4], Omar Abdul-Jawad[6], Imanol Otaegui[5], Bruno García del Blanco[5], David García-Dorado[5], Josep Reig[7], Alex Cordero[1,8] and Josep Maria de Anta[1*]

Abstract

Background: Collateral growth in patients with coronary artery disease (CAD) is highly heterogeneous. Although multiple factors are thought to play a role in collateral development, the contribution of genetic factors to coronary collateral circulation (CCC) is largely unknown. The goal of this study was to assess whether functional single nucleotide polymorphisms (SNPs) in genes involved in vascular growth are associated with CCC.

Methods: 677 consecutive CAD patients were enrolled in the study and their CCC was assessed by the Rentrop method. 22 SNPs corresponding to 10 genes involved in postischemic neovascularization were genotyped and multivariate logistic regression models were adjusted using clinically relevant variables to estimate odds ratios and used to examine associations of allelic variants, genotypes and haplotypes with CCC.

Results: Statistical analysis showed that the *HIF1A* rs11549465 and rs2057482; *VEGFA* rs2010963, rs1570360, rs699947, rs3025039 and rs833061; *KDR* rs1870377, rs2305948 and rs2071559; *CCL2* rs1024611, rs1024610, rs2857657 and rs2857654; *NOS3* rs1799983; *ICAM1* rs5498 and rs3093030; *TGFB1* rs1800469; *CD53* rs6679497; *POSTN* rs3829365 and rs1028728; and *LGALS2* rs7291467 polymorphisms, as well as their haplotype combinations, were not associated with CCC ($p < 0.05$).

Conclusions: We could not validate in our cohort the association of the *NOS3* rs1799983, *HIF1A* rs11549465, *VEGFA* rs2010963 and rs699947, and *LGALS2* rs7291467 variants with CCC reported by other authors. A validated SNP-based genome-wide association study is required to identify polymorphisms influencing CCC.

Keywords: Collateral circulation, Arteriogenesis, Postischemic neovascularization, Single nucleotide polymorphism, Genetic association study

* Correspondence: janta@ub.edu
[1]Unitat d'Anatomia i Embriologia Humanes, Departament de Patologia i Terapèutica Experimental, Facultat de Medicina, Campus de Ciències de la Salut de Bellvitge, Universitat de Barcelona, L'Hospitalet de Llobregat, Barcelona 08907, Spain
Full list of author information is available at the end of the article

Background

In patients with coronary artery disease (CAD), the perfusion of the myocardial tissue is impaired. To mitigate myocardial ischemia, a neovascularization process, which includes the creation of a capillary network in the ischemic myocardium (angiogenesis) and the growth of collateral arteries (arteriogenesis) is initiated to enhance blood flow to the myocardium. Collateral arteries are natural vascular bypasses that can significantly reduce the degree of myocardial ischemia. They develop through the growth of small pre-existing arterioles [1]. Thus, patients with good collateral circulation have a lower mortality (36 %) than patients with low levels of collateralization [1]. Patients with CAD are highly heterogeneous in their arteriogenic response, even those with totally occluded arteries [2], with this variability attributed to genetic and environmental factors [3]. Collateral vascular growth and angiogenesis are parts of the same process leading to neovascularization. They complement each other: collateral growth and arteriogenesis provide bulk flow to the tissue, and angiogenesis promotes a capillary network that salvages the ischemic area. Angiogenesis and arteriogenesis are driven by distinct, but partially overlapping, cellular and molecular pathways [4]. In this study we examine putative genetic markers of coronary collateral growth. Our group has previously reported that the p.Pro141Leu polymorphism located in the urokinase-type plasminogen activator gene (*PLAU*), a gene expressed at collateral growth sites during arteriogenesis, is associated with coronary collateral development in patients with severe CAD [5]. To this end, we performed an association study to relate coronary collateral circulation (CCC) to 22 SNPs corresponding to 10 genes with suspected or demonstrated functional involvement in the process of postischemic neovascularization, and their corresponding haplotypes, in a Spanish cohort of patients with CAD.

Methods

Study subjects

The study was conducted between 2008 and 2012. We evaluated a Spanish cohort of 677 consecutive CAD patients with severe (≥70 %) stenosis who had been scheduled to undergo diagnostic coronary angiography at the Centre Cardiovascular Sant Jordi (CCSJ) or the Hospital Universitari Vall d'Hebron (HUVH) in Barcelona, Spain. The protocol was approved by the Bioethics Committee of the two centers (Ethics Committee of Clinical Research of the HUVH and the Bioethics Committee of the CCSJ), and authorized written consent was obtained from all the subjects. The exclusion criteria were: recent (less than 1 month previously) acute myocardial infarction; anemia; recent angioplasty; prior revascularization by percutaneous coronary intervention; coronary artery bypass surgery; and renal infection, inflammation or chronic failure. Epidemiological and clinical data included hypertension, diabetes mellitus (DM), DM type, hyperlipidemia, smoking history, family history of cardiopathies (FHC), history of angina, angina type and acute myocardial infarctions (AMI); with those not referring to type recorded as present or absent.

Coronary angiography and coronary collateral artery scoring

Selective coronary angiography was performed using multiple orthogonal projections via the Judkins technique. Injection of the contrast in the donor artery was performed at a sustained high pressure with an automated controlled machine (ACIST CVi Contrast Delivery System®). CCC was assessed angiographically using a "modified" Rentrop's method [6] without occlusion of the recipient artery. The following scale was used to assess the level of filling of the channels: 0 = no visible filling of any collateral channels; 1 = collateral filling of branches of the vessel to be dilated without any dye reaching the epicardial segment of that vessel (that is, right coronary artery injection showing retrograde filling of septal branches to their origin from the left anterior descending artery, without visualization of the latter occluded artery); 2 = partial collateral filling of the epicardial segment of the vessel being dilated; and 3 = complete collateral filling of the vessel being dilated. In patients with more than one collateral vessel, the highest Rentrop score was recorded.

CAD patients were classified according to the degree of CCC as either poor CCC (Rentrop 0–1) (n = 546) or good CCC (Rentrop 2–3) (n = 131). CCC was assessed by three experienced cardiologists who were blinded to the epidemiological, clinical and genetic data. The degree of agreement in the evaluation of CCC was high among the 3 observers, as determined by the kappa coefficient: $\kappa = 0.987$; 95 % confidence interval (95 %CI), 0.953-1.000 ($P < 0.001$) using the first 100 angiograms.

SNP selection and genotype analysis

22 SNPs of genes involved in postischemic neovascularization were selected attending the following criteria: a) their suspected or proved functional or/and clinical significance regarding angiogenesis or arteriogenesis when known; b) their location within coding, 5' or 3' untranslated, or intronic sequences with known potential sites for factor binding; and c) a minor allele frequency of more than 5 % in the population studied (NCBI). We searched genes directly or indirectly involved in angiogenesis and/or arteriogenesis containing functional polymorphisms. Particularly, *HIF1A* [7–9], *VEGFA* [10–12], *KDR* [13, 14], *NOS3* [15, 16], *TGFB1* [17–19] and *LGALS2* [20, 21] have been involved in both processes.

Furthermore, *CCL2* [22] and *ICAM1* [23] play an important role in arteriogenesis, while *CD53*, which controls TNFα levels [24], also plays an important role in this process [25]; and *POSTN* has been reported to be involved in angiogenesis [26] (Table 1). The SNPs located in or near these genes that were analyzed in this study are listed in Table 1 and details of them are as follows. *HIF1A* rs11549465 and rs2057482 affect mRNA production and are associated with CAD [27]; the first is also related to collateral circulation [28]. *VEGFA* rs2010963, rs1570360 and rs699947 influence protein production [29], and along with rs3025039 and rs833061 they have also been related to VEGFA serum levels [30–32]. Moreover, *VEGFA* rs2010963 and rs699947 have been associated with collateral circulation [33] and CAD [34]. *KDR* rs1870377 and rs2305948 affect primary protein structure, whereas rs2071559 is located 5' upstream, being all related to CAD [35]. *CCL2* rs1024611 affects mRNA production [36–38]; and along with rs1024610, MCP1 plasma levels [39–41]. *CCL2* rs1024611 and rs1024610 have been associated with myocardial infarction [39, 42]. *NOS3* rs1799983 has functional consequences for the protein [43, 44] which are associated with coronary arteriogenesis [45, 46] and CAD [47]. *ICAM1* rs5498 affects the primary structure of the protein and both it and rs3093030, located near the 3' end of the gene, are related to sICAM1 plasma levels [48–51] and to coronary artery calcification [52]. *TGFB1* rs1800469 is located towards the 5' end of the gene and has been associated with coronary heart disease complications [53]. *CD53* rs6679497 is an intronic polymorphism associated with TNFα levels [24] which plays a role in modulating arteriogenesis [25]. *POSTN* rs3829365 and rs1028728 are located in the 5' UTR of the gene, with the first being associated with heart failure [54]. Finally, *LGALS2* rs7291467 is located in intron 3 and has been associated with arteriogenesis [21] and CAD [55–57].

Blood samples were drawn from patients undergoing coronary artery catheterization. Genomic DNA was isolated using the QIAmp DNA Blood kit following the manufacturer's protocol (Qiagen©, UK). TaqMan SNP genotyping assays (Applied Biosystems, Foster City, CA, USA) were performed to determine genotypes from the blood samples using a 7900HT Fast Real-Time PCR System (Applied Biosystems, Foster City, CA, USA). Genotype assessments were reproduced in three independent assays.

Statistical Analysis

Data were summarized and presented in the form of mean, standard deviation and percentage as descriptive statistics. Continuous data that were not normal-distributed were analyzed using the Mann–Whitney *U* test. In this study, age does not show a normal distribution (Shapiro-Wilk p-value <0.001). Associations among categorical data were assessed using Fisher's exact or chi-square test, and Hardy Weinberg equilibrium was assessed using the chi-square test. Multivariate logistic regression models were adjusted using clinically relevant variables to estimate odds ratios (ORs) and 95 %CIs among genotypes, haplotypes and the risk of poor CCC. Interaction terms between SNPs, haplotypes and significant covariates were also analyzed in the multivariate regression models. Statistical analysis was performed using STATA 11.2 software. The power to detect a genetic association was estimated using the same statistical package. The SNPStats software available at http://bioinfo.iconcologia.net/en/SNPStats_web was used to calculate linkage disequilibrium (measured as Lewontin's D0-values) between SNPs, to estimate haplotype frequencies, and to evaluate haplotype association with CCC.

Results

A total of 677 CAD patients (median of age 66 years, 107 females/570 males) stratified according to the level of coronary collateralization (546 poor; 131 good) were enrolled in the study. The clinical and epidemiological parameters of the patients according to CCC development are listed in Table 2. Statistical analysis showed that there were no differences among the poor and good CCC groups in terms of age, gender, hypertension or hyperlipidemia history, smoking, angina history or previous myocardial infarction (Table 2). However, the incidence of DM (55.9 %) and the percentage of patients prescribed with statins (44.3 %) were significantly higher in the poor CCC group, with p values of 0.037 and 0.035 respectively (Table 2).

None of the SNPs studied, with the exception of *NOS3* rs1799983 and *POSTN* rs3829365, showed any deviation from Hardy–Weinberg equilibrium (HWE) (tested by conventional $\chi 2$) (Table 3). Therefore, rs1799983 ($P_{HWErs1799983} = 0.0157$) and rs3829365 ($P_{HWErs3829365} = 0.0000$) were not included in further genetic association tests.

The genotype and allele distributions of all the polymorphisms in the population studied are shown in Table 2, and they did not show any differences between patients with good collateralization and patients with poor collateralization (p ≥0.05) (Table 3). Haplotype association analysis of polymorphisms in strong LD has more power than single locus tests to detect gene–disease associations. Thus, we also checked for haplotype combinations of polymorphisms in the *VEGFA*, *KDR*, *CCL2*, *ICAM1*, and *POSTN* genes to detect associations with CCC. To this end, we first estimated LD between the polymorphisms of these genes. There was a strong pairwise LD between the SNPs within these genes (data not shown), and *VEGFA*, *KDR*, *CCL2*, *ICAM1* and

Table 1 SNPs analyzed in the study

Gene	Role in angiogenesis/ arteriogenesis	SNP	Other HGVS names	Location	Functional category	FS score	Association to CCC	Association to CAD	Functional relevance
HIF1A	Both [7, 8]	rs11549465	p.Pro582Ser	Exon 2	Missense variant	0.627	[28]	[27]	Influences transactivation activity [27, 58]
		rs2057482	c.*45 T > C	3'-UTR	3' UTR variant	0	-	[27]	Influences transactivation activity [27]
VEGFA	Both [10–12]	rs2010963	c.-634C > G	Promoter	Regulatory region variant	0.257	[33]	[34]	Influences protein production [29] Related to VEGFA serum levels [30]
		rs1570360	c.-1154A > G	Promoter	Regulatory region variant	0.242	-	-	Influences protein production and related to VEGFA serum levels [31]
		rs699947	c.-2055A > C	Upstream gene	Regulatory region variant	0.176	[33]	[34]	Influences protein production and related to VEGFA serum levels [30, 31]
		rs3025039	c.*237C > T	3'-UTR	3' UTR variant	0	-	-	Related to VEGFA serum levels [32]
		rs833061	c.-958C > T	Promoter	Regulatory region variant	0.282	-	-	Related to VEGFA serum levels [30]
KDR	Both [13, 14]	rs1870377	p.Gln472His	Exon 11	Missense variant	0.103	-	[35]	-
		rs2305948	p.Val297Ile	Exon 7	Missense variant	0.621	-	[35]	-
		rs2071559	c.-906 T > C	Promoter flanking	Regulatory region variant		-	[35]	-
CCL2	Arteriogenesis [22]	rs1024611	g.2493A > G	Promoter flanking	Regulatory region variant	0.208	-	Related to myocardial infarction [39, 42]	Related to MCP1 serum levels [39–41] Influences mRNA expression [36–38]
		rs1024610	g.2936 T > A	Promoter flanking	Regulatory region variant	0.158	-	Related to myocardial infarction [39]	Related to MCP1 serum levels [39]
		rs2857657	g.5837G > C	Non coding exon	Non coding transcript exon variant	0.176	-	-	-
		rs2857654	g.2236C > A	Promoter flanking	Regulatory region variant	0	-	-	-
NOS3	Both [15, 16]	rs1799983	p.Asp298Glu	Exon 7	Missense variant	1	[45, 46]	[47]	Influences activity by different susceptibility to cleavage [43, 44]
ICAM1	Arteriogenesis [23]	rs5498	p.Lys469Glu	Exon 2	Missense variant	0.092	-	Related to coronary artery calcification [52]	Related to s-ICAM1 levels [48–50]
		rs3093030	c.-286C > T	Non coding exon	Non coding transcript exon variant	0.208	-	-	Related to s-ICAM1 levels [49, 51]
TGFB1	Both [17–19]	rs1800469	c.*309 T > C	Promoter	Regulatory region variant	0.208	-	[53]	-
CD53	-	rs6679497	c.-17-5027C > G	Intron 2	Regulatory region variant		-	-	Associated to TNFα levels [24], which has been related to arteriogenesis [25]

Table 1 SNPs analyzed in the study *(Continued)*

POSTN	Angiogenesis [26]	rs3829365	c.-33C > G	Promoter flanking	Regulatory region variant	0	-	Associated with heart failure [54]	-
		rs1028728	c.-953 T > A	Promoter flanking	Regulatory region variant	0.5	-	-	-
LGALS2	Both [20, 21]	rs7291467	c.6 + 3279C > T	Intron 1	Regulatory region variant		[21]	Related to myocardial infarction [55–57]	-

Abbreviations: CCC, coronary collateral circulation; CAD, coronary artery disease. FS score: functional effects of SNPs obtained from 16 bioinformatics tools and databases. (http://compbio.cs.queensu.ca/F-SNP/)

Table 2 Epidemiological and Clinical Characteristics of CAD patients with poor and good CCC

Characteristic	Poor CCC n = 546 (%)	Good CCC n = 131 (%)	p value
Age *(years)*	65.26 ± 10.88	66.76 ± 10.06	0.187
Gender *(male)*	460 (84.25)	110 (83.97)	0.937
Hypertension *(n)*	372 (68.13)	97 (74.05)	0.188
Diabetes mellitus *(n)*	146 (26.74)	47 (35.88)	0.037*
Hyperlipidemia *(n)*	381 (69.78)	96 (73.28)	0.430
Smoking *(n)*	126 (23.08)	33 (25.19)	0.608
Angina history *(n)*	383 (70.15)	93 (70.99)	0.849
Previous myocardial infarction *(n)*	196 (35.90)	43 (32.82)	0.509
Medication with statins *(n)*	188 (34.43)	58 (44.27)	0.035*

Abbreviations: CCC, coronary collateral circulation. Values are given as mean (S.D.) or numbers of patients (%). p <0.05 was considered as statistically significant (*)

POSTN haplotype analysis showed that the haplotype frequencies in patients with good collaterals were similar to those in patients with poor CCC (data not shown).

Discussion

An increasing number of SNPs are being accepted as underlying contributors to numerous cardiovascular disorders. Different researchers have shown the importance of several polymorphisms in CCC susceptibility [21, 28, 33, 46, 47]. *In vitro* studies have suggested that the p.Asp298Glu polymorphism plays a functional role, with the Asp 298 variant being associated with a decreased eNOS activity [43, 44], the consequences of which may include impaired collateral development. The Asp variant has been associated with poor CCC in 291 CAD patients with chronic coronary occlusions [45], and similar results have been reported in a series of 477 CAD patients with high-grade coronary stenosis ≥70 % [46]. However, because *NOS3* p.Asp298Glu deviates from HWE in our population, we could not analyze this polymorphism in our samples.

Another polymorphism which has been studied in relation to coronary arteriogenesis is p.Pro582Ser located in the *HIF1A* gene. The C/T polymorphism at nucleotide 85 of exon 12 results in a Pro/Ser polymorphism at residue 582 of HIF-1α. This substitution alters the amino acid sequence in the carboxyl-terminal domain of HIF-1α, which regulates protein stability and transcriptional activity [58]. Resar et al. demonstrated that CT or TT genotypes affecting residue 582 of the HIF-1α protein were associated with the absence of coronary collaterals in 100 patients with CAD [27]. This result indicates that p.Pro582Ser substitution could influence the expression of angiogenic growth factors, thus leading to reduced collateral formation. Although we could not validate these results in our 677 CAD patients, our results are in agreement with those published by Alidoosti et al. (2011) which found no association between rs11549465 variants and the extent of CCC (n = 196) [59]. Despite that study being conducted in Iranian CAD patients, our results support Alidoosti's observations, with our study being more robust based on a significantly higher number of patients (n = 677). Taking all this into account, the relevance of p.Pro582Ser *HIF1A* to CCC susceptibility is still under debate.

Unlike the results reported by Lin et al., 2010, showing that the *VEGFA* c.-634C > G (+405C > G) (rs2010963) and c.-2055A > C (A-2578C) (rs699947) polymorphisms were associated with the coronary arteriogenic response in 393 CAD patients [33], our results do not confirm the existence of any association between CCC and the allelic or genotypic distribution of this polymorphism. Given that the study by Lin et al. was conducted in Chinese patients, this discrepancy could be attributed to differences in population genetics.

Galectin-2, which is encoded by the *LGALS2* gene, is an inhibitor of arteriogenesis [21]. This inhibition is dependent of the gene expression on the cell surface of monocytes, acting as a modulator of monocyte/macrophage responses during collateral artery growth. CAD patients with poor CCC have increased monocytic mRNA expression of galectin-2, independent of different stimulations of these cells. Interestingly, the mRNA expression of galectin-2 was significantly associated with the *LGALS2* rs7291467 genotype, which has been associated with CCC in a small group of patients (n = 50) [21]. The same researchers also found that galectin-2 was able to inhibit collateral circulation in a mouse model of limb ischemia [21]. However, we have being unable to demonstrate an association between arteriogenic response and the allelic or genotypic distribution of this polymorphism in our cohort of patients. This may be attributable to the fact that van der Laan's study used the collateral flow index as a quantitative measure of CCC, instead of poor and good CCC based on a qualitative angiographic Rentrop score.

The most extensively studied chemokine contributing to postischemic neovascularization is the monocyte chemo-attractant protein-1 (MCP-1); a protein which is overexpressed in collateral growth, allowing for monocyte recruitment sites [60]. The crucial role of monocytes in collateral growth is exemplified by the observations that genetic targeting of the MCP-1 gene (*CCL2*) and of the MCP-1 receptor gene (*CCR2*) leads to defective collateral growth [61, 62]. However, none of the SNPs of *CCL2*, rs2857654, rs1024611, rs1024610 and rs2857657, analyzed individually or their haplotype combinations were associated with CCC development.

The main limitation of the study is that the collateralization assessment is based on the angiographic Rentrop score, which is a qualitative rather than a quantitative

Table 3 Association of genotype and allele distribution of examined polymorphisms with CAD patients with poor and good CCC

Gene	dbSNP ID	Patients	n	Genotype count (frequency)			P value[a]	Allele count (frequency)		P value[b]	HWE P
VEGFA	rs2010963			GG	GC	CC		G	C		
		Poor CCC	531	247 (46.52)	224 (42.18)	60 (11.30)	0.5760	718 (67.61)	344 (32.39)	0.495	0.8216
		Good CCC	121	50 (41.32)	58 (47.93)	13 (10.75)		158 (65.29)	84 (34.71)		
	rs1570360			GG	GA	AA		G	A		
		Poor CCC	451	207 (45.90)	197 (43.68)	47 (10.42)	0.782	611 (67.74)	291 (32.26)	0.521	0.8494
		Good CCC	97	47 (48.45)	42 (43.30)	8 (8.25)		136 (70.10)	58 (29.90)		
	rs699947			CC	AC	AA		C	A		
		Poor CCC	494	138 (27.94)	245 (49.59)	111 (22.47)	0.816	521 (52.73)	467 (47.27)	0.968	0.5199
		Good CCC	104	31 (29.81)	48 (46.15)	25 (24.04)		110 (52.90)	98 (47.12)		
	rs3025039			CC	CT	TT		C	T		
		Poor CCC	498	386 (77.51)	106 (21.29)	6 (1.20)	0.665	878 (88.15)	118 (11.85)	0.714	0.9533
		Good CCC	105	84 (80)	19 (18.10)	2 (1.90)		187 (89.05)	23 (10.95)		
	rs833061			CC	CT	TT		C	T		
		Poor CCC	526	124 (23.57)	268 (50.95)	134 (25.48)	0.471	516 (49.05)	536 (50.95)	0.232	0.6392
		Good CCC	121	33 (27.27)	63 (52.07)	25 (20.66)		129 (53.31)	113 (46.69)		
KDR	rs1870377			TT	AT	AA		T	A		
		Poor CCC	496	291 (58.67)	178 (35.89)	27 (5.44)	0.613	760 (76.61)	232 (23.39)	0.328	0.8991
		Good CCC	106	67 (63.21)	35 (33.02)	4 (3.77)		169 (79.72)	43 (20.28)		
	rs2305948			CC	CT	TT		C	T		
		Poor CCC	582	487 (83.68)	88 (15.12)	7 (1.20)	0.199	1062 (91.24)	102 (8.76)	0.207	0.3210
		Good CCC	153	120 (78.43)	32 (20.92)	1 (0.65)		272 (88.89)	34 (11.11)		
	rs2071559			TT	CT	CC		T	C		
		Poor CCC	544	147 (27.02)	276 (50.74)	121 (22.24)	0.319	570 (52.39)	518 (47.61)	0.140	0.8355
		Good CCC	129	29 (22.48)	64 (49.61)	36 (27.91)		122 (47.29)	136 (52.71)		
CCL2	rs1024611			AA	AG	GG		A	G		
		Poor CCC	576	332 (57.64)	210 (36.46)	34 (5.90)	0.221	874 (75.87)	278 (24.13)	0.826	0.3186
		Good CCC	153	94 (61.44)	46 (30.06)	13 (8.50)		234 (76.47)	72 (23.53)		
	rs1024610			AA	AT	TT		A	T		
		Poor CCC	516	312 (60.47)	180 (34.88)	24 (4.65)	0.516	804 (77.91)	228 (22.09)	0.715	0.6077
		Good CCC	112	68 (60.71)	36 (32.15)	8 (7.14)		172 (76.79)	52 (23.21)		
	rs2857657			CC	CG	GG		C	G		
		Poor CCC	511	309 (60.47)	181 (35.42)	21 (4.11)	0.365	799 (78.18)	223 (21.82)	0.832	0.8093
		Good CCC	111	71 (63.96)	33 (29.73)	7 (6.31)		175 (78.83)	47 (21.17)		
	rs2857654			CC	AC	AA		C	A		
		Poor CCC	580	336 (57.93)	211 (36.38)	33 (5.69)	0.248	883 (76.12)	277 (23.88)	0.993	0.4284
		Good CCC	153	93 (60.78)	47 (30.72)	13 (8.50)		233 (76.14)	73 (23.86)		
NOS3	rs1799983			GG	GT	TT		G	T		
		Poor CCC	513	211 (41.13)	216 (42.11)	86 (16.76)	0.596	638 (62.18)	388 (37.82)	0.686	0.0157*
		Good CCC	110	46 (41.82)	48 (43.64)	16 (14.54)		140 (63.64)	80 (36.36)		
ICAM1	rs5498			AA	AG	GG		A	G		
		Poor CCC	516	136 (26.36)	246 (47.67)	134 (25.97)	0.308	518 (50.19)	514 (49.81)	0.958	0.1039
		Good CCC	112	33 (29.46)	46 (41.08)	33 (29.46)		112 (50.00)	112 (50.00)		
	rs3093030			CC	CT	TT		C	T		
		Poor CCC	517	134 (25.92)	248 (47.97)	135 (26.11)	0.415	516 (49.90)	518 (50.10)	0.883	0.1535

Table 3 Association of genotype and allele distribution of examined polymorphisms with CAD patients with poor and good CCC *(Continued)*

		Good CCC	112	33 (29.46)	47 (41.97)	32 (28.57)		113 (50.45)	111 (49.55)		
TGFB1	rs1800469			GG	GA	AA		G	A		
		Poor CCC	483	198 (50.00)	228 (47.20)	57 (11.80)	0.696	624 (64.60)	342 (35.40)	0.979	0.8844
		Good CCC	100	43 (43.00)	43 (43.00)	14 (14.00)		129 (64.50)	71 (35.50)		
CD53	rs6679497			GG	GA	AA		G	A		
		Poor CCC	483	198 (41.00)	228 (47.20)	57 (11.80)	0.826	624 (64.60)	342 (35.40)	0.572	0.6712
		Good CCC	100	43 (43.00)	43 (43.00)	14 (14.00)		129 (64.50)	71 (35.50)		
POSTN	rs3829365			GG	GC	CC		G	C		
		Poor CCC	405	357 (88.15)	22 (5.43)	26 (6.42)	0.795	736 (90.86)	74 (9.14)	0.535	0.0000*
		Good CCC	76	69 (90.79)	3 (3.95)	4 (5.26)		141 (92.76)	11 (7.24)		
	rs1028728			AA	AT	TT		A	T		
		Poor CCC	389	242 (62.21)	128 (32.91)	19 (4.88)	0.230	612 (78.66)	166 (21.34)	0.105	0.7373
		Good CCC	77	54 (70.13)	22 (28.57)	1 (1.30)		130 (84.42)	24 (15.58)		
LGALS2	rs7291467			AA	AG	GG		A	G		
		Poor CCC	581	160 (27.54)	292 (50.26)	129 (22.20)	0.106	612 (52.67)	550 (47.33)	0.080	0.9589
		Good CCC	151	37 (24.50)	68 (45.03)	46 (30.47)		142 (47.02)	160 (52.98)		
HIF1A	rs11549465			CC	CT	TT		C	T		
		Poor CCC	518	402 (77.60)	111 (21.43)	5 (0.97)	0.563	915 (88.32)	121 (11.68)	0.474	0.4122
		Good CCC	112	84 (75)	26 (23.21)	2 (1.79)		194 (86.61)	30 (13.39)		
	rs2057482			CC	CT	TT		C	T		
		Poor CCC	497	339 (68.21)	148 (29.78)	10 (2.01)	0.490	826 (83.10)	168 (16.90)	0.328	0.1151
		Good CCC	111	70 (63.06)	38 (34.24)	3 (2.70)		178 (80.18)	44 (19.82)		

[a]Fisher's exact test was used to evaluate differences between genotype groups. [b]Pearson's chi-squared, χ^2, was used for to evaluate the allele distribution.
*p <0.05 was considered as statistically significant

technique. A modified Rentrop method without occlusion of the recipient artery was performed in the current work. This method, as well as the inclusion of a large portion of patients with subocclusive lesions (>70-100 %), probably might explain why such a relative low number of patients displayed well-developed collateral arteries in this cohort. Also, functional polymorphims in interferon-beta signaling genes, which are involved in arteriogenesis from clinical studies [63, 64], were not included in the study.

Conclusions

Despite having previously reported that *PLAU* p.Pro141-Leu (rs2227564) was associated with coronary arteriogenesis [5], none of the rs11549465, rs2057482, rs2010963, rs1570360, rs699947, rs3025039, rs833061, rs1870377, rs2305948, rs2071559, rs1024611, rs1024610, rs2857657, rs2857654, rs1799983, rs5498, rs3093030, rs1800469, rs6679497, rs3829365 or rs1028728 polymorphisms analyzed located in or close to genes involved in postischemic neovascularization (*VEGFA*, *KDR*, *CCL2*, *ICAM1* and *POSTN*) or their haplotype combinations were associated with CCC development. In addition, in our cohort of patients we could not validate the association of the *NOS3* rs1799983, *HIF1A* rs11549465, *VEGFA* rs2010963 and rs699947, and *LGALS2* rs7291467 polymorphisms with CCC development reported by other authors. We and others have demonstrated the potential role of certain polymorphisms as factors associated with CCC [5, 21, 28, 45, 46], but usually they have not been validated in other cohorts of patients. In addition, SNPs may influence collateral development not only individually, but also when acting together with other SNPs, through gene haplotype networks, as demonstrated by the role of several inflammatory gene haplotype networks in CCC [65]. In conclusion, a validated SNP-based GWAS is needed to reveal and/or confirm the SNPs that predict coronary arteriogenic response.

Competing interests

The author(s) declare that they have no competing interests.

Authors' contributions

JA and MP were responsible for study conception and design. JA and JD analyzed and interpreted the study data, and wrote the first draft of the manuscript. JD, MM, VG, AC and OA were responsible for clinical and epidemiological data collection. JD, MM and AC for DNA genotyping. JC, EM, OA, IO and BG were responsible for measurements of angiographic parameters. PS, MM, and JD were responsible for statistical analysis. JA, JD, VG, DG, BG and JR assisted in the acquisition of data and provided valuable, intellectual contributions to the manuscript draft. All authors have approved the final version of the manuscript.

Acknowledgements
We thank Montse Cairó, Eva Sánchez, Dolors Colell, Teresa Torrent, María José Fernández de Muniain, and Miquel Rugat for their valuable collaboration and technical assistance. This study was supported by the Fundació La Marató de TV3 07 (project 080810) and the Universitat de Barcelona (project ACESBELL 08).

Author details
[1]Unitat d'Anatomia i Embriologia Humanes, Departament de Patologia i Terapèutica Experimental, Facultat de Medicina, Campus de Ciències de la Salut de Bellvitge, Universitat de Barcelona, L'Hospitalet de Llobregat, Barcelona 08907, Spain. [2]Departamento de Estadística, Facultad de Ciencias, Universidad de Valparaíso, Valparaíso, Chile. [3]Neurovascular Research Group (NEUVAS), Institut Municipal d'Investigació Mèdica. Hospital del Mar, PRBB, Parc de Recerca Biomèdica de Barcelona, Barcelona, Spain. [4]Department of Cardiology and Hemodynamics, Centre Cardiovascular Sant Jordi, Barcelona, Spain. [5]Department of Cardiology, Hospital Universitari Vall d'Hebron, Barcelona, Spain. [6]Department of Cardiology, Hospital Mútua de Terrassa, Terrassa, Barcelona, Spain. [7]Departament of Morphological Sciences, Universitat Autònoma de Barcelona, Bellaterra, Cerdanyola del Vallès, Barcelona, Spain. [8]Àrea Epigenetics and Cancer Biology Area, Institut d'Investigació Biomèdica de Bellvitge (IDIBELL), L'Hospitalet de Llobregat, Barcelona, Spain.

References

1. Meier P, Hemingway H, Lansky AJ, Knapp G, Pitt B, Seiler C. The impact of the coronary collateral circulation on mortality: a meta-analysis. Eur Heart J. 2012;33(5):614–21.
2. Pohl T, Seiler C, Billinger M, Herren E, Wustmann K, Mehta H, et al. Frequency distribution of collateral flow and factors influencing collateral channel development. Functional collateral channel measurement in 450 patients with coronary artery disease. J Am Coll Cardiol. 2001;38(7):1872–8.
3. Schirmer SH, van Nooijen FC, Piek JJ, van Royen N. Stimulation of collateral artery growth: travelling further down the road to clinical application. Heart. 2009;95(3):191–7.
4. Silvestre JS, Mallat Z, Tedgui A, Levy BI. Post-ischaemic neovascularization and inflammation. Cardiovasc Res. 2008;78(2):242–9.
5. Duran J, Sánchez-Olavarría P, Mola M, Götzens V, Carballo J, Martín-Pelegrina E, et al. The PLAU P141L single nucleotide polymorphism is associated with collateral circulation in patients with coronary artery disease. Rev Esp Cardiol (Engl Ed). 2014;67(7):552–7.
6. Rentrop KP, Cohen M, Blanke H, Phillips RA. Changes in collateral channel filling immediately after controlled coronary artery occlusion by an angioplasty balloon in human subjects. J Am Coll Cardiol. 1985;5(3):587–92.
7. Coulon C, Georgiadou M, Roncal C, De Bock K, Langenberg T, Carmeliet P. From vessel sprouting to normalization: role of the prolyl hydroxylase domain protein/hypoxia-inducible factor oxygen-sensing machinery. Arterioscler, Thromb, Vasc Biol. 2010;30(12):2331–6.
8. Patel TH, Kimura H, Weiss CR, Semenza GL, Hofmann LV. Constitutively active HIF-1α improves perfusion and arterial remodeling in an endovascular model of limb ischemia. Cardiovasc Res. 2005;68(1):144–54.
9. Duran J, Götzens V, Carballo J, Martn E, Petit M, Cordero Á, et al. The HIF1A C85T single nucleotide polymorphism influences the number of branches of the human coronary tree. Cardiology. 2012;121(3):156–9.
10. Hoeben A, Landuyt B, Highley MS, Wildiers H, Van Oosterom AT, De Bruijn EA. Vascular endothelial growth factor and angiogenesis. Pharmacol Rev. 2004;56(4):549–80.
11. Clayton JA, Chalothorn D, Faber JE. Vascular endothelial growth factor-a specifies formation of native collaterals and regulates collateral growth in ischemia. Circ Res. 2008;103(9):1027–36.
12. Toyota E, Warltier DC, Brock T, Ritman E, Kolz C, O'Malley P, et al. Vascular endothelial growth factor is required for coronary collateral growth in the rat. Circulation. 2005;112(14):2108–13.
13. Hsu HW, Wall NR, Hsueh CT, Kim S, Ferris RL, Chen CS, et al. Combination antiangiogenic therapy and radiation in head and neck cancers. Oral Oncol. 2014;50(1):19–26.
14. Babiak A, Schumm AM, Wangler C, Loukas M, Wu J, Dombrowski S, et al. Coordinated activation of VEGFR-1 and VEGFR-2 is a potent arteriogenic stimulus leading to enhancement of regional perfusion. Cardiovasc Res. 2004;61(4):789–95.
15. Cooke JP, Ghebremariam YT. Endothelial nicotinic acetylcholine receptors and angiogenesis. Trends Cardiovasc Med. 2008;18(7):247–53.
16. Schaper W. Collateral circulation: past and present. Basic Res Cardiol. 2009;104(1):5–21.
17. van Royen N, Hoefer I, Buschmann I, Heil M, Kostin S, Deindl E, et al. Exogenous application of transforming growth factor beta 1 stimulates arteriogenesis in the peripheral circulation. FASEB J. 2002;16(3):432–4.
18. Peshavariya HM, Chan EC, Liu GS, Jiang F, Dusting GJ. Transforming growth factor-β1 requires NADPH oxidase 4 for angiogenesis *in vitro* and *in vivo*. J Cell Mol Med. 2014;18(6):1172–83.
19. Grundmann S, van Royen N, Pasterkamp G, Gonzalez N, Tijsma EJ, Piek JJ, et al. A New intra-arterial DeliveryPlatform for Pro-arteriogenic compounds to stimulate collateral artery growth Via transforming growth factor-beta1 release. J Am Coll Cardiol. 2007;50(4):351–8.
20. Chen C, Duckworth CA, Fu B, Pritchard DM, Rhodes JM, Yu L-G. Circulating galectins −2, −4 and −8 in cancer patients make important contributions to the increased circulation of several cytokines and chemokines that promote angiogenesis and metastasis. Br J Cancer. 2014;110(3):741–52.
21. Van der Laan AM, Schirmer SH, de Vries MR, Koning JJ, Volger OL, Fledderus JO, et al. Galectin-2 expression is dependent on the rs7291467 polymorphism and acts as an inhibitor of arteriogenesis. Eur Heart J. 2011;33(9):1076–84.
22. Keeley EC, Mehrad B, Strieter RM. Chemokines as mediators of neovascularization. Arterioscler, Thromb, Vasc Biol. 2008;28(11):1928–36.
23. Hoefer IE, van Royen N, Rectenwald JE, Deindl E, Hua J, Jost M, et al. Arteriogenesis proceeds via ICAM-1/Mac-1- mediated mechanisms. Circ Res. 2004;94(9):1179–85.
24. Bos SD, Lakenberg N, van der Breggen R, Houwing-Duistermaat JJ, Kloppenburg M, de Craen AJ, et al. A genome-wide linkage scan reveals CD53 as an important regulator of innate TNF-alpha levels. Eur J Hum Genet. 2010;18(8):953–9.
25. Hoefer IE, van Royen N, Rectenwald JE, Bray EJ, Abouhamze Z, Moldawer LL, et al. Direct evidence for tumor necrosis factor-alpha signaling in arteriogenesis. Circulation. 2002;105(14):1639–41.
26. Shao R, Bao S, Bai X, Blanchette C, Anderson RM, Dang T, et al. Acquired expression of periostin by human breast cancers promotes tumor angiogenesis through up-regulation of vascular endothelial growth factor receptor 2 expression. Mol Cell Biol. 2004;24(9):3992–4003.
27. Hlatky MA, Quertermous T, Boothroyd DB, Priest JR, Glassford AJ, Myers RM, et al. Polymorphisms in hypoxia inducible factor 1 and the initial clinical presentation of coronary disease. Am Heart J. 2007;154(6):1035–42.
28. Resar JR, Roguin A, Voner J, Nasir K, Hennebry TA, Miller JM, et al. Hypoxia-inducible factor 1alpha polymorphism and coronary collaterals in patients with ischemic heart disease. Chest. 2005;128(2):787–91.
29. Watson CJ, Webb NJ, Bottomley MJ, Brenchley PE. Identification of polymorphisms within the vascular endothelial growth factor (VEGF) gene: correlation with variation in VEGF protein production. Cytokine+. 2000;12(8):1232–5.
30. Steffensen KD, Waldstrøm M, Brandslund I, Jakobsen A. The relationship of VEGF polymorphisms with serum VEGF levels and progression-free survival in patients with epithelial ovarian cancer. Gynecol Oncol. 2010;117(1):109–16.
31. Mohammadi M, Bazrafshani MR, Day PJ, Ollier WE. Vascular endothelial growth factor production is regulated by gene polymorphisms. Iran J Immunol. 2009;6(3):119–29.
32. Al-Habboubi HH, Sater MS, Almawi AW, Al-Khateeb GM, Almawi WY. Contribution of VEGF polymorphisms to variation in VEGF serum levels in a healthy population. Eur Cytokine Netw. 2011;22(3):154–8.
33. Lin TH, Wang CL, Su HM, Hsu PC, Juo SH, Voon WC, et al. Functional vascular endothelial growth factor gene polymorphisms and diabetes: effect on coronary collaterals in patients with significant coronary artery disease. Clin Chim Acta. 2010;411(21–22):1688–93.
34. Cui QT, Li Y, Duan CH, Zhang W, Guo XL. Further evidence for the contribution of the vascular endothelial growth factor gene in coronary artery disease susceptibility. Gene. 2013;521(2):217–21.

35. Wang Y, Zheng Y, Zhang W, Yu H, Lou K, Zhang Y, et al. Polymorphisms of KDR gene are associated with coronary heart disease. J Am Coll Cardiol. 2007;50(8):760–7.
36. Rovin BH, Lu L, Saxena R. A novel polymorphism in the MCP-1 gene regulatory region that influences MCP-1 expression. Biochem Biophys Res Commun. 1999;259(2):344–8.
37. Del Guerra S, D'Aleo V, Gualtierotti G, Filipponi F, Boggi U, De Simone P, et al. A common polymorphism in the monocyte chemoattractant protein-1 (MCP-1) gene regulatory region influences MCP-1 expression and function of isolated human pancreatic islets. Transpl Proc. 2010;42(6):2247–9.
38. Pham MHT, Bonello GB, Castiblanco J, Le T, Sigala J, He W, et al. The rs1024611 regulatory region polymorphism is associated with CCL2 allelic expression imbalance. PLoS One. 2012;7(11):e49498.
39. McDermott DH, Yang Q, Kathiresan S, Cupples LA, Massaro JM, Keaney Jr JF, et al. CCL2 polymorphisms are associated with serum monocyte chemoattractant protein-1 levels and myocardial infarction in the Framingham Heart Study. Circulation. 2005;112(8):1113–20.
40. Tabara Y, Kohara K, Yamamoto Y, Igase M, Nakura J, Kondo I, et al. Polymorphism of the monocyte chemoattractant protein (MCP-1) gene is associated with the plasma level of MCP-1 but not with carotid intima-media thickness. Hypertens Res. 2003;26(9):677–83.
41. Gonzalez E, Rovin BH, Sen L, Cooke G, Dhanda R, Mummidi S, et al. HIV-1 infection and AIDS dementia are influenced by a mutant MCP-1 allele linked to increased monocyte infiltration of tissues and MCP-1 levels. Proc Natl Acad Sci U S A. 2002;99(21):13795–800.
42. Lin HL, Ueng KC, Hsieh YS, Chiang WL, Yang SF, Chu SC. Impact of MCP-1 and CCR-2 gene polymorphisms on coronary artery disease susceptibility. Mol Biol Rep. 2012;39(9):9023–30.
43. Tesauro M, Thompson WC, Rogliani P, Qi L, Chaudhary PP, Moss J. Intracellular processing of endothelial nitric oxide synthase isoforms associated with differences in severity of cardiopulmonary diseases: cleavage of proteins with aspartate vs. glutamate at position 298. Proc Natl Acad Sci U S A. 2000;97(6):2832–5.
44. Persu A, Stoenoiu MS, Messiaen T, Davila S, Robino C, El-Khattabi O, et al. Modifier effect of ENOS in autosomal dominant polycystic kidney disease. Hum Mol Genet. 2002;11(3):229–41.
45. Lamblin N, Cuilleret FJ, Helbecque N, Dallongeville J, Lablanche J-M, Amouyel P, et al. A common variant of endothelial nitric oxide synthase (Glu298Asp) is associated with collateral development in patients with chronic coronary occlusions. BMC Cardiovasc Disord. 2005;5:27.
46. Gulec S, Karabulut H, Ozdemir AO, Ozdol C, Turhan S, Altin T, et al. Glu298Asp polymorphism of the eNOS gene is associated with coronary collateral development. Atherosclerosis. 2008;198(2):354–9.
47. Abdel-Aziz TA, Mohamed RH. Association of endothelial nitric oxide synthase gene polymorphisms with classical risk factors in development of premature coronary artery disease. Mol Biol Rep. 2013;40(4):3065–71.
48. Bielinski SJ, Pankow JS, Li N, Hsu FC, Adar SD, Jenny NS, et al. ICAM1 and VCAM1 polymorphisms, coronary artery calcium, and circulating levels of soluble ICAM-1: the multi-ethnic study of atherosclerosis (MESA). Atherosclerosis. 2008;201(2):339–44.
49. Bielinski SJ, Pankow JS, Foster CL, Miller MB, Hopkins PN, Eckfeldt JH, et al. Circulating soluble ICAM-1 levels shows linkage to ICAM gene cluster region on chromosome 19: The NHLBI Family Heart Study follow-up examination. Atherosclerosis. 2008;199(1):172–8.
50. Bielinski SJ, Reiner AP, Nickerson D, Carlson C, Bailey KR, Thyagarajan B, et al. Polymorphisms in the ICAM1 gene predict circulating soluble intercellular adhesion molecule-1(sICAM-1). Atherosclerosis. 2011;216(2):390–4.
51. Barbalic M, Dupuis J, Dehghan A, Bis JC, Hoogeveen RC, Schnabel RB, et al. Large-scale genomic studies reveal central role of ABO in sP-selectin and sICAM-1 levels. Hum Mol Genet. 2010;19(9):1863–72.
52. Reilly MP, Wolfe ML, Dykhouse J, Reddy K, Localio AR, Rader DJ. Intercellular adhesion molecule 1 (ICAM-1) gene variant is associated with coronary artery calcification independent of soluble ICAM-1 levels. J Investig Med. 2004;52(8):515–22.
53. Morris DR, Moxon JV, Biros E, Krishna SM, Golledge J. Meta-analysis of the association between transforming growth Factor-Beta polymorphisms and complications of coronary heart disease. PLoS One. 2012;7(5):e37878.
54. Wang F, Song Y, Jiang Y, Yang C, Ding Z. Associations among periostin gene polymorphisms, clinical parameters and heart failure: a case–control study in 1104 Chinese individuals. J Cardiovasc Med (Hagerstown). 2011;12(7):469–74.
55. Ozaki K, Inoue K, Sato H, Iida A, Ohnishi Y, Sekine A, et al. Functional variation in LGALS2 confers risk of myocardial infarction and regulates lymphotoxin-alpha secretion *in vitro*. Nature. 2004;429(6987):72–5.
56. Ozaki K, Tanaka T. Genome-wide association study to identify SNPs conferring risk of myocardial infarction and their functional analyses. Cell Mol Life Sci. 2005;62(16):1804–13.
57. Asselbergs FW, Pai JK, Rexrode KM, Hunter DJ, Rimm EB. Effects of lymphotoxin-alpha gene and galectin-2 gene polymorphisms on inflammatory biomarkers, cellular adhesion molecules and risk of coronary heart disease. Clin Sci (Lond). 2007;112(5):291–8.
58. Tanimoto K, Yoshiga K, Eguchi H, Kaneyasu M, Ukon K, Kumazaki T, et al. Hypoxia-inducible factor-1alpha polymorphisms associated with enhanced transactivation capacity, implying clinical significance. Carcinogenesis. 2003;24(11):1779–83.
59. Alidoosti M, Ghaedi M, Soleimani A, Bakhtiyari S, Rezvanfard M, Golkhu S, et al. Study on the role of environmental parameters and HIF-1A gene polymorphism in coronary collateral formation among patients with ischemic heart disease. Clin Biochem. 2011;44(17–18):1421–4.
60. Ito WD, Arras M, Winkler B, Scholz D, Schaper J, Schaper W. Monocyte chemotactic protein-1 increases collateral and peripheral conductance after femoral artery occlusion. Circ Res. 1997;80(6):829–37.
61. Heil M, Ziegelhoeffer T, Wagner S, Fernandez B, Helisch A, Martin S, et al. Collateral artery growth (arteriogenesis) after experimental arterial occlusion is impaired in mice lacking CC-chemokine receptor-2. Circ Res. 2004;94(5):671–7.
62. Voskuil M, Hoefer IE, van Royen N, Hua J, de Graaf S, Bode C, et al. Abnormal monocyte recruitment and collateral artery formation in monocyte chemoattractant protein-1 deficient mice. Vasc Med. 2004;9(4):287–92.
63. Schirmer SH, Bot PT, Fledderus JO, van der Laan AM, Volger OL, Laufs U, et al. Blocking interferon {beta} stimulates vascular smooth muscle cell proliferation and arteriogenesis. J Biol Chem. 2010;285(45):34677–85.
64. Schirmer SH, Fledderus JO, Bot PT, Moerland PD, Hoefer IE, Baan Jr J, et al. Interferon-beta signaling is enhanced in patients with insufficient coronary collateral artery development and inhibits arteriogenesis in mice. Circ Res. 2008;102(10):1286–94.
65. Zhang J, Regieli JJ, Schipper M, Entius MM, Liang F, Koerselman J, et al. Inflammatory gene haplotype-interaction networks involved in coronary collateral formation. Hum Hered. 2008;66(4):252–64.

A cross-sectional analysis of the relationship between uric acid and coronary atherosclerosis in patients with suspected coronary artery disease in China

Yujiao Sun[1], Xin Yu[1], Ying Zhi[1], Song Geng[1], Hua Li[1], Ting Liu[2], Ke Xu[2], Ling Chen[1], Chunwei Wu[1] and Guoxian Qi[1*]

Abstract

Background: Although many studies have examined the relationship between uric acid (UA) and coronary artery disease (CAD), whether UA is an independent risk factor contributing to progression of CAD is still controversial. Whether UA plays a different role in different sexes is also unclear.

Methods: A total of 1116 individuals with suspected CAD were stratified into four groups according to their serum UA quartiles in total (men and women combined), in men, and in women. The association of UA with coronary atherosclerosis was assessed by univariable and multivariable logistic regression.

Results: In total and in women, the prevalence of any plaques and significant/severe stenosis was significantly increased with an increase in quartiles of UA (all $P < 0.05$). The proportion of triple-vessel disease and left main artery lesion was highest in the fourth quartile (both $p < 0.05$). Increasing quartiles of UA were significantly associated with a coronary artery calcium score (CACS) >10 (all $P < 0.01$). As UA levels increased in women, the incidence of double-vessel lesions ($p = 0.017$) and the proportion of mixed plaques ($p = 0.022$) were significantly increased. The proportion of a CACS of 0 in total, in men and women was highest in the first quartile (all $P < 0.01$). UA was the strongest predictor of significant stenosis, multivessel disease, and mixed plaques in women (all $p < 0.05$). UA was the only risk factor for mixed plaques in total ($P = 0.046$).

Conclusion: The level of UA was significantly associated with coronary atherosclerosis in women, but not men.

Keywords: Uric acid, Coronary atherosclerosis, Coronary computed tomography angiography, Gender, Calcium score

Background

Uric acid (UA) is the main end product of purine catabolism [1]. High UA levels are often accompanied by obesity, hyperlipidemia, hypertension, glucose intolerance, and insulin resistance [2-5], which contribute to the development of cardiovascular disease. Elevated UA levels are associated with coronary artery disease (CAD), independently of traditional CAD risk factors [6,7]. However, some studies have suggested that UA is only considered as a risk marker or an adaptive ascended to attempt to prevent atherosclerosis [8-10], and this may be due to its antioxidant properties [11]. Although studies have examined the relationship between UA and CAD, whether increased UA is an independent risk factor that contributes to early CAD is still controversial.

Sex might be an important factor involved in the relationship between UA and CAD. In a subgroup analysis of LIFE [12], the relationship between UA and CAD was significant only in women. A meta-analysis [6] found that UA was significantly correlated with CAD only in women. A strong association between UA and cardiac

* Correspondence: qigx2011@hotmail.com
[1]Department of Cardiology of Aging, Department of Cardiology, The First Affiliated Hospital of China Medical University, NO.155 Nanjing North Street, Heping Ward, Shenyang 110001, China
Full list of author information is available at the end of the article

events has been observed in both sexes in other studies [13,14]. Whether UA plays a different role in different sexes in the progression of CAD is unclear.

Therefore, in this study, we assessed the association between UA and coronary atherosclerosis in patients with suspected CAD who underwent 256-detector-row coronary computed tomographic angiography (CCTA). We further assessed these associations in sex subgroups.

Methods

Study population

This study included 5150 consecutive individuals (≥18 years) in China undergoing CCTA and coronary artery calcium score (CACS) measurements in our institution from September 2011 to February 2013. CCTA and measurement of the CACS were performed for the suspicion of CAD after clinical assessment (including cardiac symptoms, risk factors, electrocardiogram changes, and a positive stress test). Finally, 1116 individuals were enrolled (Figure 1). All patients gave written inform consent, and the study was approved by the ethics committee of the First Affiliated Hospital of China Medical University.

Assessment of CAD risk factors

All patients were systematically asked about their demographics by professionals. Body weight, height, and blood pressure were measured. Hypertension was defined as a previously established diagnosis and/or antihypertensive medication, systolic blood pressure ≥140 mmHg, and diastolic blood pressure ≥90 mmHg. Diabetes mellitus was defined as a previously established diagnosis and/or antidiabetic treatment, and fasting glucose ≥126 mg/dl. A family history of CAD was defined as a first-degree male relative aged <55 years or a first-degree female relative aged <65 years. Smoking was defined as any cigarette smoking within 1 year of CCTA. Medication use was recorded in detail.

Total cholesterol (TC), triglycerides (TG), high-density lipoprotein cholesterol (HDL-C), low-density lipoprotein cholesterol (LDL-C), creatinine and UA levels were measured after at least a 12-h fasting period within 7 days of CCTA. The contents of UA were measured with enzyme kinetics in all enrolled patients, and it was uniform throughout the study period.

Acquisition of images

Computed tomography scans were performed using 256-detector-row CCTA (Brilliance; Philips Medical System, The Netherlands). Individuals with a heart rate ≥75 beats per minute were treated orally with up to 100 mg metoprolol for several hours (except for contraindications of beta-blockers) before CCTA imaging to achieve a higher image quality. First, after a scout radiograph of the chest (lateral and anteroposterior), a non-contrast CACS scan was performed, and the image section thickness was 2.5 mm by triggering at a heart rate depending on the percentage of the R-R interval. The sections were collected from the level of the carina and proceeded to the level of the diaphragm. Thereafter, retrospective electrocardiogram-gated contrast-enhanced CCTA was performed. The CCTA scan was initiated 20 mm above the level of the left main artery to 20 mm below the inferior myocardial apex during a single

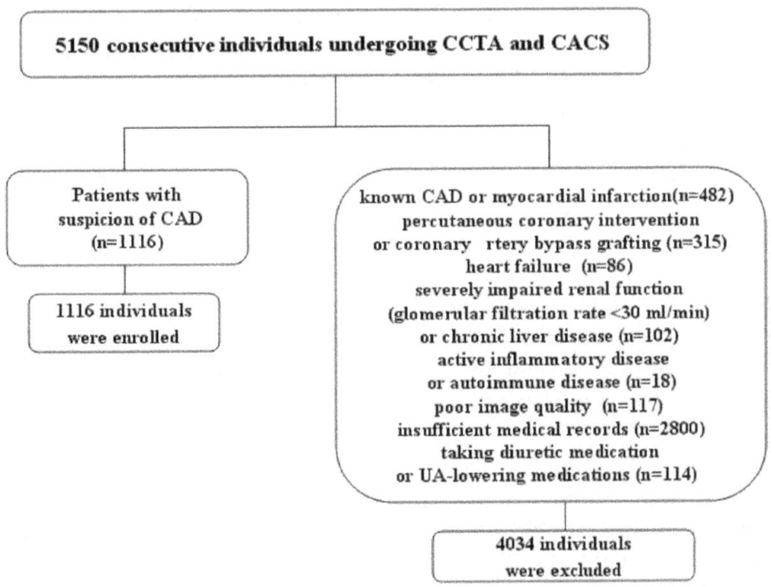

Figure 1 The path of patients enrollment.

breath-hold. Depending on the individual's weight, a bolus of 50–80 ml of iopamidol or iohexol was intravenously injected at 4–5.5 ml/s into the antecubital vein, followed by 50 ml of saline. A standard scan protocol was applied, with section collimation of 256 × 0.625 mm, 0.27 s for rotation time, 120 KV tube voltage, and 800–1100 mA tube current. In all scans, electrocardiogram-gate dose modulation was used. The electrocardiograms of individuals were simultaneously collected to allow for retrospective segmental data reconstruction. The images of all individuals were initially reconstructed at 75% of the R-R interval of the cardiac cycle. If motion artefacts were found, reconstruction of additional phases was performed. The best R-R interval image quality was chosen for interpretation. The dose range of radiation for CCTA was estimated to be 10–18 mSv.

Image analysis

All images were analysed separately by two experienced radiologists and one cardiologist who were blinded to the patients' characteristics. Consensus on interpretation was performed to achieve a final CCTA diagnosis. All scans were evaluated by a three-dimensional workstation (Brilliance; Philips Medical Systems). The CACS was measured using the scoring system previously described by Agatston et al. [15].

The three reads were permitted to use any/all available post-processing image reconstruction algorithms, including two-dimensional axial or three-dimensional maximal intensity projection, multiplanar reformat, cross-sectional analysis, or the volume-rendered technique. A 16-segment coronary artery tree model [16] was used in the analysis of coronary arteries. In each coronary segment, plaques were defined as any tissue structure >1 mm^2, which existed either within the coronary artery lumen or was adjacent to the coronary artery lumen, and could be discriminated from surrounding pericardial tissue, epicardial fat, or the vessel lumen itself. For evaluating the degree of stenosis, the coronary lumen was semi-automatically traced at the maximal stenosis site and was compared with the mean value of a proximal and distal reference site. The image quality was evaluated and classified as follows: good, with no artifact; adequate, with the presence of artifacts but feasible for evaluating the degree of stenosis and plaque characteristics; or poor, with the presence of artifacts and not feasible for evaluating the degree of stenosis and plaque characteristics. If an image was graded as poor, the image was not included.

Coronary lesions ≥50 and 70% were defined as significant and severe, respectively. Multivessel disease was defined as the presence of stenosis of more than 50% in at least two vessels. The stenosed coronary vessel of individuals was further categorized as having one-, two-, and three-vessel/left main disease. All detected plaques were classified as calcified, non-calcified, or mixed. The calcified component of a stenosis was defined as a lesion with radiodensity greater than the luminal contrast. The non-calcified component of a stenosis was defined as a lesion with radiodensity greater than that of neighbouring soft tissue and lower than the luminal contrast. Plaques that contained calcified tissue greater than 75% of the plaque area were classified as calcified plaques, less than 25% as non-calcified plaques, and 25–75% as mixed plaques [17].

Statistical analysis

Baseline characteristics are expressed as absolute counts and proportions for categorical variables, and as means ± standard deviations for continuous variables. Continuous variables were analysed by analysis of variance and categorical variables were analysed by χ^2 test.

The association of UA with coronary atherosclerosis was assessed by the χ^2 test. Univariable and multivariable logistic regression were used to assess the association of UA with significant stenosis, multivessel disease, high CACS, and plaque characteristics. Variables that showed a P value <0.1 with univariable analysis were applied to multivariate analysis. All analyses were performed using SPSS 15.0. The level of significance was set at $P < 0.05$.

Results

Baseline characteristic baseline characteristics

Among the 1116 patients in the study, 50.7% were men, and the mean age was 58.05 ± 10.69 years. All individuals were stratified into four groups according to their UA quartile, the first quartile:<259 μmmol/l (n = 278); the second quartile: 259–309 μmmol/l (n = 274); the third quartile: 310-373 μmmol/l (n = 283) and the fourth quartile: >373 μmmol/l (n = 281). With increasing UA quartiles, the prevalence of male sex, smoking, and hypertension was significantly increased (all $P < 0.01$). Body mass index (BMI) and TC level were significantly higher (all $P < 0.001$) and HDL-C level was significantly lower ($P < 0.001$, Table 1). Figure 2 showed the representative view of mixed, non-calcified and calcified plaque.

Prevalence, characteristics, and the CACS of coronary artery plaques

Men and women were stratified into four groups according to their UA quartile. The quartiles of UA in men were the first quartile: 296 μmmol/l (n = 140); the second quartile: <296-349 μmmol/l (n = 140); the third quartile: 350-406 μmmol/(n = 144) and the fourth quartile: >406 μmmol/l (n = 142). The quartiles of UA in women were the first quartile: <238 μmmol/l (n = 136); the second quartile: 238-273 μmmol/l (n = 137); the third quartile: 274-326 μmmol/l(n = 138) and the fourth quartile > 326 μmmol/l (n = 139). With increasing UA quartiles in total (men and women

Table 1 Baseline characteristics of the all study population according to the quartiles of the serum uric acid

Variables	Total (n = 1116)	1st Quartile <259 μmol/l (n = 278)	2nd Quartile 259-309 μmol/l (n = 274)	3rd Quartile 310-373 μmol/l (n = 283)	4th Quartile >373 μmol/l (n = 281)	P-value
Age(years)	58.05 ± 10.69	58.64 ± 9.19	57.86 ± 9.52	58.14 ± 11.09	57.56 ± 12.6	0.674
Male	566 (50.7)	64 (23.0)	109 (39.8)	170 (60.1)	223 (79.4)	<0.001
BMI(kg/m^2)	24.99 ± 4.00	23.46 ± 4.24	24.70 ± 3.29	25.83 ± 4.45	25.95 ± 3.38	<0.001
Smoking	279 (25.0)	40 (14.4)	59 (21.5)	89 (31.4)	91 (32.4)	<0.001
Family history of CAD	93 (8.3)	27 (9.7)	29 (10.6)	20 (7.1)	17 (6.0)	0.167
Hypertension	639 (42.7)	96 (34.5)	114 (41.6)	135 (47.7)	132 (47.0)	0.005
Diabetes Mellitus	183 (16.4)	45 (16.2)	43 (15.7)	51 (18.0)	44 (15.7)	0.861
LDL-C(mmol/l)	2.95 ± 0.88	2.93 ± 0.79	3.02 ± 1.01	2.94 ± 0.87	2.92 ± 0.87	0.544
HDL-C(mmol/l)	1.19 ± 0.37	1.33 ± 0.34	1.21 ± 0.32	1.13 ± 0.30	1.09 ± 0.46	<0.001
TC(mmol/l)	4.60 ± 1.06	4.61 ± 0.97	4.66 ± 1.22	4.58 ± 1.06	4.56 ± 0.99	0.735
TG(mmol/l)	1.64 ± 1.36	1.29 ± 0.85	1.59 ± 1.29	1.69 ± 1.47	1.98 ± 1.61	<0.001
Creatinine(μmol/l)	78.20 ± 16.32	81.47 ± 16.74	80.09 ± 14.23	74.07 ± 15.38	81.95 ± 19.17	0.121
History of Medication						
Aspirin	247 (22.1)	64 (23.0)	57 (20.8)	67 (23.7)	59 (21.0)	0.799
Beta blcker	118 (10.6)	27 (9.7)	26 (9.5)	31 (11.0)	34 (12.1)	0.733
ACEI	62 (5.6)	13 (4.7)	15 (5.5)	17 (6.0)	17 (5.6)	0.880
ARB	68 (6.1)	14 (5.0)	13 (4.7)	20 (7.1)	21 (7.5)	0.417
CCB	145 (13.0)	28 (10.1)	43 (15.7)	42 (14.8)	32 (11.4)	0.144
Statins	94 (8.4)	20 (7.2)	25 (9.1)	30 (10.6)	19 (6.8)	0.330
Antihyperglycemic	107 (9.6)	30 (10.8)	23 (8.4)	29 (10.2)	25 (8.9)	0.750
Insulin	65 (5.8)	18 (6.5)	14 (5.1)	18 (6.4)	15 (5.3)	0.863

Values are mean ± Standard deviation or n (%). The conversion of UA measuring unit: mg/dl = (μmol/l divide by 59.48).
BMI Body Mass Index, *CAD* Coronary artery disease, *LDL-C* Low-density lipoprotein Cholesterol, *HDL-C* High-density lipoprotein Cholesterol, *TC* Total Cholesterol, *TG* Triglycerides, *ACEI* Angiotensin-converting enzyme inhibitor, *ARB* Angiotensin receptor blocker, *CCB* Calcium Channel Blocker.

combined) and in women, the prevalence of plaques were significantly increased (total: 56.8% vs 62.0% vs 70.0% vs 73.0%, $P < 0.001$; women: 47.1% vs 57.7% vs 59.4% vs 69.8%, p = 0.002, (Figure 3A), significant stenosis were significantly increased (total: 25.5% vs 30.3% vs 39.6% vs 40.2%, $P < 0.001$; women: 16.9% vs 29.2% vs 30.4% vs 33.1%, $P = 0.010$, Figure 3B), and severe stenosis were significantly increased (total: 12.9% vs 18.2% vs 21.9% vs 25.6%, $P = 0.001$; women: 8.1% vs 16.8% vs 17.4% vs 19.4%, $P = 0.032$, Figure 3C).

The incidence of double-vessel lesions was only significantly increased with UA quartiles in women (9.6% vs 13.1% vs 14.5% vs 23.0%, $P = 0.017$, Figure 3E). In total and in women, the proportion of triple-vessel/left main artery lesions were highest in the fourth quartile (total: 15.8% vs 19.3% vs 26.5% vs 28.8%, $P < 0.001$; women: 13.2% vs 16.8% vs 24.6% vs 25.2%, $P = 0.027$, Figure 3F).

The proportion of a CACS of 0 in total, in men, and in women were lowest in the fourth quartile (total: 64.4% vs 59.1% vs 49.1% vs 46.6%, $P < 0.001$; men: 55.7%

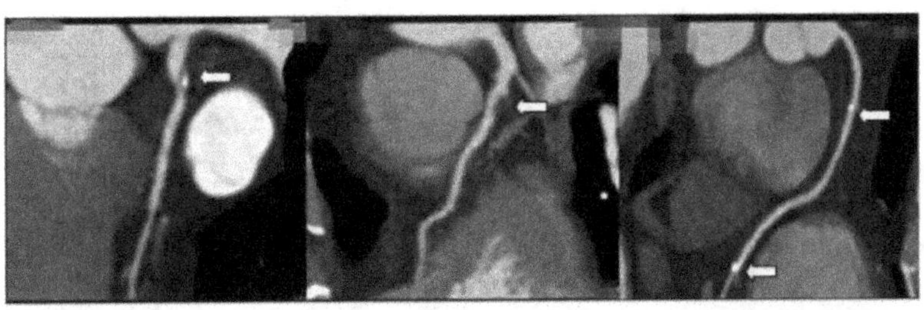

Figure 2 Showed the representative view of mixed, non-calcified plaque.

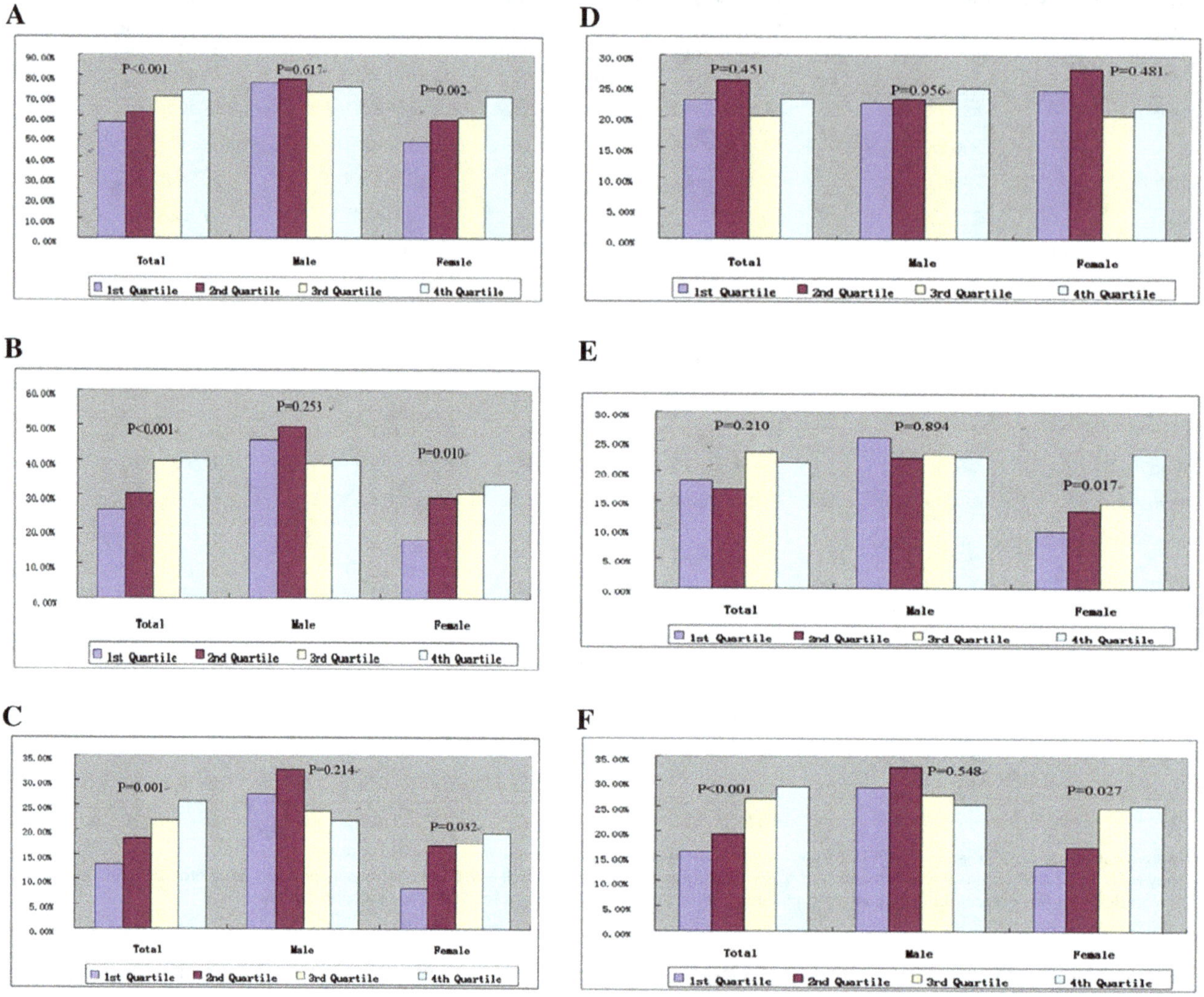

Figure 3 Relationship with anyplaque (A), significant stenosis (B) and severe stenosis (C), single vessel lesion (D), double vessel lesion (E) and triple vessel/left main artery lesion (F) across quartile of serum uric acid levels across quartile of serum uric acid levels.

vs 46.4% vs 41.0% vs 35.9%, $P = 0.006$; women: 75.7% vs 72.3% vs 60.9% vs 51.8%, $P < 0.001$, Figure 4A). The increasing quartiles of UA were significantly associated with a CACS >10 in total (30.6% vs 32.5% vs 41.7% vs 44.5%, $P = 0.001$) and in women (22.1% vs 24.1% vs 31.2% vs 41.0%, $p = 0.002$, Figure 4B.). As UA levels increased in women, the proportion of mixed plaques significantly increased (21.7% vs 22.7% vs 24.5% vs 30.5%, $P = 0.022$, Figure 5C).

Univariate and multivariate logistic regression models

In multivariate analysis for men and women combined, age, male sex, smoking, hypertension, and diabetes mellitus (DM) were significantly associated with significant stenosis, multivessel disease, and a high CACS (all $p < 0.001$). HDL-C level was only significantly associated with significant stenosis and multivessel disease (both $P \leq 0.002$). UA was the strongest predictor for significant stenosis, multivessel disease, and a high CACS in univariate analysis (all $P < 0.001$), but this association was not apparent after adjustment (Table 2).

The same analyses were performed for men and women (Tables 3 and 4). For men, significant predictors of significant stenosis were age, hypertension, and HDL-C levels after adjustment (all $p < 0.05$). Significant predictors of multivessel disease were age and hypertension after adjustment (both $P < 0.05$). The strongest risk factors for a high CACS were age and hypertension after adjustment (both $P < 0.05$, Table 3). For women, significant predictors of stenosis were age, hypertension, DM, and UA after adjustment (all $P < 0.05$). Significant predictors of multivessel disease were age, hypertension, DM, and UA after adjustment (all $P < 0.05$). The strongest risk factors for a high CACS were age, hypertension,

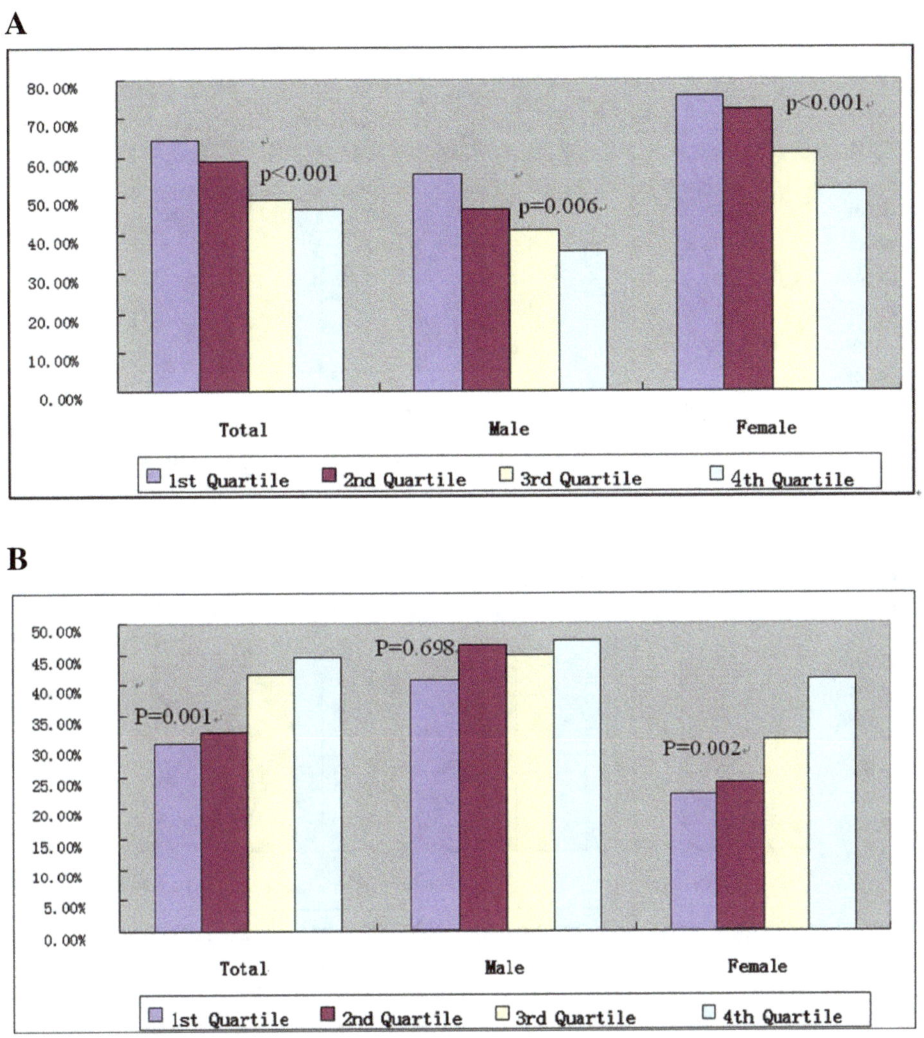

Figure 4 Prevalence of coronary artery calcium score = 0 across quartile of serum uric acid levels (A), prevalence of coronary artery calcium score >10 across quartile of serum uric acid levels (B).

DM, and HDL-C levels after adjustment (all $P < 0.05$, Table 4).

In total, significant predictors of significant stenosis were age, male sex, smoking, hypertension, and DM after adjustment (all $P < 0.05$). Significant predictors of non-calcified plaques were age, smoking, hypertension, DM, and HDL-C levels after adjustment (all $P < 0.05$). After adjustment, the strongest risk factors for mixed plaques were age, male sex, smoking, hypertension, DM, and UA (all $P < 0.05$, Table 5). For men, significant predictors of calcified plaques were age, hypertension, DM, and HDL-C after adjustment (all $P < 0.05$). The strongest risk factors for non-calcified plaques were age, smoking, DM, and HDL-C in univariate and multivariate analysis (all $P < 0.05$). The strongest risk factors for a high CACS were age, smoking, and HDL-C levels after adjustment (all $P < 0.05$, Table 6). For women, significant predictors of calcified plaques were age, hypertension, and DM after adjustment (all $P < 0.05$). Significant predictors of non-calcified plaques were age, hypertension, and HDL-C after adjustment (all $P < 0.05$). Age, hypertension, DM, and UA were significantly associated with mixed plaques in univariate and multivariate analysis (all $P < 0.05$, Table 7).

Discussion

In this study of individuals with suspected CAD using 256-detector-row CCTA, we analysed the association of UA with coronary atherosclerosis. We found the following findings. 1) Overall and in women, the prevalence of coronary atherosclerosis, severe stenosis, and triple-vessel/ left main artery lesions of plaques were significantly increased with increasing quartiles of UA. UA was significantly associated with double-vessel lesions in women. 2)

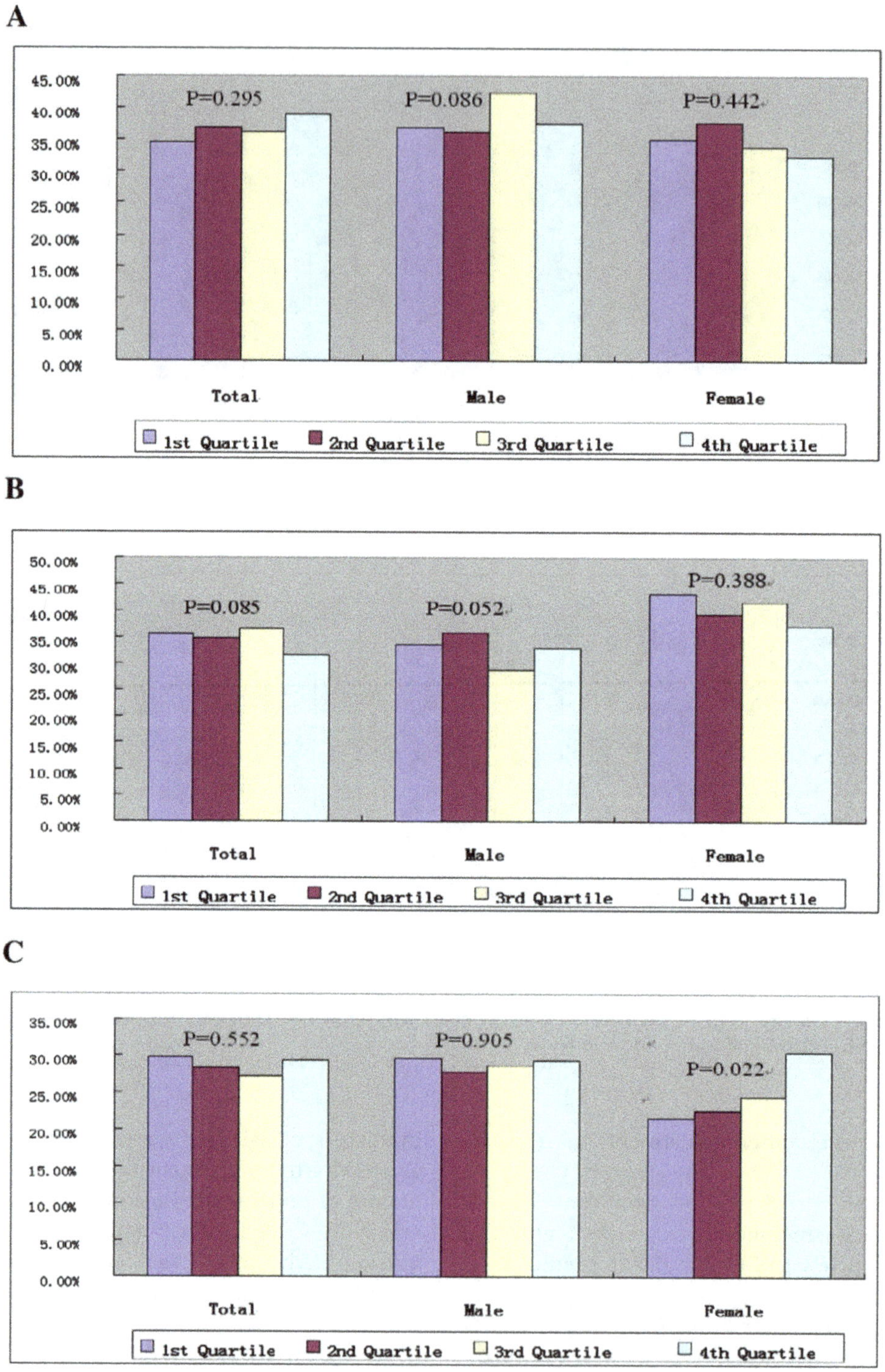

Figure 5 Relationship with (A) calcified, noncalcified (B) and mixed (C) across quartile of serum uric acid levels.

UA was significantly negatively correlated with the proportion of a CACS of 0, but was positively correlated with the proportion of a CACS >10 overall and in women. The incidence of mixed plaques was significantly increased only in women with elevated UA levels. 3) After adjustment, only UA was a significant predictor of significant stenosis, multivessel disease, and mixed plaques in women. UA was not significantly associated with coronary atherosclerosis in men.

Coronary artery angiography (CAG) is the gold standard for diagnosing CAD, but CAG cannot determine the characteristics of plaques. CAG would be difficult to use

Table 2 Univariate and multivariate logistic regression models for variables of total population associated with coronary artery lesions and high CACS (n = 1116)

V variable	Significant stenosis (>50%)				Multivessel disease				High CACS (CACS > 100)			
	Univariate		Multivariate		Univariate		Multivariate		Univariate		Multivariate	
Variable	OR (95%CI)	P	OR (95%CI)	P	OR (95%CI)	P	OR (95%CI)	P	OR (95%CI)	P	OR (95%CI)	P
Age	1.059 (1.046-1.073)	<0.001	1.070 (1.054-1.086)	<0.001	1.066 (1.052-1.081)	<0.001	1.079 (1.062-1.096)	<0. 001	1.078 (1.061-1.095)	<0.001	1.089 (1.070-1.108)	<0.001
Male	2.364 (1.830-3.054)	<0.001	2.208 (1.579-3.089)	<0.001	2.365 (1.815-3.083)	<0.001	2.320 (1.637-3.288)	<0.001	2.244 (1.653-3.047)	<0.001	2.190 (1.486-3.226)	<0.001
BMI	1.028 (0.997-1.060)	0.082	1.010 (0.975-1.047)	0.568	1.027 (0.996-1.060)	0.092	1.010. (0.974-1.047)	0.597	1.017 (0.982-1.052)	0.345	—	—
Smoking	1.789 (1.355-2.364)	<0.001	1.835 (1.306-2.578)	<0.001	1.739 (1.308-2.310)	<0.001	1.866 (1.313-2.653)	0.001	1.854 (1.352-2.542)	<0.001	2.294 (1.550-3.395)	<0.001
Family history of CAD	1.076 (0.690-1.678)	0.746	—	—	1.105 (0.701-1.742)	0.666	—	—	1.012 (0.598-1.714)	0.964	—	—
Hypertension	2.187 (1.700-2.815)	<0.001	1.856 (1.394-2.471)	<0.001	2.275 (1.754-2.950)	<0.001	1.914 (1.421-2.577)	<0.001	2.377 (1.764-3.203)	<0.001	1.939 (1.388-2.709)	<0.001
DM	2.467 (1.788-3.403)	<0.001	1.825 (1.278-2.604)	<0.001	2.823 (2.041-3.905)	<0.001	2.153 (1.501-3.089)	<0.001	2.403 (1.694-3.408)	<0.001	1.983 (1.344-2.927)	0.001
LDL-C	0.876 (0.758-1.012)	0.072	1.156 (0.812-1.645)	0.421	0.913 (0.787-1.059)	0.228	—	—	1.061 (0.900-1.251)	0.482	—	—
HDL-C	0.331 (0.202-0.477)	<0.001	0.456 (0.276-0.755)	0.002	0.311 (0.202-0.477)	<0.001	0.428 (0.256-0.717)	0.001	0.632 (0.396-1.008)	0.054	0.907 (0.559-1.471)	0.691
TC	1.802 (1.724-1.929)	0.002	0.875 (0.641-1.194)	0.399	1.845 (1.744-1.959)	0.009	1.022 (0.885-1.181)	0.765	0.943 (0.819-1.086)	0.415		
TG	0.983 (0.895-1.081)	0.726	—	—	0.992 (0.901-1.092)	0.863	—	—	0.889 (0.771-1.024)	0.145	—	—
UA	1.003 (1.002-1.004)	<0.001	1.001 (0.999-1.002)	0.535	1.003 (1.002-1.004)	<0.001	1.001 (0.999-1.002)	0.564	1.003 (1.001-1.005)	<0.001	1.001 (0.999-1.003)	0.205
Creatinine	0.980 (0.857-1.018)	0.120	—	—	1.240 (0.957-1.417)	0.258	—	—	0.760 (0.526-1.013)	0.173	—	—

Multivessel disease was defined as the present of stenosis of more than 50% in at lease two vessels.
Risk factors with $p < 0.10$ in unvariate adjusted simultaneously. Blanks indicate variables not adjusted in multivariate analyses.

Table 3 Univariate and multivariate logistic regression models for variables of male associated with coronary artery lesions and high CACS (n = 566)

V variable	Significant stenosis (>50%)				Multivessel disease				High CACS (CACS > 100)			
	Univariate		Multivariate		Univariate		Multivariate		Univariate		Multivariate	
Variable	**OR (95%CI)**	**P**	**OR (95%CI)**	**P**	**OR (95%CI)**	**P**	**OR (95%CI)**	**P**	**OR (95%CI)**	**P**	**OR(95%CI)**	**P**
Age	1.056 (1.039-1.073)	<0.001	1.052 (1.034-1.070)	<0.001	1.060 (1.043-1.077)	<0.001	1.055 (1.037-1.073)	<0.001	1.077 (1.057-1.098)	<0.001	1.071 (1.050-1.093)	<0.001
BMI	0.978 (0.937)1.020	0.296	—	—	0.979 (0.938-1.022)	0.329	—	—	0.955 (0.906-1.006)	0.084	0.996 (0.945-1.051)	0.894
Smoking	1.245 (0.889-1.743)	0.203	—	—	1.298 (0.926-1.820)	0.131	—	—	1.305 (0.896-1.900)	0.166	—	—
Family history of CAD	1.274 (0.684-2.375)	0.446	—	—	1.501 (0.805-2.798)	0.201	—	—	1.080 (0.539-2.162)	0.828	—	—
Hypertension	1.811 (1.291-2.541)	0.001	1.579 (1.098-2.270)	0.014	1.734 (1.235-2.434)	0.001	1.462 (1.016-2.104)	0.041	2.044 (1.400-2.983)	<0.001	1.731 (1.138-2.634)	0.010
DM	1.608 (1.045-2.473)	0.031	1.368 (0.862-2.172)	0.184	1.727 (1.123-2.658)	0.013	1.579 (0.998-2.499)	0.051	1.585 (1.001-2.511)	0.049	1.581 (0.952-2.624)	0.077
LDL-C	0.856 (0.694-1.054)	0.143	—	—	0.919 (0.746-1.133)	0.430	—	—	0.986 (0.782-1.243)	0.902	—	—
HDL-C	0.575 (0.317-1.044)	0.069	0.485 (0.236-0.995)	0.048	0.635 (0.350-1.152)	0.135	—	—	0.435 (0.072-0.797)	0.030	1.676 (0.813-3.453)	0.162
TC	1.764 (1.641)1.911	0.003	0.880 (0.712-1.088)	0.239	1.817 (1.688-1.971)	0.022	0.875 (0.721-1.062)	0.176	0.891 (0.738-1.075)	0.229	—	—
TG	1.868 (1.759-1.994)	0.041	0.939 (0.797-1.106)	0.451	0.874 (0.763-1.001)	0.051	0.998 (0.864-1.152)	0.973	1.754 (1.616-1.924)	0.006	0.926 (0.754-1.137)	0.464
UA	1.000 (0.998-1.002)	0.923	—	—	1.000 (0.998-1.002)	0.716	—	—	1.000 (0.998-1.002)	0.960	—	—
Creatinine	1.403 (0.549-3.073)	0.613	—	—	0.923 (0.238-1.997)	0.588	—	—	0.574 (0.185-1.236)	0.339	—	—

Multivessel disease was defined as the present of stenosis of more than 50% in at lease two vessels.
Risk factors with $p < 0.10$ in unvariate adjusted simultaneously. Blanks indicate variables not adjusted in multivariate analyses.

Table 4 Univariate and multivariate logistic regression models for variables of female associated with coronary artery lesions and high CACS (n = 550)

V variable	Significant stenosis (>50%)				Multivessel disease				High CACS (CACS > 100)			
	Univariate		Multivariate		Univariate		Multivariate		Univariate		Multivariate	
Variable	OR (95%CI)	P	OR (95%CI)	P	OR (95%CI)	P	OR (95%CI)	P	OR (95%CI)	P	OR (95%CI)	P
Age	1.096 (1.069-1.123)	<0.001	1.084 (1.055-1.113)	<0.001	1.092 (1.068-1.117)	<0.001	1.075 (1.049-1.101)	<0.001	1.100 (1.068-1.133)	<0.001	1.085 (1.049-1.122)	<0.001
BMI	1.071 (1.013-1.132)	0.015	1.024 (0.985-1.103)	0.151	1.073 (1.018-1.132)	0.009	1.036 (0.980-1.095)	0.216	1.077 (1.012-1.147)	0.020	1.060 (0.998-1.126)	0.060
Smoking	1.434 (0.723-2.845)	0.303	—	—	1.317 (0.692-2.504)	0.402	—	—	1.795 (0.822-3.918)	0.142	—	—
Family history of CAD	0.978 (0.496-1.932)	0.950	—	—	0.716 (0.376-1.363)	0.309	—	—	1.017 (0.440-2.351)	0.969	—	—
Hypertension	3.144 (2.096-4.718)	<0.001	2.229 (1.420-3.500)	<0.001	3.689 (2.550-5.336)	<0.001	2.618 (1.735-3.950)	<0.001	3.385 (2.017-5.680)	<0.001	2.162 (1.216-3.843)	0.009
DM	4.144 (2.536-6.772)	<0.001	2.669 (1.554-4.584)	<0.001	4.301 (2.620-7.061)	<0.001	2.913 (1.682-5.044)	<0.001	4.286 (2.476-7.418)	<0.001	2.958 (1.582-5.531)	0.001
LDL-C	1.049 (0.851-1.293)	0.652	—	—	1.044 (0.863-1.263)	0.654	—	—	1.381 (1.078-1.769)	0.011	2.090 (0.868-5.036)	0.100
HDL-C	0.309 (0.158-0.602)	<0.001	0.462 (0.219-0.977)	0.430	0.344 (0.192-0.618)	<0.001	0.642 (0.336-1.227)	0.180	0.265 (0.112-0.629)	0.003	0.327 (0.118-0.908)	0.032
TC	1.056 (0.878-1.271)	0.561	—	—	1.054 (0.890-1.247)	0.544	—	—	1.236 (0.991-1.541)	0.060	0.776 (0.346-1.741)	0.776
TG	1.190 (0.994-1.424)	0.058	1.043 (0.852-1.276)	0.684	1.338 (1.103-1.623)	0.003	1.131 (0.913-1.401)	0.259	1.094 (0.897-1.334)	0.374	—	—
UA	1.214 (1.101-1.407)	0.002	1.004 (1.001-1.007)	0.011	1.115 (1.103-1.134)	<0.001	11.131(0.913-1.401) 1.003(1.000-1.006)	<0.001	1.005 (1.001-1.008)	0.004	1.001 (0.997-1.004)	0.793
Creatinine	1.835 (0.511-3.164)	0.535	—	—	0.714 (0.138-2.227)	0.407	—	—	0.925 (0.238-2.764)	0.868	—	—

Multivessel disease was defined as the present of stenosis of more than 50% in at lease two vessels.
Risk factors with $p < 0.10$ in unvariate adjusted simultaneously. Blanks indicate variables not adjusted in multivariate analyses.

Table 5 Univariate and multivariate logistic regression models for variables of total population associated with calcified, non-calcified and mixed plaque (n = 1116)

V variable	Calcified plaque				Non-calcified plaque				Mixed plaque			
	Univariate		Multivariate		Univariate		Multivariate		Univariate		Multivariate	
Variable	OR (95%CI)	P	OR (95%CI)	P	OR (95%CI)	P	OR (95%CI)	P	OR (95%CI)	P	OR (95%CI)	P
Age	1.071 (1.057-1.086)	<0.001	1.052 (1.023-1.081)	<0.001	1.028 (1.016-1.040)	<0.001	1.034 (1.021-1.047)	<0.001	1.056 (1.042-1.069)	<0.001	1.066 (1.051-1.081)	<0.001
Male	2.022 (1.579-2.590)	<0.001	2.282 (1.662-3.132)	<0.001	1.666 (1.315-2.111)	<0.001	1.249 (0.925-1.686)	<0.147	2.328 (1.806-3.000)	<0.001	2.002 (1.445-2.774)	<0.001
BMI	1.017 (0.987-1.048)	0.276	———	———	1.045 (1.012-1.080)	0.008	1.023 (0.988-1.058)	0.202	1.021 (0.991-1.053)	0.173	———	———
Smoking	1.428 (1.084-1.881)	0.011	1.224 (1.036-1.467)	0.043	1.707 (1.297-2.246)	<0.001	1.729 (1.258-2.376)	0.001	2.171 (1.645-2.864)	<0.001	2.336 (1.669-3.270)	<0.001
Family history of CAD	0.825 (0.527-1.293)	0.402	———	———	1.183 (0.773-1.810)	0.438	———	———	1.022 (0.655-1.592)	0.925	———	———
Hypertension	2.180 (1.703-2.792)	<0.001	1.832 (1.393-2.409)	<0.001	1.579 (1.244-2.005)	<0.001	1.319 (1.017-1.711)	0.037	2.090 (1.627-2.683)	<0.001	1.810 (1.367-2.395)	<0.001
DM	2.538 (1.839-3.503)	<0.001	2.065 (1.524-2.265)	<0.001	1.924 (1.390-2.665)	<0.001	1.510 (1.070-2.130)	0.019	2.386 (1.731-3.291)	<0.001	1.917 (1.346-2.730)	<0.001
LDL-C	1.669 (0.930-1.227)	0.348	———	———	0.945 (0.826-1.082)	0.945	———	———	0.981 (0.852-1.129)	0.786	———	———
HDL-C	0.851 (0.601-1.206)	0.365	———	———	0.347 (0.235-0.512)	<0.001	0.493 (0.322-0.757)	0.001	0.504 (0.338-0.752)	0.001	0.763 (0.501-1.164)	0.210
TC	1.009 (0.899-1.132)	0.878	———	———	0.930 (0.831-1.041)	0.208	———	———	0.905 (0.803-1.020)	0.103	———	———
TG	0.998 (0.912-1.093)	0.969	———	———	1.113 (1.009-1.228)	0.033	1.032 (0.933-1.140)	0.542	1.044 (0.954-1.141)	0.348	———	———
UA	1.003 (1.001-1.004)	<0.001	1.002 (0.998-1.003)	0.244	1.003 (1.002-1.004)	<0.001	1.001 (0.999-1.002)	0.113	1.004 (1.002-1.005)	<0.001	1.002 (1.001-1.003)	0.046
Creatinine	1..020 (1.005-1.036)	0.005	0.823 (0.422-1.329)	0.201	1.033 (0.894-1.086)	0.165	———	———	1.157 (0.811-1.425)	0.148	———	———

Risk factors with $p < 0.10$ in unvariate adjusted simultaneously. Blanks indicate variables not adjusted in multivariate analyses.

Table 6 Univariate and multivariate logistic regression models for variables of male associated with calcified, non-calcified and mixed plaque (n = 566)

V variable	Calcified plaque				Non-calcified plaque				Mixed plaque			
	Univariate		Multivariate		Univariate		Multivariate		Univariate		Multivariate	
Variable	OR (95%CI)	P	OR (95%CI)	P	OR (95%CI)	P	OR (95%CI)	P	OR (95%CI)	P	OR (95%CI)	P
Age	1.069 (1.051-1.088)	<0.001	1.068 (1.049-1.087)	<0.001	1.018 (1.003-1.033)	0.016	1.024 (1.008-1.040)	0.003	1.048 (1.032-1.064)	<0.001	1.056 (1.038-1.075)	<0.001
BMI	0.979 (0.939-1.021)	0.315	———	———	1.009 (0.969-1.051)	0.664	———	———	0.986 (0.946-1.027)	0.500	———	———
Smoking	1.041 (0.745-1.456)	0.812	———	———	1.484 (1.058-2.082)	0.022	1.709 (1.194-2.447)	0.003	1.597 (1.140-2.237)	0.007	2.258 (1.548-3.294)	<0.001
Family history of CAD	0.771 (0.409-1.455)	0.422	———	———	1.409 (0.742-2.678)	0.295	———	———	1.488 (0.797-2.776)	0.212	———	———
Hypertension	1.745 (1.246-2.445)	0.001	1.522 (1.051-2.204)	0.026	1.291 (0.922-1.808)	0.137	———	———	1.533 (1.095-2.146)	0.013	1.411 (0.978-2.036)	0.066
DM	1.672 (1.086-2.575)	0.020	1.646 (1.027-2.637)	0.038	1.902 (1.209-2.991)	0.005	1.660 (1.043-2.642)	0.033	1.763 (1.144-2.716)	0.010	1.501 (0.942-2.393)	0.088
LDL-C	1.167 (0.948-1.436)	0.145	———	———	0.932 (0.757-1.146)	0.503	———	———	0.954 (0.775-1.173)	0.655	———	———
HDL-C	0.219 (0.094-0.344)	0.007	0.358 (0.169-0.547)	0.016	0.489 (0.271-0.882)	0.018	0.455 (0.248-0.832)	0.011	0.478 (0.261-0.874)	0.017	0.387 (0.200-0.749)	0.005
TC	1.058 (0.900-1.244)	0.496	———	———	0.970 (0.825-1.141)	0.717	———	———	0.851 (0.719-1.006)	0.059	0.946 (0.785-1.140)	0.561
TG	0.893 (0.787-1.013)	0.080	1.046 (0.925-1.182)	0.476	1.092 (0.967-1.233)	0.158	———	———	0.990 (0.890-1.102)	0.855	———	———
UA	0.999 (0.998-1.001)	0.601	———	———	1.001 (0.999-1.003)	0.232	———	———	1.001 (0.999-1.003)	0.498	———	———
Creatinine	1.061 (0.777-1.321)	0.543	———	———	1.980 (0.860-4.522)	0.126	———	———	0.631 (0.483-1.376)	0.194	———	———

Risk factors with $p < 0.10$ in unvariate adjusted simultaneously. Blanks indicate variables not adjusted in multivariate analyses.

Table 7 Univariate and multivariate logistic regression models for variables of female associated with calcified, non-calcified and mixed plaque (n = 550)

V variable	Calcified plaque				Non-calcified plaque				Mixed plaque			
	Univariate		Multivariate		Univariate		Multivariate		Univariate		Multivariate	
Variable	**OR (95%CI)**	**P**	**OR (95%CI)**	**P**	**OR (95%CI)**	**P**	**OR (95%CI)**	**P**	**OR (95%CI)**	**P**	**OR (95%CI)**	**P**
Age	1.101 (1.075-1.127)	<0.001	1.083 (1.056-1.111)	<0.001	1.057 (1.036-1.078)	<0.001	1.048 (1.026-1.070)	<0.001	1.101 (1.074-1.128)	<0.001	1.086 (1.058-1.115)	<0.001
BMI	1.041 (0.991-1.093)	0.110	—	—	1.073 (1.018-1.131)	0.008	1.047 (0.992-1.106)	0.098	1.038 (0.987-1.090)	0.145	—	—
Smoking	1.101 (0.557-2.177)	0.782	—	—	1.259 (0.670-2.366)	0.474	—	—	1.702 (0.877-3.302)	0.116	—	—
Family history of CAD	0.943 (0.494-1.800)	0.859	—	—	1.076 (0.599-1.933)	0.806	—	—	0.712 (0.346-1.464)	0.355	—	—
Hypertension	3.078 (2.101-4.508)	<0.001	2.216 (1.453-3.380)	<0.001	1.991 (1.411-2.810)	<0.001	1.506 (1.037-2. 188)	0.032	3.503 (2.340-5.244)	<0.001	2.720 (1.759-4.206)	<0.001
DM	4.093 (2.513-6.665)	<0.001	2.845 (1.666-4.858)	<0.001	1.868 (1.161-3.006)	0.010	1.287 (0.772-2.146)	0.333	3.383 (2.076-5.513)	<0.001	2.192 (1.281-3.750)	0.004
LDL-C	1.132 (0.930-1.379)	0.216	—	—	1.046 (0.870-1.257)	0.633	—	—	1.186 (0.967-1.455)	0.101	—	—
HDL-C	0.693 (0.404-1.188)	0.182	—	—	0.358 (0.206-0.622)	<0.001	0.486 (0.272-0.870)	0.015	0.965 (0.596-1.561)	0.884	—	—
TC	1.104 (0.926-1.315)	0.270	—	—	0.982 (0.834-1.156)	0.824	—	—	1.157 (0.965-1.388)	0.115	—	—
TG	1.202 (1.005-1.438)	0.044	1.111 (0.919-1.343)	0.277	1.111 (0.941-1.312)	0.215	—	—	1.112 (0.937-1.320)	0.224	—	—
UA	1.004 (1.002-1.007)	0.001	1.001 (0.998-1.434)	0.393	1.004 (1.001-1.006)	0.002	1.001 (0.998-1.004)	0.500	1.004 (1.002-1.007)	0.001	1.003 (0.001-1.006)	0.015
Creatinine	1.119 (0.866-1.288)	0.274	—	—	1.026 (0.687-1.537)	0.253	—	—	0.498 (0.173-2.051)	0.341	—	—

Risk factors with $p < 0.10$ in unvariate adjusted simultaneously. Blanks indicate variables not adjusted in multivariate analyses.

as a general screening tool in China because of its highly invasive nature, radiation exposure, and cost. The technique of 256-detector-row CCTA with a shorter scanning time can improve image quality and it has a minimal radiation dose [18]. Use of CCTA in a general routine health evaluation is not discouraged [19]. Therefore, healthy subjects were not included in our study. We enrolled those patients with suspected CAD who needed to have a CCTA examination while undergoing a clinician's assessment. CCTA is a screening tool for assessing individuals of suspected CAD, and is the most feasible and effective method to reflect widespread epidemiology and characteristics of early CAD in China.

Many studies have assessed the association of UA with CAD and clinical outcome, but the results were still controversial. Kocaman et al. found that UA was an independent predictor of CAD in individuals undergoing CAG [20]. However, the Framingham studies showed that UA was not an independent predictor of CAD and cardiovascular outcomes [21], and similar results were found in the ARIC study [22] and a study by Strask et al. [23]. Carotid intima-media thickness (C-IMT) measured by ultrasonography is widely used as a surrogate marker for atherosclerotic disease and directly associated with increased risk of cardiovascular disease. The higher UA levels were associated with higher C-IMT independent from hypertension, UA levels were independently associated with C-IMT [24,25]. But a study shown UA was not significantly associated with C-IMT, UA was associated with Internal carotid artery resistive index in hypertensive women, suggesting that there might gender-related differences in the relationship between UA and vascular damage [26]. In our study, although the prevalence and degree of plaques were significantly increased with UA overall, UA was not a significant independent predictor. Several studies have shown conflicting results on the association between UA and CAD in men and women. Some studies have demonstrated that UA was an independent risk factor for CAD in both sexes [13,14]. A high UA level was found to be an independent predictor for cardiovascular mortality in men [27]. In the LIFE study, the significant association of UA with CAD was found only in women [12]. Cardiovascular death was increased by 1.77 times in men and 3.0 times in women in the upper UA quartile in the NHANES I study [28]. A previous study reported that UA levels only in women were associated with CAD [29]. Our study supported the opinion that UA was an independent predictor for the prevalence and severity of early CAD only in women.

Previous reports have proven the highly predictive value of the CACS on cardiovascular outcomes [30,31]. Some studies have shown a significant relationship between UA and the CACS [32-34], and a recent study showed that UA was an independent factor predictive of the CACS [34]. However, some studies did not support these previous findings [7,35]. In our study, we found that UA was significantly associated with the CACS, but UA was not an independent risk factor for a high CACS overall, in men and women. The relationship between UA and CACS, and the concrete mechanisms are still unclear. Few studies have focused on the role of UA in characterization of plaques as shown by CCTA. One study showed that UA was only significantly associated with calcified plaques [36]. In our study, only UA was an independent predictor for mixed plaques overall and in women. The relationship between UA and mixed plaques was likely caused by the female subgroup. Many studies have indicated that mixed plaques might be the biggest risk of plaque rupture, causing acute coronary events [37,38]. This may be a rational explanation for why high UA level was associated with an increase in the prevalence of mixed plaques in women, which causes an increase in the incidence of adverse cardiovascular outcomes. However, there are too few studies on the relationship between UA and plaque characteristics, and further studies are required.

UA is a general antioxidant in the body, and a high UA level is suggestive of oxidative stress, endothelial dysfunction, and slow coronary artery flow [39,40]. UA promotes vascular smooth muscle proliferation, and upregulates the expression of monocyte chemoattractant protein-1 and platelet-derived growth factor [41]. Endothelial dysfunction is an important step in the development of atherosclerosis. A recent study showed a relationship between UA and endothelial dysfunction of coronary microvasculature only in women [42], which may be a possible explanation for the significant association between UA and CAD in women. The underlying mechanisms behind the significant relationship between UA and CAD in women but not men remain enigmatic. Our study suggests that UA plays an important role in coronary atherosclerosis in women.

The incidence of cardiovascular events is still high after controlling for traditional risk factors. Our study suggests that UA should be considered as an additional risk factor beyond traditional factors for CAD in women. However, a randomized study still needs to be performed to determine the effect of UA-lowering therapies on cardiovascular prevention. In the GREACE study, decreased UA levels by atorvastatin were independently correlated with a reduced risk of cardiovascular outcomes [43]. The LIFE study showed an association between UA and cardiovascular events in hypertensive women, the unique results may be due in part to the specific feature of reduction of UA by losartan, but it did not mean that the beneficial effects observed with losartan were contributed to decreasing UA levels [12]. The relationship between low UA level and cardiovascular benefits is still uncertain. Therefore, further research should be performed to assess the direct relationship between decreasing UA level and cardiovascular benefits.

There were several limitations to our study. All individuals were suspected of having CAD, we mainly want to explore the relationship between UA and early CAD in the study. Patients with known CAD may implement lifestyle modifications and drugs intervention to some extent, the real relationship between UA and CAD may be influenced by those confounding factors, So, we exclude the patients who had known CAD. There was a possible selection bias and this could restrict generalizability of our results to similar care settings. Unmeasured confounders may have affected our results. In our study, almost 90% of women were post-menopausal and few women received oestrogen-replacement therapy. Therefore, we did not analyse the potential effects of oestrogen on the relationship between UA and CAD. In cross-sectional analysis, we did not find a longitudinal relationship between UA and cardiovascular outcomes. In spite of these limitations, the strong association of UA with early CAD in women had an important clinical significance in prevention and treatment of CAD. Longitudinal studies are required to confirm the association of UA with CAD and cardiovascular outcome.

Conclusion

UA is a significant predictor of significant stenosis, multivessel disease, and mixed plaques in women. Importantly, our study suggests that UA level may play an important role in the occurrence and development of coronary atherosclerosis in women but not men.

Abbreviations

UA: Uric acid; CAD: Coronary artery disease; CCTA: Coronary computed tomography angiography; CACS: Calcium score; BMI: Body mass index; TC: Total cholesterol; TG: Triglyceride; HDL-C: High-density lipoprotein cholesterol; LDL-C: Low-density lipoprotein cholesterol; CAG: Coronary artery angiography.

Competing interests

The authors declare that they have no competing interest.

Authors' contribution

SYJ participated in the design of the study, collected and organized datas, analysed images, performed the statistical analysis and drafted the manuscript. YX collected, organized and analysed datas. ZY, GS and LH collected and organized datas. LT and XK analysed images. CL and WCW collected datas. QGX conceived of the study, and participated in its design and coordination and helped to draft the manuscript. All authors read and approved the final manuscript.

Acknowledgements

We acknowledge Professor Qi Guoxian who contributed towards the article by making substantial contributions to conception, design, drafting the manuscript and revising it critically for important intellectual content.

Author details

[1]Department of Cardiology of Aging, Department of Cardiology, The First Affiliated Hospital of China Medical University, NO.155 Nanjing North Street, Heping Ward, Shenyang 110001, China. [2]Department of Radiology, The First Affiliated Hospital of China Medical University, Shenyang, China.

References

1. Saugstad OD: **Role of xanthine oxidase and its inhibitor in hypoxia: reoxygenation injury.** *Pediatrics* 1996, **98**:103–107.
2. Lee J, Sparrow D, Vokonas PS, Landsberg L, Weiss ST: **Uric acid and coronary heart disease risk: evidence for a role of uric acid in the obesity-insulin resistance syndrome: the normative aging study.** *Am J Epidemiol* 1995, **142**:288–294.
3. Puig JG, Michán AD, Jiménez ML, Pérez De Ayala C, Mateos FA, Capitán CF, De Miguel E, Gijón JB: **Female gout: clinical spectrum and uric acid metabolism.** *Arch Intern Med* 1991, **151**:726–732.
4. Puig JG, Ruilope LM: **Uric acid as a cardiovascular risk factor in arterial hypertension.** *J Hypertens* 1999, **17**:869–872.
5. Chu NF, Wang DJ, Liou SH, Shieh SM: **Relationship between hyperuricemia and other cardiovascular disease risk factors among adult males in Taiwan.** *Eur J Epidemiol* 2000, **16**:13–17.
6. Kim SY, Guevara JP, Kim KM, Choi HK, Heitjan DF, Albert DA: **Hyperuricemia and coronary heart disease: a systematic review and meta-analysis.** *Arthritis Care Res (Hoboken)* 2010, **62**:170–180.
7. Yildiz A, Kaya Z: **A crucial marker of cardiovascular diseases?** *Int J Cardiol* 2012, **159**:158.
8. Culleton BF, Larson MG, Kannel WB, Levy D: **Serum uric acid and risk for cardiovascular disease and death: the Framingham heart study.** *Ann Intern Med* 1999, **131**:7–13.
9. Dutta A, Henley W, Pilling LC, Wallace RB, Melzer D: **Uric acid measurement improves prediction of cardiovascular mortality in later life.** *J Am Geriatr Soc* 2013, **61**:319–326.
10. Niskanen LK, Laaksonen DE, Nyyssonen K, Alfthan G, Lakka HM, Lakka TA: **Uric acid level as a risk factor for cardiovascular and all-cause mortality in middle-aged men: a prospective cohort study.** *Arch Intern Med* 2004, **164**:1546–1551.
11. Davies KJ, Sevanian A, Muakkassah-Kelly SF, Hochstein P: **Uric acid-iron ion complexes. A new aspect of the antioxidant functions of uric acid.** *Biochem J* 1986, **235**:747–754.
12. Hoieggen A, Alderman MH, Kjeldsen SE, Julius S, Devereux RB, De Faire U, Fyhrquist F, Ibsen H, Kristianson K, Lederballe-Pedersen O, Lindholm LH, Nieminen MS, Omvik P, Oparil S, Wedel H, Chen C, Dahlöf B, LIFE Study Group: **LIFE study group. The impact of serum uric acid on cardiovascular outcomes in the LIFE study.** *Kidney Int* 2004, **65**:1041–1049.
13. Ndrepepa G, Braun S, King L, Fusaro M, Tada T, Cassese S, Hadamitzky M, Haase HU, Schömig A, Kastrati A: **Uric acid and prognosis in angiography-proven coronary artery disease.** *Eur J Clin Invest* 2013, **43**:256–266.
14. Sinan Deveci O, Kabakci G, Okutucu S, Tulumen E, Aksoy H, Baris Kaya E, Evranos B, Aytemir K, Tokgozoglu L, Oto A: **The association between serum uric acid level and coronary artery disease.** *Int J Clin Pract* 2010, **64**:900–907.
15. Agatston AS, Janowitz WR, Hildner FJ, Zusmer NR, Viamonte M Jr, Detrano R: **Quantification of coronary artery calcium using ultrafast computed tomography.** *J Am Coll Cardiol* 1990, **15**:827–832.
16. Austen WG, Edwards JE, Frye RL, Gensini GG, Gott VL, Griffith LS, McGoon DC, Murphy ML, Roe BB: **A reporting system on patients evaluated for coronary artery disease. Report of the *Ad Hoc* committee for grading of coronary artery disease, council on cardiovascular surgery. American heart association.** *Circulation* 1975, **51**(suppl):5–40.
17. Cheng VY, Wolak A, Gutstein A, Gransar H, Wong ND, Dey D, Thomson LE, Hayes SW, Friedman JD, Slomka PJ, Berman DS: **Low-density lipoprotein and noncalcified coronary plaque composition in patients with newly diagnosed coronary artery disease on computed tomographic angiography.** *Am J Cardiol* 2010, **105**:761–766.
18. Abada HT, Larchez C, Daoud B, Sigal-Cinqualbre A, Paul JF: **MDCT of the coronary arteries: feasibility of low-dose CT with ECG-pulsed tube**

current modulation to reduce radiation dose. *Am J Roentgenl* 2006, **186**:S387–S390.
19. Mark DB, Berman DS, Budoff MJ, Carr JJ, Gerber TC, Hecht HS, Hlatky MA, Hodgson JM, Lauer MS, Miller JM, Morin RL, Mukherjee D, Poon M, Rubin GD, Schwartz RS: **ACCF/ACR/AHA/NASCI/SAIP/SCAI/SCCT2010 expert consensus document on coronary computed tomographic angiography: a report of the American college of cardiology foundation task force on expert consensus documents.** *Circulation* 2010, **121**:2509–2543.
20. Kocaman SA, Sahinarslan A, Cemri M, Timurkaynak T, Boyaci B, Cengel A: **Independent relationship of serum uric acid levels with leukocytes and coronary atheroscleroticburden.** *Nutr Metab Cardiovasc Dis* 2009, **19**:729–735.
21. Ioachimescu AG, Brennan DM, Hoar BM, Hazen SL, Hoogwerf BJ: **Serum uric acid is an independent predictor of all-cause mortality in patients at high risk of cardiovascular disease: a preventive cardiology information system (PreCIS) database cohort study.** *Arthritis Rheum* 2008, **58**:623–630.
22. Moriarity JT, Folsom AR, Iribarren C, Nieto FJ, Rosamond WD: **Serum acid uric and risk of coronary heart disease: atherosclerosis risk in communities (ARIC) study.** *Ann Epidemiol* 2000, **10**:136–143.
23. Strasak A, Ruttmann E, Brant L, Kelleher C, Klenk J, Concin H, Diem G, Pfeiffer K, Ulmer H, VHM&PP Study Group: **Serum uric acid and risk of cardiovascular mortality: a prospective long-term study of 83,683 Austrian men.** *Clin Chem* 2008, **54**:273–284.
24. Tavil Y, Kaya MG, Oktar SO, Sen N, Okyay K, Yazici HU, Cengel A: **Uric acid level and its association with carotid intima-media thickness in patients with hypertension.** *Atherosclerosis* 2008, **197**:159–163.
25. Mutluay R, Deger SM, Bahadir E, Durmaz AO, Citil R, Sindel S: **Uric acid is an important predictor for hypertensive early atherosclerosis.** *Adv Ther* 2012, **29**:276–286.
26. Cipolli JA, Ferreira-Sae MC, Martins RP, Pio-Magalhães JA, Bellinazzi VR, Matos-Souza JR, Junior WN: **Relationship between serum uric acid and internal carotid resistive index in hypertensive women: a cross-sectional study.** *BMC Cardiovasc Disord* 2012, **12**:52.
27. Liese AD, Hense HW, Löwel H, Döring A, Tietze M, Keil U: **Association of serum uric acid with all-cause and cardiovascular disease mortality and inci-dent myocardial infarction in the MONICA Augsburg cohort world health organization monitoring trends and determinants in cardiovascular diseases.** *Epidemiology* 1999, **10**:391–397.
28. Fang J, Alderman MH: **Serum uric acid and cardiovascular mortal-ity the NHANES I epidemiologic follow-up study, 1971–1992 national health and nutrition examination survey.** *JAMA* 2000, **283**:2404–2410.
29. Tuttle KR, Short RA, Johnson RJ: **Sex differences in uric acid and risk factors for coronary artery disease.** *Am J Cardiol* 2001, **87**:1411–1414.
30. Detrano R, Guerci AD, Carr JJ, Bild DE, Burke G, Folsom AR, Liu K, Shea S, Szklo M, Bluemke DA, O'Leary DH, Tracy R, Watson K, Wong ND, Kronmal RA: **Coronary calcium as a predictor of coronary events in four racial or ethnic groups.** *N Engl J Med* 2008, **358**:1336–1345.
31. Pletcher MJ, Tice JA, Pignone M: **Using the coronary artery calcium score to predict coronary heart disease events: a systematic review and meta-analysis.** *Arch Internmed* 2004, **164**:1285–1292.
32. Rodrigues TC, Maahs DM, Johnson RJ, Jalal DI, Kinney GL, Rivard C, Rewers M, Snell-Bergeon JK: **Serum uric acid predicts progression of subclinical coronary atherosclerosis in individuals without renal disease.** *Diabetes Care* 2010, **33**:2471–2473.
33. Mitsutake R, Miura S, Saku K: **Association between coronary artery calcification score as assessed by multi-detector row computed tomography and upstroke time of pulse wave.** *Intern Med* 2007, **46**:1833–1836.
34. Coutinho Tde A, Turner ST, Peyser PA, Bielak LF, Sheedy PF, Kullo IJ: **Associations of serum uric acid with markers of inflammation, metabolic syndrome, and subclinical coronary atherosclerosis.** *Am J Hypertens* 2007, **20**:83–89.
35. Atar AI, Yilmaz OC, Akin K, Selcoki Y, Er O, Eryonucu B: **Association between gamma-glutamyltransferase and coronary artery calcification.** *Int J Cardiol* 2012, Epub ahead of print.
36. Kaya EB, Yorgun H, Canpolat U, Hazırolan T, Sunman H, Ülgen A, Ates AH, Aytemir K, Tokgözoğlu L, Kabakcı G, Akata D, Oto A: **Serum uric acid levels predict the severity and morphology of coronary atherosclerosis detected by multidetector computed tomography.** *Atherosclerosis* 2010, **213**:178–183.
37. Sano K, Kawasaki M, Ishihara Y, Okubo M, Tsuchiya K, Nishigaki K, Zhou X, Minatoguchi S, Fujita H, Fujiwara H: **Assessment of vulnerable plaques causing acute coronary syndrome using integrated backscatter intravascular ultrasound.** *J Am Coll Cardiol* 2006, **47**:734–741.
38. Pundziute G, Schuijf JD, Jukema JW, Decramer I, Sarno G, Vanhoenacker PK, Boersma E, Reiber JH, Schalij MJ, Wijns W, Bax JJ: **Evaluation of plaque characteristics in acute coronary syndrome: non-invasive assessment with multi-slice computed tomography and invasive evaluation with intravascular ultrasound radiofrequency data analysis.** *Eur Heart J* 2008, **29**:2373–2381.
39. Gagliardi AC, Miname MH, Santos RD: **Uric acid: a marker of increased cardiovascular risk.** *Atherosclerosis* 2009, **202**:11–17.
40. Yildiz A, Yilmaz R, Demirbag R, Gur M, Bas MM, Erel O: **Association of serum uric acid level and coronary blood flow.** *Coron Artery Dis* 2007, **18**:607–613.
41. Kanellis J, Watanabe S, Li JH, Kang DH, Li P, Nakagawa T, Wamsley A, Sheikh-Hamad D, Lan HY, Feng L, Johnson RJ: **Uric acid stimulates monocyte chemoattractant protein-1 production in vascular smooth muscle cells via mitogen-activated protein kinase and cyclooxygenase-2.** *Hypertension* 2003, **41**:1287–1293.
42. Kuwahata S, Hamasaki S, Ishida S, Kataoka T, Yoshikawa A, Orihara K, Ogawa M, Oketani N, Saihara K, Okui H, Shinsato T, Kubozono T, Ichiki H, Fujita S, Takumi T, Yoshino S, Nakazaki M, Miyata M, Tei C: **Effect of uric acid on coronary microvascular endothelial function in women: association with eGFR and ADMA.** *J Atheroscler Thromb* 2010, **17**:259–269.
43. Athyros VG, Mikhailidis DP, Liberopoulos EN, Kakafika AI, Karagiannis A, Papageorgiou AA, Tziomalos K, Ganotakis ES, Elisaf M: **Effect of statin treatment on renal function and serum uric acid levels and their relation to vascular events in patients with coronary heart disease and metabolic syndrome: a subgroup analysis of the Greek atorvastatin and coronary heart disease evaluation (GREACE) study.** *Nephrol Dial Transplant* 2007, **22**:118–127.

14

Rationale and Design of the CREDENCE Trial: computed TomogRaphic evaluation of atherosclerotic DEtermiNants of myocardial IsChEmia

Asim Rizvi[1], Bríain ó. Hartaigh[1], Paul Knaapen[2], Jonathon Leipsic[3], Leslee J. Shaw[4], Daniele Andreini[5], Gianluca Pontone[6], Subha Raman[7], Muhammad Akram Khan[8], Michael Ridner[9], Faisal Nabi[10], Alessia Gimelli[11], James Jang[12], Jason Cole[13], Ryo Nakazato[14], Christopher Zarins[15,16], Donghee Han[1], Ji Hyun Lee[1], Jackie Szymonifika[1], Millie J. Gomez[1], Quynh A. Truong[1,17,18], Hyuk-Jae Chang[19], Fay Y. Lin[1,18] and James K. Min[1,17,18,20*]

Abstract

Background: Coronary computed tomography angiography (CCTA) allows for non-invasive assessment of obstructive coronary artery disease (CAD) beyond measures of stenosis severity alone. This assessment includes atherosclerotic plaque characteristics (APCs) and calculation of fractional flow reserve (FFR) from CCTA (FFR_{CT}). Similarly, stress imaging by myocardial perfusion scintigraphy (MPS) provides vital information. To date, the diagnostic performance of integrated CCTA assessment versus integrated MPS assessment for diagnosis of vessel-specific ischemia remains underexplored.

Methods: CREDENCE will enroll adult individuals with symptoms suspicious of CAD referred for non-emergent invasive coronary angiography (ICA), but without known CAD. All participants will undergo CCTA, MPS, ICA and FFR. FFR will be performed for lesions identified at the time of ICA to be ≥40 and <90 % stenosis, or those clinically indicated for evaluation. Study analyses will focus on diagnostic performance of CCTA versus MPS against invasive FFR reference standard. An integrated stenosis-APC-FFR_{CT} metric by CCTA for vessel-specific ischemia will be developed from derivation cohort and tested against a validation cohort. Similarly, integrated metric by MPS for vessel-specific ischemia will be developed, validated and compared. An FFR value of ≤0.80 will be considered as ischemia causing. The primary endpoint will be the diagnostic accuracy of vessel territory-specific ischemia of integrated stenosis-APC-FFR_{CT} measure by CCTA, compared with perfusion or perfusion–myocardial blood flow stress imaging testing, against invasive FFR.

Discussion: CREDENCE will determine the performance of integrated CCTA metric compared to integrated MPS measure for diagnosis of vessel-specific ischemia. If proven successful, this study may reduce the number of missed diagnoses and help to optimally predict ischemia-causing lesions.

Keywords: Coronary computed tomography angiography, Coronary artery disease, Fractional flow reserve, Myocardial blood flow, Myocardial perfusion scintigraphy

* Correspondence: jkm2001@med.cornell.edu
[1]Dalio Institute of Cardiovascular Imaging, NewYork-Presbyterian Hospital, New York, NY, USA
[17]Department of Medicine, Weill Cornell Medical College, New York, NY, USA
Full list of author information is available at the end of the article

Background

Coronary revascularization remains a mainstay of treatment for coronary artery disease (CAD), which continues to affect more than 16 million US adults. Functional myocardial ischemia may result from anatomically obstructive CAD and strongly determines prognosis, and thus is useful for guiding decisions of revascularization [1, 2]. Invasive fractional flow reserve (FFR) is the reference standard for determining the physiologic significance of CAD for vessel-specific ischemia among patients with multi-vessel CAD. However, the invasive nature of FFR measurement limits this evaluation to only high-risk patients with indications for ICA.

Until now, for the vast numbers of patients at low or intermediate risk for CAD, numerous non-invasive stress imaging modalities including echocardiography, cardiac magnetic resonance (CMR), and myocardial perfusion scintigraphy (MPS) have served as a mainstay for identifying ischemia by detecting stress-induced regional myocardial perfusion defects, of which the most commonly employed is MPS [3, 4]. At a per-patient level, MPS by single photon emission computed tomography (SPECT) or positron emission tomography (PET) is capable of determining the severity and extent of myocardial ischemia with high performance [5, 6]. However, the ability of MPS to correctly discriminate ischemia on a per-vessel basis is less robust [7]. Further, the accuracy of MPS is compromised in patients with multi-vessel CAD [8]. These findings therefore raise questions regarding the ability of MPS to correctly identify coronary lesions that would benefit from revascularization [9].

In the recent past, coronary computed tomography angiography (CCTA) has emerged as a promising non-invasive imaging modality for the diagnosis of anatomically obstructive CAD, with high sensitivity and negative predictive value compared to ICA [10, 11]. Although CCTA enables discrimination of stenosis with high accuracy, it can overestimate stenosis, and similar to ICA, may misidentify ischemia [12]. These findings have led to the emergence of several methods using CCTA-specific data beyond luminal stenosis severity alone for the diagnosis of lesion-specific ischemia. These methods include additional atherosclerotic plaque characteristics (APCs) and calculation of FFR from CCTA (FFR_{CT}).

APCs assessment by CCTA has demonstrated high agreement with invasive methods of plaque assessment and has shown to improve discrimination of ischemia-causing coronary lesions [13]. These include plaque burden and composition, and arterial remodeling [14, 15]. Previous studies have reported that selected APCs are also associated with ischemia by MPS [16, 17]. Yet, the entirety of APCs to optimize the precise identification of ischemia-causing culprit lesions has not been examined to date.

FFR_{CT} represents a novel non-invasive imaging technique that can evaluate the physiologic significance of CAD and enables the calculation of vessel-specific FFR [18]. Further still, given the computational modeling technique in FFR_{CT} calculations, it is possible to place a "virtual stent" by modeling the resolution of luminal compromise. In a recent prospective multicenter study, FFR_{CT} was found to be superior to CCTA stenosis alone for diagnosis of ischemia-causing lesions, and demonstrated good correlation with FFR [19].

Similar to CCTA, which can provide important information beyond luminal stenosis severity alone, stress imaging testing can also do so by an array of prognostically and diagnostically important factors. These include high-risk imaging features (e.g., transient ischemic dilation, stress-induced lung uptake of radiotracer, increased right ventricular uptake), myocardial blood flow (MBF), exercise electrocardiographic (ECG) findings, functional capacity, stress-induced symptom complexes. Even within these categories, other more granular data are available, e.g., in ECG data, extent of ST-segment depression, rate-pressure product, heart rate recovery, and other variables are well known to augment CAD diagnosis.

The overall objective of the CREDENCE trial is to determine the utility of a novel diagnostic integrated approach by integrating anatomic APCs with physiologic FFR_{CT} to optimize the precise identification of vessel-specific ischemia by CCTA, and to compare this measure against the totality of relevant variables by MPS.

Methods/Design

The Computed TomogRaphic Evaluation of Atherosclerotic DEtermiNants of Myocardial IsChEmia (CREDENCE) trial (clinicaltrials.gov NCT02173275) is a prospective multicenter cross-sectional study of 618 individuals ($n = 309$ [derivation cohort]; $n = 309$ [validation cohort]) wherein eligible participants will undergo CCTA, MPS, ICA and FFR. For the purposes of the study, either MPS, CCTA, and/or FFR will have been performed for clinical purposes, with the other test being performed as part of the trial procedure. Study analyses will focus on the diagnostic performance of MPS versus CCTA against the gold standard of invasively determined FFR for vessel-specific ischemia.

The relationships of anatomic APCs and physiologic FFR_{CT} by CCTA will be assessed according to measures of vessel-specific ischemia, referenced to an invasive FFR standard. An integrated anatomic-physiologic metric by CCTA for vessel-specific ischemia will be developed from a derivation cohort and tested against a validation cohort, both of which will undergo CCTA, MPS, ICA and FFR. Similarly, an integrated metric by MPS for vessel-specific ischemia will be developed and validated. The performance of this integrated CCTA measure will be directly compared with MPS for diagnosis of vessels that manifest ischemia. The schematic summary of the trial design is depicted in Fig. 1.

Importantly, for reasons of safety, all FFRs to be performed will be limited to lesions identified at the time of ICA to be ≥40 and <90 % stenosis, or those that should be clinically indicated for evaluation. As lesions <40 % in diameter stenosis severity are almost uniformly non-ischemic and those ≥90 % are typically ischemic, these lesions should be avoided for interrogation with an FFR guidewire for reasons of patient safety, unless deemed medically necessary. In contrast, coronary stenoses between 40 and 90 % demonstrate variable rates of ischemia and may be appropriately interrogated for clinical indications. If FFR interrogation of a coronary lesion between 40 and 90 % is considered as imparting excess risk to a study subject for anatomical or other reasons, it will be avoided. In keeping with prior studies, vessel territories will be comprised of the left anterior descending artery [LAD] (and diagonal branches), the left circumflex artery [LCx] (and obtuse marginal branches), and the right coronary artery [RCA] (and posterolateral branch and posterior descending artery). Patients who undergo percutaneous coronary intervention (PCI) by intracoronary stenting of ≥1 coronary lesions after the ICA and FFR measurements may have repeat measurements of FFR after the completion of stent deployment, as clinically indicated.

The CREDENCE study will be performed in 19 investigative sites in USA, Canada, Netherlands, Japan, China, Latvia, Italy, and South Korea (ClinicalTrials.gov, NCT02173275). Each center may not enroll more than 40 % of the total number of subjects. The shortest time duration between noninvasive and invasive testing will be at the discretion of the local physician. The maximum time permitted between noninvasive and invasive tests will be 60 days.

Study objectives

Primary objective

The primary objective is to determine the diagnostic accuracy of vessel territory-specific ischemia by use of an integrated stenosis-APC-FFR_{CT} measure determined by CCTA, when compared with perfusion or perfusion–MBF stress imaging testing, against invasive FFR. Stress imaging will also include additional characteristics, as described above, which do not exhibit co-linearity with other variables. CCTA and stress imaging features will be hierarchically evaluated: CCTA will be evaluated by stenosis, then FFR_{CT}, then APCs; while stress imaging will be evaluated by perfusion, then MBF, then ECG features and finally, functional capacity.

Secondary objectives

The secondary objective is to compare the accuracy of the individual components of the CCTA and MPS measures to detect ischemia by invasive FFR: APC components; FFR_{CT}; MPS vessel-specific perfusion deficits; and reduced MBF. Another objective is to determine the accuracy of FFR_{CT} "virtual stenting" with a post-PCI FFR value of >0.80 in an effort to assess the correlation between FFR_{CT} "virtual stenting" to post-PCI FFR.

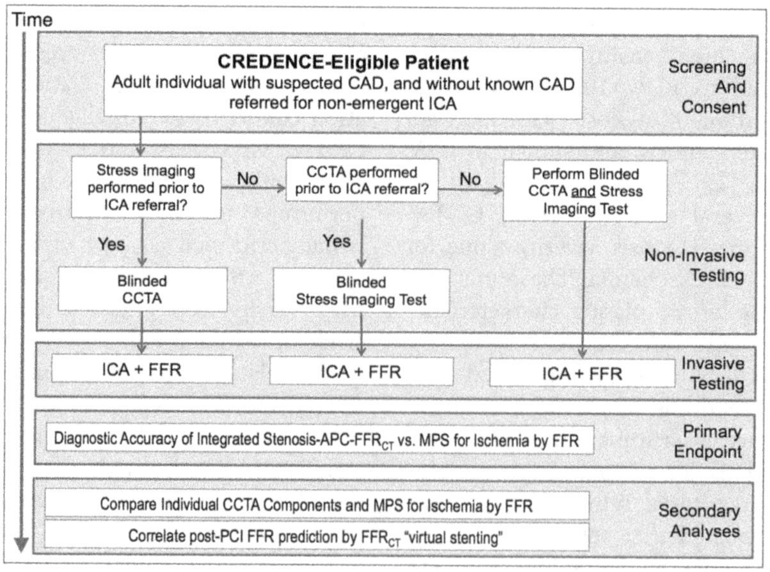

Fig. 1 CREDENCE study design. CAD, coronary artery disease; ICA, invasive coronary angiography; CCTA, coronary computed tomography angiography; MPS, myocardial perfusion scintigraphy; FFR, fractional flow reserve; FFR_{CT}, fractional flow reserve derived from coronary computed tomography angiography; APCs, atherosclerotic plaque characteristics; PCI, percutaneous coronary intervention

Target population

The CREDENCE target population will comprise a large and representative sample of individuals for whom CCTA and MPS testing confer the largest potential benefit; that is, for those with suspected CAD who are being referred for non-emergent clinically indicated ICA based upon an imaging study (either MPS or CCTA). In this regard, CREDENCE will enroll adult individuals who meet the inclusion criteria and none of the exclusion criteria, as detailed in Table 1. The study is considered non-significant risk because all subjects will undergo clinically-indicated ICA as planned, with FFR performed in vessel territories with >40 % stenosis for which there is equipoise of ischemia presence [20].

Efficacy analyses and sample size

Primary efficacy analysis

The primary statistical analysis will be diagnostic accuracy of vessel territory-specific ischemia using an integrated APC-FFR_{CT} metric by CCTA, as compared with territory-specific ischemia on perfusion or perfusion-MBF stress imaging, against invasive FFR. Three vessel territories including the LAD, LCx, and RCA will be examined. The non-ischemic vessels will serve as controls to ischemic vessels. An FFR measurement cutoff value of ≤0.80 will be considered as ischemia-causing, and >0.80 as non ischemia-causing.

Table 1 CREDENCE trial inclusion and exclusion criteria

Inclusion criteria
(1) Age ≥18 years
(2) Patients scheduled to undergo clinically-indicated non-emergent invasive coronary angiography
Exclusion criteria
(1) Known coronary artery disease (myocardial infarction, percutaneous coronary interventions, coronary artery bypass graft)
(2) Hemodynamic instability
(3) Inability to provide written informed consent
(4) Concomitant participation in another clinical trial in which an individual is subject to investigational drug or device
(5) Pregnancy or unknown pregnancy status
(6) Absolute contraindication to iodinated contrast due to prior near-fatal anaphylactoid reaction (laryngospasm, bronchospasm, cardiorespiratory collapse, or equivalent)
(7) Impaired chronic renal function (serum creatinine ≥1.7 mg/dl or Glomerular Filtration Rate <30 ml/min)
(8) Baseline irregular heart rhythm (e.g., atrial fibrillation, etc.)
(9) Heart rate ≥100 beats per minute
(10) Systolic blood pressure ≤90 mm Hg
(11) Contraindications to β blockers or nitroglycerin or adenosine

Analysis of APCs and FFR_{CT} against an invasive FFR standard

APCs and FFR_{CT} will be assessed against an invasive FFR standard for diagnosis of lesion-specific ischemia. Direct comparison of an integrated APC-FFR_{CT} metric to a non-invasive gold standard by a composite perfusion, MBF, ECG, and functional capacity metric will then be made.

(A) Assessment of APCs for diagnosis of lesion-specific ischemia

Coronary vessels from 309 patients (927 vessels) with moderate or severe ischemia by MPS and who undergo ICA will be studied, so as to determine the physiologically most relevant APCs. If there is no ischemia in a vessel, then the angiographically most severe lesion measured by invasive FFR will be chosen for APC assessment. For these vessels, associations of the APC measures will be examined in relation to vessel-based ischemia.

Within-subject comparison of APCs of ischemia-causing versus non ischemia-causing coronary lesions

APCs within ischemia-causing lesions will be compared with within-subject control lesions. Matched analysis will be performed to predict the likelihood of a vessel being ischemic based on APCs for lesions (e.g., matched 1:1 within persons); with an ischemic vessel--that possess the angiographically most severe stenosis and is measured by invasive FFR--matched to one of the remaining arteries (LAD, LCx or RCA).

Moreover, additional ischemic:nonischemic vessel combinations will be considered. For any patient with one ischemic vessel, an analysis will be performed using a 1:2 case:control match to compare results with the 1:1 matched analysis. For individuals with two ischemic vessels, a 2:1 case:control match will be performed for each ischemic vessel to the same non-ischemic control vessel, and then comparing these results with the 1:1 matched analysis.

(B) Assessment of FFR_{CT} for diagnosis of lesion-specific ischemia

In individuals who experience ischemia, coronary lesions from 309 patients will be studied, and ischemic vessels will be identified by invasive FFR. The region within the same coronary vessel will be identified distal to the most angiographically obstructive stenosis on the CCTA image that was measured by FFR. The agreement between measured FFR_{CT} and invasive FFR will be examined for these vessels, both as dichotomous (≤ versus >0.80) and continuous (ranging from 0 to 1) variables. In addition, the diagnostic performance of FFR_{CT} to invasive FFR will be tested by measures of sensitivity, specificity, positive predictive value (PPV), and negative predictive value (NPV).

Within-subject comparison of FFR_{CT} of ischemia-causing lesions to non-ischemia causing coronary lesions

FFR_{CT} for ischemic vessels will be compared with within-subject controls. Matched analysis will be performed to predict the likelihood of a vessel to be ischemic based on FFR_{CT} for lesions matched 1:1 within a person. Within-subject matched comparisons will be performed as discussed earlier for the APCs.

(C) Derivation and validation of an integrated anatomic-physiologic CCTA metric for diagnosis of ischemia

An integrated CCTA metric will then be developed that will represent the most parsimonious set of APCs for improving diagnosis of vessel-specific ischemia. The weighted APC set will be combined to FFR_{CT} values using information derived from (A) and (B). Multivariate mixed-effects logistic regression analyses will be conducted with APC-FFR_{CT} measures as a predictor of ischemia. A backward stepwise selection method will be used so that only significant variables at $p < 0.05$ level will be included in the final model. Since these analyses are on a per-vessel basis, a random effects model will be used to account for within-patient clustering. Finally, a summary APC-FFR_{CT} metric as a predictor of ischemia, accounting for the weighted contribution of APCs and FFR_{CT}, will be obtained. This summary APC-FFR_{CT} metric will be tested for its ability to diagnose vessel-based ischemia in a validation cohort of 309 patients who will also undergo CCTA, MPS, ICA, and FFR.

(D) Comparison of an integrated anatomic-physiologic CCTA metric to vessel-territory specific ischemia by MPS

In the validation cohort, the integrated APC-FFR_{CT} metric will be directly compared against MPS for the diagnosis of vessel-specific ischemia, using invasive FFR as a reference standard. This integrated metric will be compared against a combined perfusion-MBF-ECG-functional capacity measure by MPS so as to assure the highest diagnostic performance of both CCTA and MPS in comparison. MBF is anticipated to be most useful in the presence of balanced reduction of perfusion (i.e., in the absence of relative perfusion differences) and thus, is expected to increase specificity when a regional vessel-based territory appears normal by perfusion.

Secondary efficacy analysis

The secondary statistical analysis will compare the accuracy of the individual components of the CCTA and MPS measures to detect ischemia by invasive FFR: APC components; FFR_{CT}; MPS vessel-specific perfusion deficits; and reduced MBF. Another analysis will compare the accuracy of FFR_{CT} "virtual stenting" with a post-PCI FFR value of >0.80, and to determine the correlation between the FFR_{CT} "virtual stenting" and post-PCI FFR. For segments that were treated with coronary stent and underwent FFR, the post-PCI FFR value will be measured. On a per-segment analysis, "virtual stenting" will be performed and post-"virtual stent" FFR_{CT} will be predicted. The diagnostic accuracy of FFR_{CT} "virtual stenting" to post-PCI FFR will then be calculated, using a cutoff value of >0.80 to be considered non-ischemic and a successful intervention. Further, the correlation between post-FFR_{CT} "virtual stenting" and post-PCI FFR will be performed using Pearson's correlation or Spearman's rank correlation, as appropriate.

Sample size calculation and statistical power

A total of 618 participants will be enrolled in this study. The sample size determination of the primary endpoint was based upon a sequential derivation-validation design for APCs and FFR_{CT}. For a logistic regression of a binary response variable, a sample size of 618 patients is needed for a 90 % power at a 0.05 significance level to detect a 30 % increase in the probability that a vessel manifest ischemia. This change corresponds to an odds ratio of 2.0. The study expects to have 309 patients available that will provide more than sufficient sample for variation in the estimated parameters for sample size. To ensure statistical validity, a post hoc power analysis will be run and the actual power achieved by the analysis will be reported.

Quality assurance

CCTA image acquisition and interpretation

All CCTA scans will be performed with single- or dual source CCTA scanners with a minimum of 64 detector rows. Detector row width will be ≤0.75 mm. At a minimum, single-head power injectors allowing fast injection rates of 4–7 mL/s will be required. Laboratories will follow local CCTA scanning protocols as long as they are consistent with quality standards defined by the Society of Cardiovascular Computed Tomography (SCCT) guidelines [21]. CCTA interpretation has also been detailed elsewhere, and will conform to SCCT guidelines [21].

CCTA images will be transmitted to independent masked readers at the CCTA Core Laboratory, who will use dedicated 3-dimensional workstations to evaluate the CCTA images. The 18-segment SCCT model of the coronary tree will be used for the coronary evaluation [21]. Coronary atherosclerosis will be defined as any tissue >1 mm^2 within or adjacent to the lumen that can be discriminated from surrounding pericardial tissue, epicardial fat, or lumen; and identified in ≥2 planes. Stenoses will be graded in accordance with the SCCT segmental 5-point scale: 0 %; 1–24 %; 25–49 %, 50–69 %, and 70–100 % [21]. Plaque will be measured on 3days workstations, with reconstructions at the smallest slice thickness (~500 μm). All CCTA scans will be interpreted by a minimum of 2 readers, with 20 % randomly repeated to test for inter- and intra-observer variability. APCs and FFR_{CT} analyses will be performed using the already-acquired CCTA data set. CCTA core lab readers and automated software will perform interpretation of APCs. APCs will be studied by multiplanar reconstructions (MPR) and cross-sections using optimal phases, and by automated software with manual correction, with segments classified by an 18-segment SCCT model [21].

Atherosclerotic plaque characteristics

Given their association to myocardial ischemia in prior studies, six coronary APCs will be selected and will include 1) low attenuation plaque (LAP); 2) positive remodeling (PR); 3) mixed plaque (MP); 4) plaque burden (PB); 5) minimal luminal area (MLA); and 6) transluminal attenuation gradient (TAG) [12, 16, 17, 22]. To determine the incremental value of APCs beyond conventional CCTA measures of CAD, baseline CAD burden by the CAD index and CAD complexity by the SYNTAX score will also be determined [23].

Briefly, a Hounsfield unit (HU) <30 will signify LAP, as this threshold exhibits the best performance compared to intravascular ultrasound (IVUS) [15]. A remodeling index (RI) >1.10 will be defined as PR and a RI <0.95 will be defined as negative remodeling, with in-between values categorized as intermediate remodeling [13]. Plaque composition will be classified on a 5-level scale: non-calcified (0 % calcified plaque [CP]), mostly non-calcified (1–30 % CP), mixed (30–70 % CP), mostly calcified (70–99 % CP), and calcified (100 % CP). Plaque composition scores will be made by summing the number of segments with each type of plaque composition. Finally, TAG will be defined as the change in HU per mm of artery, and will be calculated from the coefficient of linear regression between luminal attenuation and length from vessel ostium [24]. An automated plaque analysis will also be performed with a validated software (QAngio CT, Medis medical imaging systems, Leiden, the Netherlands).

FFR_{CT} and virtual stenting

FFR_{CT} will be performed by applying a computational fluid dynamics (CFD) approach to typically-acquired CCTA scans for calculation of coronary artery pressure and flow by HeartFlow, Inc. (Redwood City, CA). More detailed information regarding FFR_{CT} and virtual stenting is provided in the online supplementary material, Additional file 1.

Myocardial perfusion scintigraphy

MPS will be performed by a variety of methods, including PET, SPECT, or CMR. Standard acquisition and analysis protocols will be agreed on for each technique covering patient preparation, cardiovascular stress, administration of radiopharmaceutical or contrast medium, image acquisition and quality control, image processing and interpretation. These procedures will be based on available international guidelines [25, 26].

As such, all MPS studies in this investigation will employ PET when possible. Briefly, dynamic MPS will be performed at rest and during vasodilator stress by 13 N-ammonia (13-NH3) or rubidium-82 (Rb-82) PET using a high-resolution PET/CT scanner, in accordance with societal guidelines [27]. Data will be reconstructed with attenuation correction, based on a validated model from our lab to quantify radionuclide signal attenuation and peak absolute MBF as well as MBF reserve in the territory of the LAD, LCx, and RCA. Time-activity curves will be constructed beginning with initiation of 13-N-NH3 or Rb-82 infusion, using spillover correction [28, 29]. Radionuclide signal in each territory from stress and rest will be compared for calculation of regional (per-vessel) total perfusion defect (rTPD, amount of hypoperfused myocardium as % of total myocardium). Stress-induced perfusion in each territory will be defined as [stress rTPD – rest rTPD], or "reversible" rTPD (REVrTPD), which will be examined continuously for regional myocardial ischemia [30]. In cases when PET cannot be performed, MPS by SPECT will be done and will evaluate perfusion as described above.

For MPS, perfusion in each of the 17 segments will be classified as normal, mild reduction, moderate reduction, severe reduction, or absent perfusion, and the segmental scores were summed for the stress and rest images. An inducible perfusion abnormality will be defined as a summed segmental difference score between stress and rest images ≥2, either from a score ≥1 in ≥2 contiguous segments, or ≥2 in ≥1 segment. Scarring will be defined similarly from the summed segmental rest score. For wall motion abnormalities (WMA), segmental myocardial wall motion will be scored at rest and during stress as normal, hypokinetic, akinetic, or dyskinetic. Inducible ischemia will be defined as an increase in segmental wall motion score ≥1 from rest to stress in ≥2 contiguous segments. Scarring will be defined similarly from the resting wall motion score [31]. The angiographic dominance of the vascular territories will be used for designation of territories during MPS as previously described [32, 33]. In patients with left coronary dominance, the inferior and infero-lateral segments will be assigned to the LCx territory, and all 4 apical segments will be assigned to the LAD territory [33]. In the case of RCA dominance, the inferior, infero-lateral, and apical inferior segments will be assigned to the RCA territory, with the remaining 3 apical segments assigned to the LAD territory [33].

Invasive coronary angiography and fractional flow reserve

Patients will undergo diagnostic ICA in accordance with usual clinical indications and by imaging standards set forth by the American College of Cardiology/Society for Cardiac Angiography and Interventions [34]. Further detailed information about ICA and FFR procedure is outlined in the online supplementary material, Additional file 1.

Integration of FFR, CCTA and FFR_{CT} measurements

For suitable comparison of CCTA APCs, FFR_{CT}, and FFR, accurate alignment of CCTA and ICA must be performed. An integration process will be performed in a masked fashion by a study investigator not responsible for CCTA, FFR_{CT}, or MPS evaluation in order to identify the location of a lesion by CCTA that corresponds to the location where the distal pressure sensor of the wire is located at the time of FFR. The latter integration approach will ensure complete masking of the interpretation of CCTA APCs, FFR_{CT}, and ICA and FFR results. On this model, the cardiologist will demarcate the location of the FFR wire, and will refer the model to investigators responsible for interpretation of the CCTA APCs and FFR_{CT}.

Organization and data management

This study will be coordinated by the Dalio Institute of Cardiovascular Imaging Clinical and Data Coordinating Center (DICI CDCC). The DICI CDCC will be responsible for the processing and quality control of the data. The study protocol will be approved at each participating center by the local institutional review board. Completed electronic case report forms (eCRFs) will be entered by trained site personnel, and will be transmitted to a central data repository at the DCC. At regular intervals, all data will be transferred from electronic case report form (REDCAP) to SAS for statistical summarization, data description, and data analysis. Further cross-checking of the data will be performed in SAS.

Site qualification will be issued by the DICI CDCC for each modality before subject enrollment. Before beginning enrollment, eligible sites will be qualified by the imaging Core Laboratories based on site surveys and on successful transfer of one or more complete datasets with sufficient image quality and completeness for each modality. During the study, technical quality assessment of image and test acquisition will be accomplished on all studies by central repository research technicians trained by the CDCC. This ongoing review will ensure the adequate quality and completeness of datasets.

Discussion

The CREDENCE study aims to integrate the anatomic and physiologic information derived from CCTA for the precise identification of ischemia-causing coronary lesions, and to compare this measure against an integrated metric for MPS. To date, no non-invasive imaging modality has been routinely capable of a "one-stop shop," wherein anatomic identification of stenoses and physiologic determination of ischemia are derived from a single test, thus resulting in layered testing and increased complexity and cost of clinical care. Specifically, this study will assess the performance of anatomic APCs by CCTA and physiologic FFR_{CT} for diagnosis of vessel-specific ischemia. An integrated APC-FFR_{CT} metric by CCTA will then be directly compared to a perfusion-MBF-ECG-functional capacity metric by MPS for diagnosis of vessel-specific ischemia. As such, we hypothesize that an integrated assessment by CCTA will be superior to an integrated assessment by MPS for the diagnosis of vessel-specific ischemia.

Prior studies have established that MPS is capable of determining the severity and extent of myocardial ischemia with high performance at a per-patient level, and that MPS evaluation is augmented by MBF, ECG, and functional capacity findings [5, 6]. Nevertheless, the "real world" accuracy of MPS is less assertive despite its high reported diagnostic performance [35]. To date, no study has included the totality of information imparted by MPS—including MBF, ECG, and functional capacity—rendering comparisons of CCTA to MPS incomplete and, in general, skewed towards improved CCTA diagnostic performance.

CCTA has demonstrated high performance for diagnosis of obstructive CAD compared to ICA, and predicts adverse prognosis [36]. In the prospective multicenter ACCURACY trial, CCTA demonstrated a sensitivity, specificity, PPV and NPV of 94, 83, 48, and 99 %, respectively, compared with ICA. The results of this ACCURACY trial are in agreement with two subsequent multicenter studies that demonstrated high accuracy of CCTA [10, 11]. On the contrary, even though CCTA can discriminate stenosis with high accuracy, the ability to identify ischemia-causing coronary lesions is suboptimal at present [12]. In a study of 79 patients undergoing CCTA and ICA with FFR, high rates of false positive CCTAs were noted, with an overall specificity for ischemia of 40 % [12]. Similar findings have been observed from pooled analyses comparing CCTA to MPS wherein CCTA stenoses were associated with ischemia less than half of the time [37, 38].

The PROMISE trial demonstrated equivalent outcomes between functional imaging by multiple modalities, including PET, and anatomic evaluation of stenosis severity by CCTA [39]. The CREDENCE trial posits that stenosis evaluation alone discards important anatomic and functional data in routinely performed CCTA, and that a combined assessment may be superior for vessel ischemia. Similarly, the CREDENCE trial posits that perfusion evaluation alone by MPS discards important functional information, and that combined assessment may be superior for vessel ischemia. Prior studies have shown that CCTA enables assessment of several coronary APCs with generally high accuracy beyond luminal diameter stenosis, and similar to invasive studies by intravascular ultrasound, APCs visualized on CCTA have been associated with ischemia-causing culprit lesions [40] [14, 15, 17]. Further still, the accuracy of FFR_{CT} for diagnosing coronary ischemia has been reported in several studies [19, 41, 42]. In the DISCOVER-FLOW (Diagnosis of Ischemia-Causing Stenoses Obtained Via Noninvasive Fractional Flow Reserve) trial, compared with invasive FFR, non-invasive FFR_{CT} demonstrated per-vessel accuracy, sensitivity, specificity, PPV, and NPV for ischemia-causing lesions of 84.3 %, 87.9 %, 82.2 %, 73.9 %, 92.2 %, respectively [19]. Further, in a more recent HeartFlow NXT study, the FFR_{CT} data matched closely with invasively measured FFR [42].

To date, however, clinical reporting of CCTA has been limited to stenosis severity, with relative neglect of APCs and unavailability of FFR_{CT}. The aversion to incorporate APC findings may originate from the fact that APC quantification is time-intensive with per-patient evaluation taking 8–10 h for comprehensive APC evaluation. This study will facilitate widespread applicability by assessing co-linearity of APCs to develop the most parsimonious set of APCs that offers the greatest diagnostic value; and validate the diagnostic utility of the APCs in a separate cohort of individuals. We have ensured that APC measures will be accurate by several safeguards. We will use images only from CCTA scanners with 64-rows or more, the threshold for adequate coronary imaging by CCTA. Further, APCs will be interpreted at a state-of-the-art laboratory by ≥2 readers with inter- and intra-observer assessment for a 20 % of CCTAs for assurances of reliability. Similarly, this study will assess FFR_{CT}, referenced against both invasive FFR and non-invasive stress test "gold" standards. Furthermore, this study will perform APC and FFR_{CT} evaluation with automated software that will facilitate time-efficient evaluation of both APCs and FFR_{CT}.

Similar to CCTA, we will perform a comprehensive assessment of MPS. By a dedicated and blinded core laboratory, we will examine factors beyond regional myocardial perfusion, and will include imaging high-risk features of CAD (including transient ischemic dilatation, and increased lung uptake of radiotracer), as well as high-risk ECG features (such as ST-segment depression, hypotensive response to stress, heart rate recovery, and rate-pressure product). Functional capacity and MBF will also be assessed.

If proven successful and the superiority of a combined anatomic-physiologic approach is shown, this trial will provide the rationale in developing and establishing a novel diagnostic paradigm that not only identifies patients who manifest ischemia, but also specify ischemia-causing coronary lesions that may be more accurate than conventional stress imaging. If the strategies are equivalent, there will still be information gain in determining the most efficient means to determine lesion-specific ischemia by CCTA and MPS. The results of this approach may reduce the number of missed diagnoses and help to optimally predict ischemia-causing lesions, considering the fact that millions of patients are tested for CAD each year in the US alone. Further, this novel diagnostic paradigm may help promote avoidance of unnecessary invasive procedures and procedure-related complications in the future, and allow for improved clinical decision-making to identify patients who are versus who are not eligible for coronary revascularization. Finally, the proposed trial will potentially reduce downstream care related to these invasive procedures as well as the cost burden, and directly impacts annual healthcare savings.

New knowledge gained

The CREDENCE study aims to fill many gaps in knowledge and is distinctive from other prior studies in determining which coronary vessels can be non-invasively determined as manifesting ischemia. By comparing an integrated CCTA measure directly against an integrated measure for MPS, this study will provide unavailable comparative effectiveness data for CCTA and stress testing for diagnosis of lesion-specific ischemia. Moreover, the proposed trial will potentially provide improved patient care and may directly impact clinical practice by reducing rates of unnecessary invasive procedures as well as health care costs.

Abbreviations

13-NH3: 13 N-ammonia; APCs: Atherosclerotic plaque characteristics; CAD: Coronary artery disease; CCTA: Coronary computed tomography angiography; CFD: Computational fluid dynamics; CMR: Cardiac magnetic resonance; CREDENCE: Computed TomogRaphic Evaluation of Atherosclerotic DEtermiNants of Myocardial IsChEmia; DICI CDCC: Dalio Institute of Cardiovascular Imaging Clinical and Data Coordinating Center; DISCOVER-FLOW: Diagnosis of Ischemia-causing stenoses obtained via noninvasive fractional flow reserve; ECG: Electrocardiography; eCRFs: Electronic case report forms; FFR: Fractional flow reserve; FFR_{CT}: Fractional flow reserve from coronary computed tomography angiography; HU: Hounsfield unit; ICA: Invasive coronary angiography; IVUS: Intravascular ultrasound; LAD: Left anterior descending artery; LAP: Low attenuation plaque; LCx: Left circumflex artery; MBF: Myocardial blood flow; MLA: Minimal luminal area; MP: Mixed plaque; MPR: Multiplanar reconstructions; MPS: Myocardial perfusion scintigraphy; PB: Plaque burden; PCI: Percutaneous coronary intervention; PET: Positron emission tomography; PR: Positive remodeling; Rb-82: Rubidium-82; RCA: Right coronary artery; REVrTPD: Reversible regional total perfusion defect; RI: Remodeling index; rTPD: Regional total perfusion defect; SCCT: Society of Cardiovascular Computed Tomography; SPECT: Single photon emission computed tomography; TAG: Transluminal attenuation gradient; WMA: Wall motion abnormalities

Acknowledgements

We would like to acknowledge and thank all the members of the laboratory teams.

Principal Investigators: Andrejs Erglis, MD, Paul Stradins Clinical University Hospital, Riga, Latvia; Erick Avelar, MD, Oconee Heart and Vascular Center at St Mary's Hospital, Athens, GA; U Joseph Schoepf, MD, Medical University of South Carolina, Charleston, SC; Randall Thompson, MD, St. Luke's Mid America Heart Institute, Kansas City, MO; Bin Lu, MD, State Key Laboratory of Cardiovascular Disease, Fuwai Hospital, Beijing, China; Atizazul Mansoor, MD, PinnacleHealth Cardiovascular Institute, Wormleysburg, PA; Chris Rowan, MD, Renown Heart and Vascular, Reno, NV; Philippe Généreux, MD, Cardiovascular Research Foundation, New York, NY.

Other Investigators: Hiroyuki Niinuma, MD PhD, Cardiovascular Imaging Lab, St. Luke's International Hospital, Tokyo, Japan; Ae-Young Her, MD, Severance Cardiovascular Hospital, Yonsei University Health System, Seoul, South Korea; Joon-Hyung Doh, MD, Severance Cardiovascular Hospital, Yonsei University Health System, Seoul, South Korea; Jung Hyun Choi, MD, Severance Cardiovascular Hospital, Yonsei University Health System, Seoul, South Korea; So-Yeon Choi, MD PhD, Severance Cardiovascular Hospital, Yonsei University Health System, Seoul, South Korea; Bon-Kwon Koo, MD PhD, Severance Cardiovascular Hospital, Yonsei University Health System, Seoul, South Korea; Chang-Wook Nam, MD PhD, Severance Cardiovascular Hospital, Yonsei University Health System, Seoul, South Korea; Sanghoon Shin, MD, Severance Cardiovascular Hospital, Yonsei University Health System, Seoul, South Korea; Hyung-Bok Park, MD, Severance Cardiovascular Hospital, Yonsei University Health System, Seoul, South Korea; Daniel H. Steinberg, MD, Medical University of South Carolina, Charleston, SC; Irfan Ullah, MD CCRP, Cardiac Center of Texas, Mczkinney, TX; Ahmed Ladak, MD CCRP, Cardiac Center of Texas, Mczkinney, TX; Venkata S. Chilakapati, MD FACC, Cardiac Center of Texas, Mczkinney, TX; Dante Chiappino, MD, Fondazione Toscana/CNR Gabriele Monasterio, Pisa PI, Italy; Yang Gao, MD, State Key Laboratory of Cardiovascular Disease, Fuwai Hospital, Beijing, China; Chaowei Mu, MD, State Key Laboratory of Cardiovascular Disease, Fuwai Hospital, Beijing, China.

Funding

This study was supported in part by a grant from the National Institutes of Health (R01HL118019). This study was also funded, in part, by a generous gift from the Dalio Institute of Cardiovascular Imaging and the Michael Wolk Foundation.

Authors' contributions

AR drafted the manuscript. BH, FL, and JM critically revised the manuscript. JS contributed to the statistical analysis. All authors made a contribution to the design and conception of the study. All authors read and approved the final manuscript.

Competing interests

Dr. Min serves as a consultant to HeartFlow, is on the scientific advisory board of Arineta, has ownership in Autoplaq and MDDX, and has a research agreement with GE Healthcare. All other authors have no disclosures to report.

Author details

[1]Dalio Institute of Cardiovascular Imaging, NewYork-Presbyterian Hospital, New York, NY, USA. [2]Department of Cardiology, VU University Medical Center, Amsterdam, The Netherlands. [3]Department of Medical Imaging, University of British Columbia, St. Paul's Hospital, Vancouver, BC, Canada. [4]Emory University School of Medicine, Atlanta, GA, USA. [5]Centro Cardiologico Monzino, IRCCS, Milan, Italy. [6]Istituto di Ricovero e Cura a Carattere Scientifico, Centro Cardiologico Monzino, Milan, Italy. [7]Davis Heart and Lung Research Institute and Heart Center, The Ohio State University, Columbus, OH, USA. [8]The Cardiac Center of Texas, McKinney, TX, USA. [9]Heart Center Research, LLC, Huntsville, AL, USA. [10]Houston Methodist DeBakey Heart & Vascular Center, Houston Methodist Hospital, Houston, TX, USA. [11]Fondazione Toscana/CNR Gabriele Monasterio, Pisa, Italy. [12]Division of Cardiology, Kaiser Permanente San Jose Medical Center, San Jose, CA, USA. [13]Mobile Cardiology Associates, Mobile, AL, USA. [14]Cardiovascular Imaging Lab, St. Luke's International Hospital, Tokyo, Japan. [15]Heart Flow, Inc., Redwood City, CA, USA. [16]Department of Surgery, Stanford University, Stanford, CA, USA. [17]Department of Medicine, Weill Cornell Medical College, New York, NY, USA. [18]Department of Radiology, Weill Cornell Medical College, New York, NY, USA. [19]Division of Cardiology, Severance Cardiovascular Hospital, Yonsei University Health System, Seoul, South Korea. [20]Radiology and Medicine, New York-Presbyterian Hospital and Weill Cornell Medical College, 413 E. 69th Street, Suite 108, New York, NY 10021, USA.

References

1. Uren NG, Melin JA, De Bruyne B, Wijns W, Baudhuin T, Camici PG. Relation between myocardial blood flow and the severity of coronary-artery stenosis. N Engl J Med. 1994;330(25):1782–8. doi:10.1056/NEJM199406233302503.
2. Pijls NH, Fearon WF, Tonino PA, Siebert U, Ikeno F, Bornschein B, et al. Fractional flow reserve versus angiography for guiding percutaneous coronary intervention in patients with multivessel coronary artery disease: 2-year follow-up of the FAME (Fractional Flow Reserve Versus Angiography for Multivessel Evaluation) study. J Am Coll Cardiol. 2010; 56(3):177–84. doi:10.1016/j.jacc.2010.04.012.
3. Fraker Jr TD, Fihn SD, Gibbons RJ, Abrams J, Chatterjee K, Daley J, et al. 2007 chronic angina focused update of the ACC/AHA 2002 Guidelines for the management of patients with chronic stable angina: a report of the American College of Cardiology/American Heart Association Task Force on Practice Guidelines Writing Group to develop the focused update of the 2002 Guidelines for the management of patients with chronic stable angina. Circulation. 2007;116(23):2762–72. doi:10.1161/CIRCULATIONAHA.107.187930.
4. Klocke FJ, Baird MG, Lorell BH, Bateman TM, Messer JV, Berman DS, et al. ACC/AHA/ASNC guidelines for the clinical use of cardiac radionuclide imaging–executive summary: a report of the American College of Cardiology/American Heart Association Task Force on Practice Guidelines (ACC/AHA/ASNC Committee to Revise the 1995 Guidelines for the Clinical Use of Cardiac Radionuclide Imaging). J Am Coll Cardiol. 2003;42(7):1318–33.
5. Klocke FJ, Baird MG, Lorell BH, Bateman TM, Messer JV, Berman DS, et al. ACC/AHA/ASNC guidelines for the clinical use of cardiac radionuclide imaging–executive summary: a report of the American College of Cardiology/American Heart Association Task Force on Practice Guidelines (ACC/AHA/ASNC Committee to Revise the 1995 Guidelines for the Clinical Use of Cardiac Radionuclide Imaging). Circulation. 2003;108(11):1404–18. doi:10.1161/01.CIR.0000080946.42225.4D.
6. Kim C, Kwok YS, Heagerty P, Redberg R. Pharmacologic stress testing for coronary disease diagnosis: a meta-analysis. Am Heart J. 2001;142(6):934–44. doi:10.1067/mhj.2001.119761.
7. Elhendy A, Schinkel AF, Bax JJ, van Domburg RT, Valkema R, Biagini E, et al. Accuracy of stress Tc-99 m tetrofosmin myocardial perfusion tomography for the diagnosis and localization of coronary artery disease in women. J Nucl Cardiol. 2006;13(5):629–34. doi:10.1016/j.nuclcard.2006.06.128.
8. Melikian N, De Bondt P, Tonino P, De Winter O, Wyffels E, Bartunek J, et al. Fractional flow reserve and myocardial perfusion imaging in patients with angiographic multivessel coronary artery disease. JACC Cardiovasc Interv. 2010;3(3):307–14. doi:10.1016/j.jcin.2009.12.010.
9. Beller GA, Ragosta M. Decision making in multivessel coronary disease: the need for physiological lesion assessment. JACC Cardiovasc Interv. 2010;3(3): 315–7. doi:10.1016/j.jcin.2010.01.007.
10. Miller JM, Rochitte CE, Dewey M, Arbab-Zadeh A, Niinuma H, Gottlieb I, et al. Diagnostic performance of coronary angiography by 64-row CT. N Engl J Med. 2008;359(22):2324–36. doi:10.1056/NEJMoa0806576.
11. Meijboom WB, Meijs MF, Schuijf JD, Cramer MJ, Mollet NR, van Mieghem CA, et al. Diagnostic accuracy of 64-slice computed tomography coronary

angiography: a prospective, multicenter, multivendor study. J Am Coll Cardiol. 2008;52(25):2135–44. doi:10.1016/j.jacc.2008.08.058.

12. Meijboom WB, Van Mieghem CA, van Pelt N, Weustink A, Pugliese F, Mollet NR, et al. Comprehensive assessment of coronary artery stenoses: computed tomography coronary angiography versus conventional coronary angiography and correlation with fractional flow reserve in patients with stable angina. J Am Coll Cardiol. 2008;52(8):636–43. doi:10.1016/j.jacc.2008.05.024.
13. Voros S, Rinehart S, Qian Z, Joshi P, Vazquez G, Fischer C, et al. Coronary atherosclerosis imaging by coronary CT angiography: current status, correlation with intravascular interrogation and meta-analysis. JACC Cardiovasc Imaging. 2011;4(5):537–48. doi:10.1016/j.jcmg.2011.03.006.
14. Motoyama S, Sarai M, Harigaya H, Anno H, Inoue K, Hara T, et al. Computed tomographic angiography characteristics of atherosclerotic plaques subsequently resulting in acute coronary syndrome. J Am Coll Cardiol. 2009;54(1):49–57. doi:10.1016/j.jacc.2009.02.068.
15. Motoyama S, Kondo T, Sarai M, Sugiura A, Harigaya H, Sato T, et al. Multislice computed tomographic characteristics of coronary lesions in acute coronary syndromes. J Am Coll Cardiol. 2007;50(4):319–26. doi:10.1016/j.jacc.2007.03.044.
16. Lin F, Shaw LJ, Berman DS, Callister TQ, Weinsaft JW, Wong FJ, et al. Multidetector computed tomography coronary artery plaque predictors of stress-induced myocardial ischemia by SPECT. Atherosclerosis. 2008;197(2): 700–9. doi:10.1016/j.atherosclerosis.2007.07.002.
17. Shmilovich H, Cheng VY, Tamarappoo BK, Dey D, Nakazato R, Gransar H, et al. Vulnerable plaque features on coronary CT angiography as markers of inducible regional myocardial hypoperfusion from severe coronary artery stenoses. Atherosclerosis. 2011;219(2):588–95. doi:10.1016/j.atherosclerosis.2011.07.128.
18. Kim HJ, Vignon-Clementel IE, Coogan JS, Figueroa CA, Jansen KE, Taylor CA. Patient-specific modeling of blood flow and pressure in human coronary arteries. Ann Biomed Eng. 2010;38(10):3195–209. doi:10.1007/s10439-010-0083-6.
19. Koo BK, Erglis A, Doh JH, Daniels DV, Jegere S, Kim HS, et al. Diagnosis of ischemia-causing coronary stenoses by noninvasive fractional flow reserve computed from coronary computed tomographic angiograms. Results from the prospective multicenter DISCOVER-FLOW (Diagnosis of Ischemia-Causing Stenoses Obtained Via Noninvasive Fractional Flow Reserve) study. J Am Coll Cardiol. 2011;58(19):1989–97. doi:10.1016/j.jacc.2011.06.066.
20. Tobis J, Azarbal B, Slavin L. Assessment of intermediate severity coronary lesions in the catheterization laboratory. J Am Coll Cardiol. 2007;49(8):839–48. doi:10.1016/j.jacc.2006.10.055.
21. Raff GL, Abidov A, Achenbach S, Berman DS, Boxt LM, Budoff MJ, et al. SCCT guidelines for the interpretation and reporting of coronary computed tomographic angiography. J Cardiovasc Comput Tomogr. 2009;3(2):122–36. doi:10.1016/j.jcct.2009.01.001.
22. Wong DT, Ko BS, Cameron JD, Nerlekar N, Leung MC, Malaiapan Y et al. Transluminal attenuation gradient in coronary computed tomography angiography is a novel noninvasive approach to the identification of functionally significant coronary artery stenosis: a comparison with fractional flow reserve. J Am Coll Cardiol. 2013;61(12):1271–9. doi:10.1016/j.jacc.2012.12.029.
23. Min JK, Shaw LJ, Devereux RB, Okin PM, Weinsaft JW, Russo DJ, et al. Prognostic value of multidetector coronary computed tomographic angiography for prediction of all-cause mortality. J Am Coll Cardiol. 2007; 50(12):1161–70. doi:10.1016/j.jacc.2007.03.067.
24. Choi JH, Min JK, Labounty TM, Lin FY, Mendoza DD, Shin DH, et al. Intracoronary transluminal attenuation gradient in coronary CT angiography for determining coronary artery stenosis. JACC Cardiovasc Imaging. 2011; 4(11):1149–57. doi:10.1016/j.jcmg.2011.09.006.
25. Hesse B, Tagil K, Cuocolo A, Anagnostopoulos C, Bardies M, Bax J, et al. EANM/ESC procedural guidelines for myocardial perfusion imaging in nuclear cardiology. Eur J Nucl Med Mol Imaging. 2005;32(7):855–97. doi:10.1007/s00259-005-1779-y.
26. Bluemke DA, Achenbach S, Budoff M, Gerber TC, Gersh B, Hillis LD, et al. Noninvasive coronary artery imaging: magnetic resonance angiography and multidetector computed tomography angiography: a scientific statement from the american heart association committee on cardiovascular imaging and intervention of the council on cardiovascular radiology and intervention, and the councils on clinical cardiology and cardiovascular disease in the young. Circulation. 2008;118(5):586–606. doi:10.1161/CIRCULATIONAHA.108.189695.
27. Bacharach SL, Bax JJ, Case J, Delbeke D, Kurdziel KA, Martin WH, et al. PET myocardial glucose metabolism and perfusion imaging: part 1-guidelines for data acquisition and patient preparation. J Nucl Cardiol. 2003;10(5):543–56.
28. Coxson PG, Brennan KM, Huesman RH, Lim S, Budinger TF. Variability and reproducibility of rubidium-82 kinetic parameters in the myocardium of the anesthetized canine. J Nucl Med. 1995;36(2):287–96.
29. Yoshida K, Mullani N, Gould KL. Coronary flow and flow reserve by PET simplified for clinical applications using rubidium-82 or nitrogen-13-ammonia. J Nucl Med. 1996;37(10):1701–12.
30. Hachamovitch R, Berman DS, Shaw LJ, Kiat H, Cohen I, Cabico JA, et al. Incremental prognostic value of myocardial perfusion single photon emission computed tomography for the prediction of cardiac death: differential stratification for risk of cardiac death and myocardial infarction. Circulation. 1998;97(6):535–43.
31. Neglia D, Rovai D, Caselli C, Pietila M, Teresinska A, Aguade-Bruix S, et al. Detection of significant coronary artery disease by noninvasive anatomical and functional imaging. Circ Cardiovasc Imaging. 2015;8(3). doi:10.1161/CIRCIMAGING.114.002179.
32. Cerqueira MD, Weissman NJ, Dilsizian V, Jacobs AK, Kaul S, Laskey WK, et al. Standardized myocardial segmentation and nomenclature for tomographic imaging of the heart. A statement for healthcare professionals from the Cardiac Imaging Committee of the Council on Clinical Cardiology of the American Heart Association. Circulation. 2002;105(4):539–42.
33. Pereztol-Valdes O, Candell-Riera J, Santana-Boado C, Angel J, Aguade-Bruix S, Castell-Conesa J, et al. Correspondence between left ventricular 17 myocardial segments and coronary arteries. Eur Heart J. 2005;26(24):2637–43. doi:10.1093/eurheartj/ehi496.
34. Smith Jr SC, Feldman TE, Hirshfeld Jr JW, Jacobs AK, Kern MJ, King 3rd SB, et al. ACC/AHA/SCAI 2005 guideline update for percutaneous coronary intervention: a report of the American College of Cardiology/American Heart Association Task Force on Practice Guidelines (ACC/AHA/SCAI Writing Committee to Update the 2001 Guidelines for Percutaneous Coronary Intervention). J Am Coll Cardiol. 2006;47(1):e1–121. doi:10.1016/j.jacc.2005.12.001.
35. Miller TD, Hodge DO, Christian TF, Milavetz JJ, Bailey KR, Gibbons RJ. Effects of adjustment for referral bias on the sensitivity and specificity of single photon emission computed tomography for the diagnosis of coronary artery disease. Am J Med. 2002;112(4):290–7.
36. Min JK, Shaw LJ, Berman DS. The present state of coronary computed tomography angiography a process in evolution. J Am Coll Cardiol. 2010; 55(10):957–65. doi:10.1016/j.jacc.2009.08.087.
37. Rispler S, Keidar Z, Ghersin E, Roguin A, Soil A, Dragu R, et al. Integrated single-photon emission computed tomography and computed tomography coronary angiography for the assessment of hemodynamically significant coronary artery lesions. J Am Coll Cardiol. 2007;49(10):1059–67. doi:10.1016/j.jacc.2006.10.069.
38. Schuijf JD, Wijns W, Jukema JW, Atsma DE, de Roos A, Lamb HJ, et al. Relationship between noninvasive coronary angiography with multi-slice computed tomography and myocardial perfusion imaging. J Am Coll Cardiol. 2006;48(12):2508–14. doi:10.1016/j.jacc.2006.05.080.
39. Douglas PS, Hoffmann U, Patel MR, Mark DB, Al-Khalidi HR, Cavanaugh B, et al. Outcomes of anatomical versus functional testing for coronary artery disease. N Engl J Med. 2015;372(14):1291–300. doi:10.1056/NEJMoa1415516.
40. Nakazato R, Shalev A, Doh JH, Koo BK, Dey D, Berman DS, et al. Quantification and characterisation of coronary artery plaque volume and adverse plaque features by coronary computed tomographic angiography: a direct comparison to intravascular ultrasound. Eur Radiol. 2013;23(8):2109–17. doi:10.1007/s00330-013-2822-1.
41. Min JK, Leipsic J, Pencina MJ, Berman DS, Koo BK, van Mieghem C, et al. Diagnostic accuracy of fractional flow reserve from anatomic CT angiography. JAMA. 2012;308(12):1237–45. doi:10.1001/2012.jama.11274.
42. Norgaard BL, Leipsic J, Gaur S, Seneviratne S, Ko BS, Ito H, et al. Diagnostic performance of noninvasive fractional flow reserve derived from coronary computed tomography angiography in suspected coronary artery disease: the NXT trial (Analysis of Coronary Blood Flow Using CT Angiography: Next Steps). J Am Coll Cardiol. 2014;63(12):1145–55. doi:10.1016/j.jacc.2013.11.043.

15

Differential association between metabolic syndrome and coronary artery disease evaluated with cardiac computed tomography according to the presence of diabetes in a symptomatic Korean population

Ki-Bum Won[1,2], Hyuk-Jae Chang[1,5,6*], Jimin Sung[3], Sanghoon Shin[1], In-Jeong Cho[1], Chi-Young Shim[1], Geu-Ru Hong[1], Young Jin Kim[4], Byung-Wook Choi[4] and Namsik Chung[1]

Abstract

Background: Metabolic syndrome (MetS) is associated with increased risks of diabetes and coronary artery disease (CAD). Despite the controversial inclusion of established diabetes in MetS, the association between MetS and CAD according to diabetes status has not been elucidated in the Asian population.

Methods: We evaluated the association between MetS and CAD using the parameters including any plaque, obstructive plaque, and coronary artery calcium score (CACS) >100 according to diabetes status in 2,869 symptomatic Korean subjects who underwent cardiac computed tomographic angiography.

Results: The prevalence of MetS was significantly higher in the diabetic subjects than in the non-diabetic subjects (69% vs. 34%, P <0.001). The incidence of any plaque (64% vs. 43%, P <0.001), obstructive plaque (26% vs. 13%, P = 0.006), and CACS >100 (23% vs. 12%, P = 0.012) was significantly higher in diabetic subjects than in non-diabetic subjects. Among the MetS components, decreased high-density lipoprotein level was significantly associated with any plaque (odds ratio [OR] 1.35), obstructive plaque (OR 1.55), and CACS >100 (OR 1.57) in the non-diabetic subjects (P <0.01, respectively). However, none of the MetS components were associated with all the parameters in the diabetic subjects. Multivariate regression analysis revealed that MetS and the number of MetS components (MetSN) were independently associated with any plaque (MetS: OR 1.55, P <0.001; MetSN: OR 1.22, P <0.001), obstructive plaque (MetS: OR 1.52, P = 0.003; MetSN: OR 1.25, P <0.001), and CACS >100 (MetS: OR 1.46, P = 0.015; MetSN: OR 1.21, P = 0.004) only in the non-diabetic subjects, respectively.

Conclusions: MetS was independently associated with the presence and severity of CAD only in the non-diabetic subjects among the symptomatic Korean population.

Keywords: Metabolic syndrome, Diabetes, Coronary artery disease, Coronary computed tomographic angiography

* Correspondence: hjchang@yuhs.ac
[1]Division of Cardiology, Yonsei Cardiovascular Center, Yonsei University College of Medicine, Seoul, Republic of Korea
[5]Severance Biomedical Science Institute, Seoul, Republic of Korea
Full list of author information is available at the end of the article

Background

Metabolic syndrome (MetS) is a clustering condition of several cardiovascular (CV) risk factors, and it represents insulin resistance as a major characteristic [1]. MetS is associated with the development of coronary artery disease (CAD) and increased risk of CV morbidity and mortality [2]. MetS also increases the risk of diabetes development because its components represent major risk factors for impaired glucose metabolism [3]. Accordingly, MetS has been promoted as a means for identifying the risk of diabetes development in clinical practice. Recently, it has been strongly recommended that conditions with established diabetes should be excluded from the definition of MS [4]. However, data supporting this recommendation are limited, especially regarding coronary atherosclerosis.

A previous study reported that the prevalence of coronary heart disease (CHD) was significantly higher in diabetic subjects with MetS than in those without MetS [2]. However, this study defined CHD with only self-reported myocardial infarction or a positive response to the angina pectoris section of the Rose Questionnaire without an imaging approach for evaluating coronary atherosclerosis [5]. Accordingly, this study might underestimate the prevalence of CHD. In addition, this study was performed only in a Western (U.S) population, including African Americans and Mexican Americans.

Diabetes is a chronic, complex, and progressive illness that requires persistent medical care to prevent major CV complications. Diabetes significantly influences the development of CAD, and most diabetic subjects have MetS, which represents a major phenotype of insulin resistance. Although deterioration of insulin secretion and aggravation of insulin resistance are two major defects in the pathogenesis of diabetes [6,7], the clinical features of type 2 diabetes cases in Asia are explicitly different from those of type 2 diabetes cases in other parts of the world [8]. Several recent studies have reported that impaired insulin secretion was more prominent than insulin resistance, even in the status of impaired glucose tolerance, in Asian subjects [9,10]. Considering that MetS represents insulin resistance as a major characteristic, the impact of MetS on coronary atherosclerosis in diabetic subjects may be different in the Asian population compared with the Western population. However, the association between MetS, individual MetS components, and coronary atherosclerosis according to the presence of diabetes is not elucidated in an Asian population.

Coronary computed tomographic angiography (cCTA) was recently introduced as a novel noninvasive imaging approach for evaluating coronary atherosclerosis and for predicting CAD [11,12]. cCTA has high diagnostic accuracy in detecting CAD [13,14], and the coronary artery calcium score (CACS) is known as a good marker of CAD, representing the degree of atheromatous plaque burden [15,16].

In this study, we aim to evaluate the association between MetS, individual MetS components, and coronary atherosclerosis according to the presence of diabetes in symptomatic Korean subjects who underwent cardiac computed tomographic angiography.

Methods

Study population

This was a cross-sectional study analyzing single-center data collected from 3,159 consecutive symptomatic South Korean subjects who underwent cCTA evaluation with 64-slice multidetector computed tomography (MDCT) at Yonsei Cardiovascular Hospital between January 2005 and April 2009. All participants were referred for evaluation of CAD who had at least one of the symptoms, including typical angina, atypical angina, dyspnea, and excessive fatigue, but were not patients with acute coronary syndrome who required emergent coronary intervention or surgery. Subjects who were younger than 30 years (n = 26), or had an estimated modification of diet in renal disease (MDRD) glomerular filtration rate (GFR) <60 mL/min/1.73m^2 (n = 264) were excluded from the present study according to the study protocol. As a result, 2,869 participants were finally included. All patients provided written informed consent, and ethical approval was obtained from the Institutional Review Board of Severance Hospital, Yonsei University Health System.

MDCT protocol

Subjects with an initial heart rate ≥65 beats/min before MDCT examination received a single oral dose of 50 mg metoprolol tartrate (Betaloc, Yuhan, Seoul, South Korea) 1 h before CT examination unless beta-adrenergic blocking agents were contraindicated owing to overt heart failure, atrioventricular conduction abnormalities, and bronchial asthma. In patients with atrial fibrillation, patients with a mean heart rate >100 beats/min received beta-adrenergic blocking agents orally 1 h before cCTA. If the mean heart rate remained >100 beats/min at the time of scanning, we withdraw the scan. A contrast-enhanced volume data set was acquired with retrospective electrocardiogram gating without using tube current modulation to allow reconstructions during all phases of the cardiac cycle. In subjects with a mild allergy to the contrast material such as drug eruption or urticaria, we used a prophylactic IV steroid. However, we did not allow a scan for the patients with severe allergic reactions such as shock or laryngeal edema.

Imaging was performed for all the subjects using a 64-slice CT scanner (Sensation 64; Siemens Medical System, Forchheim, Germany). All CT examinations were performed during breath holding in inspiration. Initially, a non-enhanced prospective electrocardiogram-gated scan to evaluate CACS was performed with the following parameters: rotation time of 330 ms, slice collimation of 0.6 mm, slice width of 3.0 mm, tube voltage of 100–120 kV, tube current of 50 mA, and table feed/scan of 18 mm. Thereafter, cCTA was performed using retrospective electrocardiographic gating with the following scan parameters: rotation time of 330 ms, slice collimation of 64 × 0.6 mm, tube voltage of 100–120 kV, tube current of 400–800 mA (depending on patient size), table feed/scan of 3.8 mm, and pitch factor of 0.2. ECG-based tube current modulation was applied to 65% of the R–R interval. A real-time bolus-tracking technique was applied to trigger scan initiation. The total estimated average radiation dose for the multislice CT protocol was 8.8 ± 1.6 mSv. Contrast enhancement was achieved with 60 mL iopamidol (370 mg/mL iodine, Iopamiro; Bracco, Milan, Italy) injected at 5 mL/s, followed by an injection of 30 mL of diluted contrast medium (saline-to-contrast agent ratio, 7:3) and then 30 mL saline at 5 mL/s, with a power injector (Envision CT; Medrad, Indianola, PA) via an antecubital vein. The estimated volume CT dose index (CTDIvol) was recorded for each patient. The product of CTDIvol and scanning length (dose–length product, mGy × cm) was calculated, and effective dose was estimated using a normalization factor for the adult chest (0.017 mSv × mGy^{-1} × cm^{-1}). Image reconstruction was performed in the scanner workstation using commercially available software (Wizard, Siemens Medical Solutions). Axial images were reconstructed retrospectively at 65% of the R–R interval for each cardiac cycle. If artifacts were present, additional data sets were obtained for various points of the cardiac cycle, and the data set with the minimum artifact was selected for further analysis. The reconstructed image data sets were transferred to an off-line workstation (Aquar-ius Workstation, TeraRecon, Inc., San Mateo, CA). Each lesion identified was examined using maximum intensity projection and multiplanar reconstruction techniques on a short axis and along multiple longitudinal axes. Lesions were classified by the maximal stenosis of luminal diameter observed on any plane.

Measurement of coronary parameters

All cCTA were evaluated by 2 experienced cardiac radiologists (Y.J.K. and B.W.C., who respectively had 6 and 9 years of experience in cardiac CT). In case of disagreement, a joint reading was performed to reach a consensus. This study primarily evaluated the presence of any plaque, obstructive plaque, and a CACS >100. Both any plaque and obstructive plaque were divided into 2 subtypes according to the presence of coronary calcification as follows: calcified or mixed plaque (CMP) and non-calcified plaque (NCP). CACS was measured with the scoring system using a previously described method [17]. Because the frequency of CACS >100 in the Asian population is known to be low compared with that in Caucasians, African-Americans, and Hispanics [18], and few subjects had a CACS >400 (5%) in the present study, consequently, we used CACS >100 as the parameter for estimating severe coronary calcification. Plaque was defined as structures >1 mm^2 within and/or adjacent to the vessel lumen that were clearly distinguished from the lumen and surrounding pericardial tissue; obstructive plaque was defined as plaque with ≥50% luminal diameter stenosis. CAD was defined as the presence of any coronary plaque identified in cCTA (both non-obstructive and obstructive lesions, including non-calcified plaques).

Measurement of biochemical and clinical parameters

Information on medical history of hypertension, diabetes, and smoking status were systematically collected. Height, weight, and blood pressure were measured during hospital visits. All blood samples were obtained after a minimum 8-h fast and analyzed for triglycerides, high-density lipoprotein (HDL) cholesterol, low-density lipoprotein (LDL) cholesterol, and glucose levels. Body mass index (BMI) was calculated as weight (kg) ÷ height (m^2), and obesity was defined as a BMI ≥25 kg/m^2. Kidney function was assessed based on the estimated GFR calculated using the formula validated in the Modification of Diet in Renal Disease study [19]. Current smoking history was considered present if the subject consistently smoked or smoked within 1 month before the study. MetS was defined as the presence of ≥3 of the following: (a) blood pressure ≥130 mmHg systolic or ≥85 mmHg diastolic, or on antihypertensive treatment; (b) HDL cholesterol level <40 mg/dL in men or <50 mg/dL in women; (c) fasting triglycerides level ≥150 mg/dL; (d) BMI ≥25 kg/m^2; and (e) impaired fasting glucose, defined as a fasting glucose level ≥100 mg/dL, a referral diagnosis of diabetes, or diabetes treatment according to the National Cholesterol Education Program–Adult Treatment Panel III definition [1]. Diabetes was defined as a fasting glucose level ≥126 mg/dL, undergoing an antidiabetic treatment, or a referral diagnosis of diabetes.

Statistical analysis

Clinical, biochemical, and coronary characteristics are described according to the presence of MetS and diabetes. Values are expressed as mean ± SD or n (%). Continuous variables were compared using the Student t-test, and categorical variables were compared using the χ^2 test. The associations between the individual MetS components and the coronary parameters, namely plaque, obstructive plaque, and CACS >100, were analyzed in the subjects with and without diabetes after adjusting for confounding risk factors. Univariate and multivariate logistic regression analyses for identifying the association between MetS and coronary parameters were performed according to diabetes status. These analyses were also performed to identify the association between the increase in number of MetS components (MetSN) and coronary parameters according to diabetes status. The covariate-adjusted odds ratios (OR) and 95% confidence intervals (CI) for each coronary parameter were calculated. Statistical Package for the Social Sciences version 18 (SPSS Inc., Chicago, IL) was used for all the analyses. All the statistical tests were 2-tailed, and P <0.05 was considered significant.

Results

Clinical characteristics

The clinical characteristics of the 2,869 subjects (58 ± 9 years, 51% male) are listed in Table 1. Of the subjects, 2,308 were non-diabetic subjects (80%) and 561 were diabetic subjects (20%). The prevalence of MetS was significantly higher in the diabetic subjects than in the non-diabetic subjects (69% vs. 34%, P <0.001). The incidence of any plaque (64% vs. 43%, P <0.001), obstructive plaque (26% vs. 13%, P = 0.006), and CACS >100 (23% vs. 12%, P = 0.012) was also significantly higher in diabetic subjects than in non-diabetic subjects (Figure 1). The incidence of any plaque (48% vs. 39%, P <0.001), obstructive plaque (15% vs. 11%, P = 0.006), and CACS >100 (14% vs. 10%, P = 0.012), was significantly higher in the non-diabetic subjects with MetS than in those without MetS. However, the incidence of all these parameters was not significantly different in the diabetic subjects according to the presence of MetS (Figure 2).

Association individual MetS component and coronary parameters according to diabetes status

The association between the individual MetS components and the coronary parameters according to the presence of diabetes is presented in Table 2. After adjusting for age, sex, current smoking status, LDL, and GFR, obesity

Table 1 Baseline characteristics

Characteristics	No diabetes			P	Type 2 diabetes			P
	Total (n = 2,308)	No MetS (n = 1,515)	MetS (n = 793)		Total (n = 561)	No MetS (n = 176)	MetS (n = 385)	
Subjects								
Age (years)	57 ± 9	57 ± 9	57 ± 9	0.526	60 ± 9*	61 ± 9	60 ± 8	0.219
Men, n (%)	1,155 (50)	749 (49)	406 (51)	0.430	313 (56)†	105 (60)	208 (54)	0.234
Body mass index (kg/m^2)	24.4 ± 2.8	23.6 ± 2.6	25.9 ± 2.5	<0.001	25.0 ± 3.0*	23.1 ± 2.3	25.9 ± 3.0	<0.001
Current smoking, n (%)	277 (12)	176 (12)	101 (13)	0.500	76 (14)	23 (14)	53 (14)	0.876
SBP (mmHg)	126 ± 15	124 ± 14	130 ± 15	<0.001	128 ± 15†	123 ± 13	130 ± 16	<0.001
DBP (mmHg)	79 ± 10	78 ± 9	81 ± 10	<0.001	78 ± 10	76 ± 9	79 ± 10	<0.001
Antihypertensive treatment, n (%)	1,098 (49)	628 (43)	470 (61)	<0.001	298 (54)†	61 (36)	237 (63)	<0.001
Total cholesterol (mg/dL)	188 ± 35	187 ± 34	190 ± 37	0.047	181 ± 37*	176 ± 36	183 ± 38	0.045
Triglyceride (mg/dL)	140 ± 91	115 ± 61	190 ± 114	<0.001	160 ± 102*	105 ± 50	185 ± 109	<0.001
HDL cholesterol (mg/dL)	51 ± 12	54 ± 12	45 ± 10	<0.001	48 ± 11*	54 ± 11	46 ± 10	<0.001
LDL cholesterol (mg/dL)	120 ± 33	120 ± 32	120 ± 34	0.850	114 ± 38*	115 ± 42	114 ± 36	0.670
Creatinine (mg/dL)	0.90 ± 0.16	0.90 ± 0.16	0.91 ± 0.16	0.182	0.91 ± 0.16	0.91 ± 0.17	0.90 ± 0.16	0.779
GFR (mL/min/1.73 m^2)	82 ± 13	82 ± 13	82 ± 13	0.235	83 ± 14	83 ± 14	82 ± 14	0.513
FBS (mg/dL)	95 ± 10	93 ± 9	100 ± 11	<0.001	135 ± 43*	133 ± 42	135 ± 44	0.584
Duration of diabetes (years)	-	-	-	-	11 ± 7	12 ± 7	10 ± 7	0.094
Anti-diabetic treatment, n (%)	-	-	-	-	433 (77)	133 (76)	300 (78)	0.588
Coronary atherosclerosis parameters, n (%)								
Any plaque	981 (43)	597 (26)	384 (48)	<0.001	359 (64)*	104 (59)	255 (66)	0.108
CMP	797 (35)	480 (32)	317 (40)	<0.001	311 (55)*	96 (55)	215 (56)	0.784
NCP	184 (8)	117 (8)	67 (8)	0.571	48 (9)	8 (5)	40 (10)	0.022
Obstructive plaque	292 (13)	171 (11)	121 (15)	0.007	145 (26)*	44 (25)	101 (26)	0.835
Obstructive CMP	244 (11)	140 (9)	104 (13)	0.005	122 (22)*	39 (22)	83 (22)	0.912
Obstructive NCP	48 (2)	31 (2)	17 (2)	0.876	23 (4)†	5 (3)	18 (5)	0.366
CACS ≥ 100	264 (12)	155 (10)	109 (14)	0.013	129 (23)*	41 (23)	88 (23)	0.946

Data are expressed as n (%) or mean ± SD. CACS, coronary artery calcium score; CAD, coronary artery disease; CMP, calcified or mixed plaque; DBP, diastolic blood pressure; FBS, fasting blood sugar; GFR, glomerular filtration rate; HDL, high-density lipoprotein; LDL, low-density lipoprotein; MetS, metabolic syndrome; NCP, non-calcified plaque; SBP, systolic blood pressure. *P <0.001 vs. no diabetes. †P <0.05 vs. no diabetes.

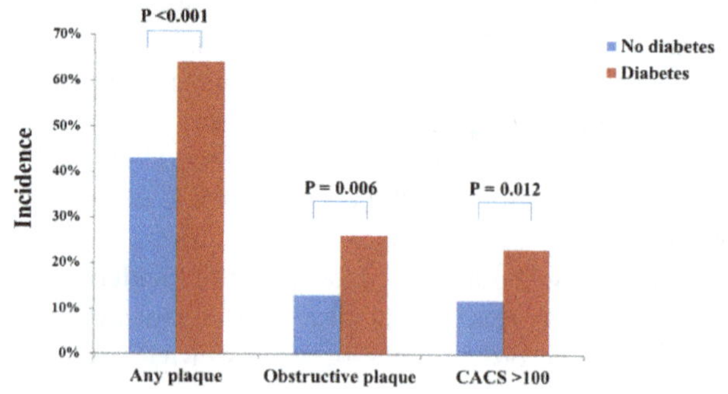

Figure 1 Comparison of the incidence of coronary parameters according to diabetes status.

was significantly associated with any plaque (OR 1.27, 95% CI 1.05–1.55, P = 0.016). Increased blood pressure and increased triglycerides were significantly associated with any plaque (increased blood pressure: OR 1.25, 95% CI 1.01–1.55, P = 0.045; increased triglycerides: OR 1.37, 95% CI 1.12–1.68, P = 0.002) and obstructive plaque (increased blood pressure: OR 1.59, 95% CI 1.14–2.23, P = 0.006; increased triglycerides: OR 1.56, 95% CI 1.18–2.06, P = 0.002). Decreased HDL level was significantly associated with any plaque (OR 1.35, 95% CI 1.09–1.68, P = 0.007), obstructive plaque (OR 1.55, 95% CI 1.14–2.10, P = 0.005), and CACS >100 (OR 1.57, 95% CI 1.12–2.19, P = 0.008) in the non-diabetic subjects. However, no MetS components were significantly associated with all the coronary parameters in the diabetic subjects.

Association between MetS, MetSN, and coronary parameters according to diabetes status

The association between MetS, the MetSN, and the coronary parameters, including any plaque, obstructive plaque, and CACS >100 according to the presence of diabetes are presented in Table 3. The univariate logistic regression analysis revealed that MetS was significantly associated with increased risks of all coronary parameters in the non-diabetic subjects (any plaque: OR 1.44, 95% CI 1.21–1.72, P <0.001; obstructive plaque: OR 1.42, 95% CI 1.10–1.82, P = 0.007; CACS >100: OR 1.40, 95% CI 1.08–1.82, P = 0.012). However, MetS was not significantly associated with any of these parameters in the diabetic subjects. The MetSN was significantly associated with increased risks of all coronary parameters in the non-diabetic subjects (any plaque: OR 1.19, 95% CI 1.11–1.28, P <0.001; obstructive plaque: OR 1.22, 95% CI 1.10–1.35, P <0.001; CACS >100: OR 1.18, 95% CI 1.06–1.32, P = 0.002) but not in the diabetic subjects. After adjusting for age, sex, current smoking status, LDL, and GFR, MetS was significantly associated with increased risks of all the coronary parameters in the non-diabetic subjects (any plaque: OR 1.55, 95% CI 1.27–1.89, P <0.001; obstructive plaque: OR 1.52, 95% CI 1.15–2.01, P = 0.003; CACS >100: OR 1.46, 95% CI 1.08–1.99, P = 0.015). However, MetS was not significantly associated with any of these parameters in the diabetic subjects. The MetSN was significantly associated with increased risks of all the coronary parameters in the non-diabetic subjects (any plaque: OR 1.22, 95% CI 1.12–1.32, P <0.001; obstructive plaque: OR 1.25, 95% CI 1.11–1.41, P <0.001; CACS >100: OR 1.21, 95% CI 1.06–1.37, P = 0.004) but not in the diabetic subjects (Figure 3).

Discussion

To the best of our knowledge, these are the first findings on the differential association between MetS and CAD according to diabetes status in a symptomatic Asian population. We identified that both MetS and MetSN were independently associated with the presence of plaque, obstructive plaque, and CACS >100 in the subjects without established diabetes. However, despite the significantly higher incidence of all the coronary parameters in the diabetic subjects than in the non-diabetic subjects, MetS, the individual MetS components, and the MetSN were not significantly associated with all these parameters in diabetic subjects.

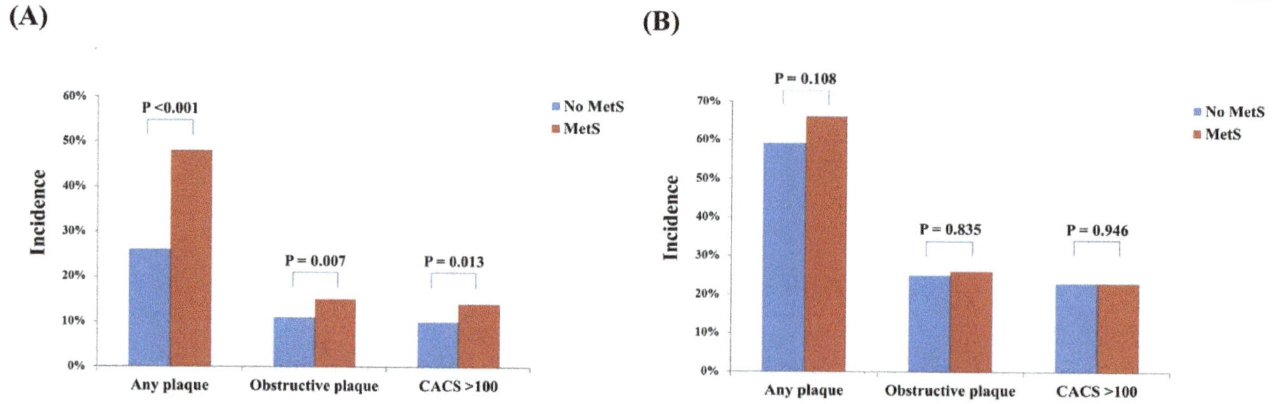

Figure 2 Comparison of the incidence of coronary parameters according to MetS status. (A) Non-diabetes and (B) diabetes.

Table 2 Association between individual MetS component and coronary parameters according to diabetes status

Characteristic	n	Any plaque OR (95% CI)	Obstructive plaque OR (95% CI)	CACS >100 OR (95% CI)
No diabetes	2308			
Obesity				
No	1383	1.00	1.00	1.00
Yes	925	1.27 (1.05–1.55) ‡	1.20 (0.91–1.59)	1.19 (0.88–1.62)
Increased blood pressure				
No	664	1.00	1.00	1.00
Yes	1644	1.25 (1.01–1.55)‡	1.59 (1.14–2.23)†	1.27 (0.89–1.81)
Increased triglycerides				
No	1522	1.00	1.00	1.00
Yes	786	1.37 (1.12–1.68)†	1.56 (1.18–2.06)†	1.18 (0.87–1.62)
Decreased HDL				
No	1616	1.00	1.00	1.00
Yes	692	1.35 (1.09–1.68)†	1.55 (1.14–2.10)†	1.57 (1.12–2.19)†
Increased fasting glucose				
No	1640	1.00	1.00	1.00
Yes	668	1.22 (0.99–1.50)	0.97 (0.72–1.31)	1.24 (0.90–1.69)
Type 2 diabetes	561			
Obesity				
No	288	1.00	1.00	1.00
Yes	273	1.27 (0.85–1.90)	0.86 (0.57–1.31)	1.12 (0.72–1.75)
Increased blood pressure				
No	140	1.00	1.00	1.00
Yes	421	1.03 (0.65–1.63)	0.76 (0.48–1.21)	1.11 (0.66–1.86)
Increased triglycerides				
No	315	1.00	1.00	1.00
Yes	246	1.34 (0.89–2.02)	1.00 (0.65–1.53)	0.93 (0.59–1.47)
Decreased HDL				
No	347	1.00	1.00	1.00
Yes	214	0.92 (0.60–1.40)	1.44 (0.93–2.24)	1.13 (0.70–1.82)

All models are adjusted for age, sex, current smoking, LDL, and GFR. CACS, coronary artery calcium score; CI, confidence intervals; GFR, glomerular filtration rate; HDL, high-density lipoprotein; LDL, low-density lipoprotein, MetS, metabolic syndrome; OR, odds ratios. *P <0.001; †P <0.01; ‡P <0.05.

Table 3 Association between MetS, MetSN, and coronary parameters according to diabetes status

	Any plaque				Obstructive plaque				CACS >100			
	Univariate		Multivariate		Univariate		Multivariate		Univariate		Multivariate	
	OR	95% CI	OR	95% CI	OR	95% CI	OR	95% CI	OR	95% CI	OR	95% CI
No diabetes												
MetS	1.44	1.21–1.72*	1.55	1.27–1.89*	1.42	1.10–1.82†	1.52	1.15–2.01†	1.40	1.08–1.82‡	1.46	1.08–1.99‡
MetSN	1.19	1.11–1.28*	1.22	1.12–1.32*	1.22	1.10–1.35*	1.25	1.11–1.41*	1.18	1.06–1.32†	1.21	1.06–1.37†
Diabetes												
MetS	1.36	0.94–1.96	1.38	0.90–2.12	1.07	0.71–1.61	0.98	0.63–1.52	0.99	0.65–1.50	1.10	0.69–1.77
MetSN	1.06	0.89–1.25	1.11	0.92–1.35	1.01	0.84–1.21	0.99	0.81–1.21	0.94	0.78–1.14	1.05	0.85–1.30

CACS, coronary artery calcium score; CI, confidence intervals; LDL, low-density lipoprotein; MetS, metabolic syndrome; MetSN, number of metabolic syndrome components; OR, odd ratios.
Multivariate models are adjusted for age, sex, current smoking, LDL, and GFR. *P <0.001; †P <0.01; ‡P <0.05

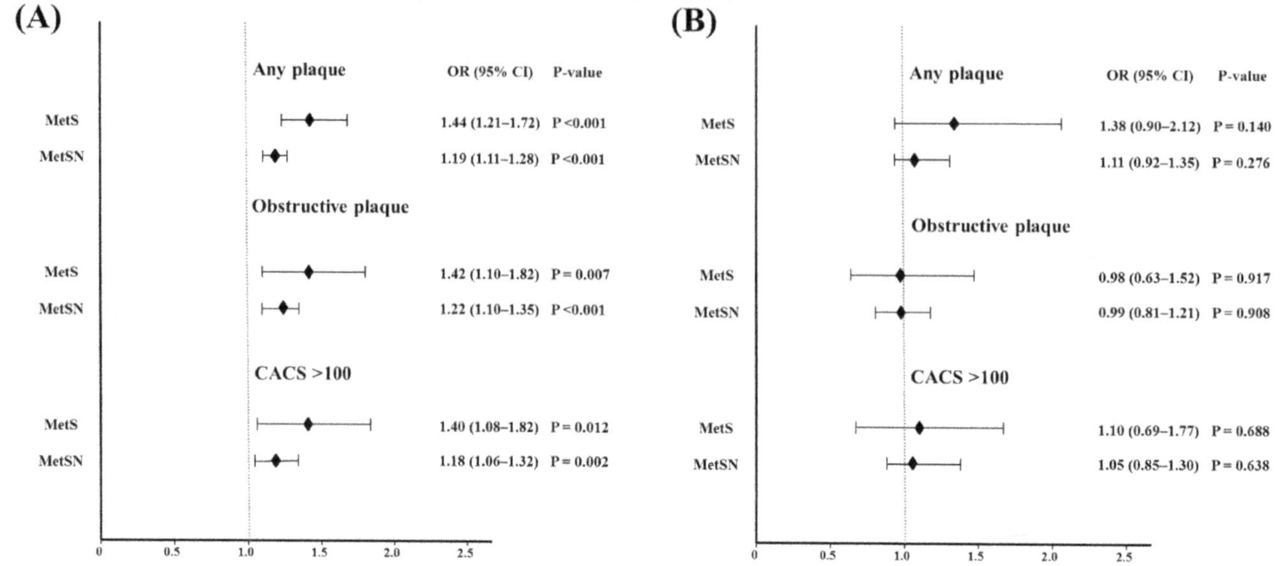

Figure 3 Impact of MetS and MetSN on the coronary parameters (multivariate analysis). (A) Non-diabetes and (B) diabetes.

The prevalence of MetS is rapidly increasing worldwide [20,21], and is affecting approximately 31% of adults in South Korea [22]. MetS and diabetes share many common characteristics, and 65–85% of diabetic patients have MetS [23,24]. Despite the similarities, MetS is considered as a pre-morbid condition rather than a clinical diagnosis and has been promoted as a means of identifying the risk of diabetes development [25]. However, most definitions of MetS simultaneously include diabetes in the diagnostic criteria as a component of impaired fasting glucose. The World Health Organization (WHO) strongly recommends that the conditions of established diabetes or CV disease should be excluded from MetS [4], but data supporting this recommendation are limited.

Previous studies have reported that the progression of atherosclerosis is independently associated with long-term hyperglycemia in patients with established diabetes [26,27]. Recently, Church et al. [28] reported that the presence of diabetes in the Aerobics Center Longitudinal Study was associated with a threefold greater mortality risk from CV disease and that MetS status did not modify this risk. Won et al. [29] reported that MetS was significantly associated with subclinical atherosclerosis, which is evaluated with brachial-ankle pulse wave velocity and carotid intima-media thickness and plaque, in conditions without diabetes and that a concurrent diagnosis of MetS might be of little value for predicting subclinical atherosclerosis in diabetic subjects. These results suggest the clinical usefulness of MetS for CV risk stratification only in subjects without established diabetes. Although MetS and diabetes are associated with an increased risk of major CV events, recent studies have suggested that people with these conditions face a wide range of increased risks of CV events and that coronary artery calcium is a good parameter for predicting CV events in people with MetS and diabetes [30-32]. Although these studies identified the strong influence of MetS and diabetes on coronary calcification, they did not evaluate the differential impact of MetS on coronary calcification according to diabetes status. Moreover, there is a paucity of data on the association between MetS and coronary plaque according to the presence of diabetes. The present study identified the different association between MetS and coronary atherosclerosis according to diabetes status. MetS was independently associated with any plaque, obstructive plaque, and CACS >100 only in the non-diabetic subjects after adjusting for confounding risk factors. In addition, although the incidence of these coronary parameters tended to increase according to the increase of MetSN in all participants (Additional file 1: Table S1), the MetSN was also independently associated with these coronary parameters only in the non-diabetic subjects. These results suggest that the progression of coronary atherosclerosis may be influenced by multiple metabolic risk factors in non-diabetic subjects but may be predominantly dependent on long-term hyperglycemia in subjects with established diabetes status [26,27].

The present study evaluated the association between the individual MetS component and coronary atherosclerosis according to the presence of diabetes. Among all the coronary atherosclerotic parameters, the identification of obstructive plaque might be the most important because this study was performed in symptomatic subjects. Although the measurement of CACS was not recommended in symptomatic subjects, the incidence of obstructive plaque was similar with that of CACS >100 in both the non-diabetic and diabetic subjects among the symptomatic

Korean population. Interestingly, the components of increased blood pressure, increased triglycerides level, and decreased HDL level were independently associated with obstructive plaque in the non-diabetic subjects, but no MetS components were associated with obstructive plaque in the diabetic subjects. In the multivariate regression analysis for identifying the association between the individual MetS component and subtypes of obstructive plaque according to diabetes status, increased blood pressure, increased triglycerides level, and decreased HDL level were associated with obstructive CMP, not obstructive NCP, in the non-diabetic subjects. However, none of MetS components were associated with either obstructive CMP or obstructive NCP in the diabetic subjects (Additional file 2: Table S2). In the present study, we could not evaluate the association between impaired fasting glucose and obstructive plaque in the diabetic subjects because all of them had impaired fasting glucose. The component of impaired fasting glucose was unable to reflect differences in degree of hyperglycemic control, diabetes duration, and diabetes treatment in the diabetic subjects. Considering the significantly higher incidence of obstructive plaque in diabetic subjects than in non-diabetic subjects, these factors might be more closely related to obstructive plaque compared with the other MetS components in an established diabetic condition.

The present study has some limitations. First, we did not involve asymptomatic subjects in the present study. However, the application of cCTA for CV risk stratification in asymptomatic or low CV risk subjects has not been justified [33]. Second, we could not eliminate the possible effects of underlying medication on CAD because of the observational design of this study. Third, although we analyzed the association between MetS, individual MetS components, and plaque subtype, the incidence of NCP and obstructive NCP was too low to identify the impact of MetS and its individual component on these coronary parameters. Lastly, in the present study, we identified only the differential impact of MetS and its individual components on CAD, focusing on the presence of plaque, obstructive plaque, and coronary calcification, using MDCT according to diabetes status. Recent CT studies investigating patients with acute coronary syndrome have identified high-risk plaque features characteristic of culprit lesions, such as low plaque attenuation, positive remodeling, and spotty calcification [34,35]. Further large-scale investigations for identifying the impact of MetS and diabetes on plaque vulnerability may be necessary in subjects with suspected CAD.

Despite the several limitations of the present study, it was unique in that we identified the association between MetS and CAD according to the diabetic status of the subjects of Asian ethnicity only. Considering the clinical features of diabetic subjects in the Asian population might be explicitly different compared with those in a Western population, identification of the impact of MetS and its individual components on coronary atherosclerosis according to diabetes status in the Asian population might be important. The present study identified that MetS and the MetSN were independently associated with the presence and severity of CAD only in the non-diabetic subjects, despite the significant impact of diabetes on CAD in symptomatic Korean subjects. Moreover, this might provide clinical evidence related to the WHO recommendation that established diabetes should be excluded from MetS.

Conclusions

In conclusion, MetS was independently associated with the presence and severity of CAD only in the non-diabetic subjects among the symptomatic Korean population. However, despite the significantly higher incidence of all the coronary parameters in the diabetic subjects than in the non-diabetic subjects, MetS, the individual MetS components, and the MetSN were not significantly associated with the presence and severity CAD in the diabetic subjects.

Abbreviations

BMI: Body mass index (BMI); CACS: Coronary artery calcium score; CAD: Coronary artery disease; cCTA: Coronary computed tomographic angiography; CHD: Coronary heart disease; CI: Confidence intervals (CI); CMP: Calcified or mixed plaque; CV: Cardiovascular; GFR: Glomerular filtration rate; HDL: High-density lipoprotein; LDL: Low-density lipoprotein; MetS: Metabolic syndrome; MetSN: Number of MetS components; MDCT: Multidetector computed tomography; NCP: Non-calcified plaque; OR: Odds ratios.

Competing interests

The authors declare that they have no competing interests.

Authors' contributions

All authors have made substantial contributions. KW and HC conducted the design of the study. SS, IC, CS, and GH conducted all clinical measurements. YK and BC conducted all image measurements. KW and JS conducted the statistical analyses. NC reviewed, corrected and helped finalize the manuscript. All authors read and approved the final manuscript.

Acknowledgment

This research was supported by the Leading Foreign Research Institute Recruitment Program through the National Research Foundation of Korea, funded by the Ministry of Education, Science and Technology (2012027176).

Author details

[1]Division of Cardiology, Yonsei Cardiovascular Center, Yonsei University College of Medicine, Seoul, Republic of Korea. [2]Division of Cardiology, St. Luke's International Hospital, Tokyo, Japan. [3]Graduate School of Health and Welfare CHA University, Seongnam, Republic of Korea. [4]Division of Radiology, Yonsei Cardiovascular Center, Yonsei University College of Medicine, Seoul, Republic of Korea. [5]Severance Biomedical Science Institute, Seoul, Republic of

Korea. [6]Yonsei Cardiovascular Center, Yonsei University College of Medicine, 50 Yonsei-ro, Seodaemun-gu, Seoul 120-752, Republic of Korea.

References

1. NCEP: **Executive summary of the third report of the national cholesterol education program (NCEP) expert panel on detection, evaluation, and treatment of high blood cholesterol in adults (adult treatment panel III.** *JAMA* 2001, **285:**2486–2497.
2. Alexander CM, Landsman PB, Teutsch SM, Haffner SM: **NCEP-defined metabolic syndrome, diabetes, and prevalence of coronary heart disease among NHANES III participants age 50 years and older.** *Diabetes* 2003, **52:**1210–1214.
3. Haffner SM, Valdez RA, Hazuda HP, Mitchell BD, Morales PA, Stern MP: **Prospective analysis of the insulin-resistance syndrome (syndrome X).** *Diabetes* 1992, **41:**715–722.
4. Simmons RK, Alberti KG, Gale EA, Colagiuri S, Tuomilehto J, Qiao Q, Ramachandran A, Tajima N, Brajkovich Mirchov I, Ben-Nakhi A, Reaven G, Hama Sambo B, Mendis S, Roglic G: **The metabolic syndrome: useful concept or clinical tool? Report of a WHO expert consultation.** *Diabetologia* 2010, **53:**600–605.
5. Rose GA, Blackburn H, Gillium RF, Prineas RJ: *Cardiovascular Survey Methods.* 2nd edition. Geneva: Switzerland, World Health Organization; 1982.
6. Welsh M, Mares J, Oberg C, Karlsson T: **Genetic factors of importance for beta-cell proliferation.** *Diabetes Metab Rev* 1993, **9:**25–36.
7. DeFronzo RA: **Pathogenesis of type 2 diabetes mellitus.** *Med clin North Am* 2004, **88:**787–835.
8. Yoon KH, Lee JH, Kim JW, Cho JH, Choi YH, Ko SH, Zimmet P, Son HY: **Epidemic obesity and type 2 diabetes in Asia.** *Lancet* 2006, **368:**1681–1688.
9. Shin CS, Lee HK, Koh CS, Kim YI, Shin YS, Yoo KY, Paik HY, Park YS, Yang BG: **Risk factors for the development of NIDDM in Yonchon County, Korea.** *Diabetes Care* 1997, **20:**1842–1846.
10. Kim DJ, Lee MS, Kim KW, Lee MK: **Insulin secretory dysfunction and insulin resistance in the pathogenesis of korean type 2 diabetes mellitus.** *Metabolism* 2001, **50:**590–593.
11. Budoff MJ, Dowe D, Jollis JG, Gitter M, Sutherland J, Halamert E, Scherer M, Bellinger R, Martin A, Benton R, Delago A, Min JK: **Diagnostic performance of 64-multidetector row coronary computed tomographic angiography for evaluation of coronary artery stenosis in individuals without known coronary artery disease: results from the prospective multicenter ACCURACY (assessment by coronary computed tomographic angiography of individuals undergoing invasive coronary angiography) trial.** *J Am Coll Cardiol* 2008, **52:**1724–1732.
12. Miller JM, Rochitte CE, Dewey M, Arbab-Zadeh A, Niinuma H, Gottlieb I, Paul N, Clouse ME, Shapiro EP, Hoe J, Lardo AC, Bush DE, de Roos A, Cox C, Brinker J, Lima JA: **Diagnostic performance of coronary angiography by 64-row CT.** *N Engl J Med* 2008, **359:**2324–2336.
13. Hoffmann MH, Shi H, Schmitz BL, Schmid FT, Lieberknecht M, Schulze R, Ludwig B, Kroschel U, Jahnke N, Haerer W, Brambs HJ, Aschoff AJ: **Noninvasive coronary angiography with multislice computed tomography.** *JAMA* 2005, **293:**2471–2478.
14. Cho I, Min HS, Chun EJ, Park SK, Choi Y, Blumenthal RS, Rivera JJ, Nasir K, Kim YJ, Sohn DW, Oh BH, Park YB, Chang HJ: **Coronary atherosclerosis detected by coronary CT angiography in asymptomatic subjects with early chronic kidney disease.** *Atherosclerosis* 2010, **208:**406–411.
15. Budoff MJ, Shaw LJ, Liu ST, Weinstein SR, Mosler TP, Tseng PH, Flores FR, Callister TQ, Raggi P, Berman DS: **Long-term prognosis associated with coronary calcification: observations from a registry of 25,253 patients.** *J Am Coll Cardiol* 2007, **49:**1860–1870.
16. Detrano R, Guerci AD, Carr JJ, Bild DE, Burke G, Folsom AR, Liu K, Shea S, Szklo M, Bluemke DA, O'Leary DH, Tracy R, Watson K, Wong ND, Kronmal RA: **Coronary calcium as a predictor of coronary events in four racial or ethnic groups.** *N Engl J Med* 2008, **358:**1336–1345.
17. Agatston AS, Janowitz WR, Hildner FJ, Zusmer NR, Viamonte M Jr, Detrano R: **Quantification of coronary artery calcium using ultrafast computed tomography.** *J Am Coll Cardiol* 1990, **15:**827–832.
18. Nasir K, Shaw LJ, Liu ST, Weinstein SR, Mosler TR, Flores PR, Flores FR, Raggi P, Berman DS, Blumenthal RS, Budoff MJ: **Ethnic differences in the prognostic value of coronary artery calcification for all-cause mortality.** *J Am Coll Cardiol* 2007, **50:**953–960.
19. Levey AS, Coresh J, Balk E, Kausz AT, Levin A, Steffes MW, Hogg RJ, Perrone RD, Lau J, Eknoyan G: **National Kidney Foundation practice guidelines for chronic kidney disease: evaluation, classification, and stratification.** *Ann Intern Med* 2003, **139:**137–147.
20. Mozumdar A, Liguori G: **Persistent increase of prevalence of metabolic syndrome among U.S. adults: NHANES III to NHANES 1999–2006.** *Diabetes Care* 2011, **34:**216–219.
21. Nestel P, Lyu R, Low LP, Sheu WH, Nitiyanant W, Saito I, Tan CE: **Metabolic syndrome: recent prevalence in East and Southeast Asian populations.** *Asia Pac J Clin Nutr* 2007, **16:**362–367.
22. Lim S, Shin H, Song JH, Kwak SH, Kang SM, Won YJ, Choi SH, Cho SI, Park KS, Lee HK, Jang HC, Koh KK: **Increasing prevalence of metabolic syndrome in Korea: the Korean National Health and Nutrition Examination Survey for 1998–2007.** *Diabetes Care* 2011, **34:**1323–1328.
23. Koehler C, Ott P, Benke I, Hanefeld M: **Comparison of the prevalence of the metabolic syndrome by WHO, AHA/NHLBI, and IDF definitions in a German population with type 2 diabetes: the diabetes in Germany (DIG) study.** *Horm Metab Res* 2007, **39:**632–635.
24. Tong PC, Kong AP, So WY, Yang X, Ho CS, Ma RC, Ozaki R, Chow CC, Lam CW, Chan JC, Cockram CS: **The usefulness of the international diabetes federation and the national cholesterol education Program's adult treatment panel III definitions of the metabolic syndrome in predicting coronary heart disease in subjects with type 2 diabetes.** *Diabetes Care* 2007, **30:**1206–1211.
25. Gupta AK, Prieto-Merino D, Dahlöf B, Sever PS, Poulter NR: **Metabolic syndrome, impaired fasting glucose and obesity, as predictors of incident diabetes in 14120 hypertensive patients of ASCOT-BPLA: comparison of their relative predictability using a novel approach.** *Diabet Med* 2011, **28:**941–947.
26. Sander D, Schulze-Horn C, Bickel H, Gnahn H, Bartels E, Conrad B: **Combined effects of hemoglobin A1c and C-reactive protein on the progression of subclinical carotid atherosclerosis: the INVADE study.** *Stroke* 2006, **37:**351–357.
27. Larsen JR, Brekke M, Bergengen L, Sandvik L, Arnesen H, Hanssen KF, Dahl-Jorgensen K: **Mean HbA1c over 18 years predicts carotid intima media thickness in women with type 1 diabetes.** *Diabetologia* 2005, **48:**776–779.
28. Church TS, Thompson AM, Katzmarzyk PT, Sui X, Johannsen N, Earnest CP, Blair SN: **Metabolic syndrome and diabetes, alone and in combination, as predictors of cardiovascular disease mortality among men.** *Diabetes Care* 2009, **32:**1289–1294.
29. Won KB, Chang HJ, Kim HC, Jeon K, Lee H, Shin S, Cho IJ, Park SH, Lee SH, Jang Y: **Differential impact of metabolic syndrome on subclinical atherosclerosis according to the presence of diabetes.** *Cardiovasc Diabetol* 2013, **12:**41.
30. Bulugahapitiya U, Siyambalapitiya S, Sithole J, Idris I: **Is diabetes a coronary risk equivalent? systematic review and metaanalysis.** *Diabet Med* 2009, **26:**142–148.
31. Wong ND, Nelson JC, Granston T, Bertoni AG, Blumenthal RS, Carr JJ, Guerci A, Jacobs DR Jr, Kronmal R, Liu K, Saad M, Selvin E, Tracy R, Detrano R: **Metabolic syndrome, diabetes, and incidence and progression of coronary calcium: the Multiethnic Study of Atherosclerosis study.** *JACC Cardiovasc Imaging* 2012, **5:**358–366.
32. Malik S, Budoff MJ, Katz R, Blumenthal RS, Bertoni AG, Nasir K, Szklo M, Barr RG, Wong ND: **Impact of subclinical atherosclerosis on cardiovascular disease events in individuals with metabolic syndrome and diabetes: the multi-ethnic study of atherosclerosis.** *Diabetes Care* 2011, **34:**2285–2290.
33. Cho I, Chang HJ, Sung JM, Pencina MJ, Lin FY, Dunning AM, Achenbach S, Al-Mallah M, Berman DS, Budoff MJ, Callister TQ, Chow BJ, Delago A, Hadamitzky M, Hausleiter J, Maffei E, Cademartiri F, Kaufmann P, Shaw LJ, Raff GL, Chinnaiyan KM, Villines TC, Cheng V, Nasir K, Gomez M, Min JK: **Coronary computed tomographic angiography and risk of all-cause mortality and nonfatal myocardial infarction in subjects without chest pain syndrome from the CONFIRM Registry (coronary CT angiography evaluation for clinical outcomes: an international multicenter registry).** *Circulation* 2012, **126:**304–313.

16

Dual-time-point myocardial ^{18}F-FDG imaging in the detection of coronary artery disease

Ke-Fei Dou[1*†], Xiao-Jin Gao[1,2], Bo-Qia Xie[3], Yan Li[4], Zuo-Xiang He[4] and Min-Fu Yang[5*†]

Abstract

Background: Myocardial ^{18}F-deoxyglucose (^{18}F-FDG) uptake has been observed to be enhanced in patients with coronary artery disease (CAD) under fasting conditions. However, whether the increased ^{18}F-FDG is induced by myocardial ischemia and how to discriminate ischemic from physiological ^{18}F-FDG uptake have rarely been investigated.

Methods: Under fasting conditions, ^{18}F-FDG PET imaging was performed in 52 patients with suspected CAD. Two ^{18}F-FDG imaging sessions were conducted within two hours after a single administration of ^{18}F-FDG (dual-time-point imaging), and with an intervention of an exercise test after the first imaging. Abnormal ^{18}F-FDG uptake was determined by the classification of the ^{18}F-FDG distribution pattern, and the changes of the ^{18}F-FDG distribution between the two PET imaging sessions were analyzed. ^{99m}Tc-sestamibi was injected at peak exercise and myocardial perfusion imaging (MPI) was conducted after ^{18}F-FDG imaging. Coronary angiography was considered the reference for diagnosing CAD.

Results: Overall, 54.8% (17/31) of CAD patients and 36.2% (21/58) of stenotic coronaries showed exercise-induced abnormal uptake of ^{18}F-FDG. Based on the classification of the ^{18}F-FDG distribution pattern, the sensitivity and specificity of exercise ^{18}F-FDG imaging to diagnose CAD was 80.6% and 95.2% by patient analysis, 56.9% and 98.0% by vascular analysis, respectively. Compared with MPI, ^{18}F-FDG imaging had a tendency to have higher sensitivity (80.6% vs 64.5%, $P = 0.06$) on the patient level.

Conclusion: Myocardial ischemia can induce ^{18}F-FDG uptake. With the classification of the ^{18}F-FDG distribution pattern, dual-time-point ^{18}F-FDG imaging under fasting conditions is efficient in diagnosing CAD.

Keywords: Dual-time-point imaging, ^{18}F-FDG, Coronary artery disease, Myocardial ischemia

Background

Glucose uptake in normal myocardium is suppressed under fasting conditions, nevertheless myocardial ischemia results in a dramatic switch of metabolic substrate to glucose uptake. Hence, the ischemic and normal myocardium have significant difference in glucose uptake [1, 2]. Therefore, myocardial ^{18}F-deoxyglucose (^{18}F-FDG) imaging under fasting conditions is in theory a potential method to detect myocardial ischemia. Previous studies have observed enhanced ^{18}F-FDG uptake in myocardium supplied by stenotic coronaries or in myocardium with perfusion abnormalities [3–11]. However, whether the enhanced ^{18}F-FDG uptake is induced by myocardial ischemia is controversial [12], since non-ischemic myocardium can also exhibit varying extents of ^{18}F-FDG uptake even under strict dietary control [13–15]. In the present study, we performed dual-time-point imaging within two hours after a single administration of ^{18}F-FDG, and myocardial ischemia was induced using an exercise test after the first imaging. We speculated that most factors that presumably affect myocardial ^{18}F-FDG uptake would not significantly change in such a short time, and thus we could evaluate whether exercise-induced myocardial ischemia would induce myocardial ^{18}F-FDG uptake.

Moreover, even if myocardial ischemia can induce ^{18}F-FDG uptake, another issue that comes along is

* Correspondence: drdoukefei@126.com; minfuyang@126.com
†Equal contributors
1 State Key Laboratory of Cardiovascular Disease, Department of Cardiology, Cardiovascular Institute, Fuwai Hospital and National Center for Cardiovascular Diseases, Chinese Academy of Medical Sciences and Peking Union Medical College, Beijing, China
5 Department of Nuclear Medicine, Beijing Chaoyang Hospital, Capital Medical University, 8th Gongtinanlu Rd, Chaoyang District, Beijing 100020, China
Full list of author information is available at the end of the article

how to differentiate the ischemic uptake from the uptake in non-ischemic myocardium, which was considered physiological. Several studies have investigated the distribution pattern of ^{18}F-FDG in patients without heart disease [11, 16, 17]. These studies found that most individuals had no obvious ^{18}F-FDG uptake, or had diffuse but homogenous uptake. Contrarily, 'focal' or 'focal on diffuse' uptake was rarely observed. Even if some patients showed focal uptake, the uptake was usually located on the basal segments, including the papillary muscle. We had adopted these classification methods to differentiate ischemic from physiological uptake in patients with suspected unstable angina who underwent resting ^{18}F-FDG imaging, and obtained favorable diagnostic results [11]. In this study, we evaluated the diagnostic performance of ^{18}F-FDG imaging in patients with suspected CAD using the classification of ^{18}F-FDG distribution pattern.

Methods

Study population

This prospective study was approved by the Institutional Ethics Committee of Fuwai Hospital, and written consent was obtained from all patients before study entry. Fifty-five patients with suspected stable angina (37 patients) or unstable angina (18 patients) were recruited. Patients with suspected unstable angina were simultaneously included in the other study aiming at investigating the value of ^{18}F-FDG imaging in the diagnosis of unstable angina [11]. Angina was well controlled in all patients and no new onset of angina occurred for > 40 h before the entry to the present study. Patients with the following conditions were not recruited: prior myocardial infarction (history of previously documented myocardial infarction or Q waves on electrocardiogram), acute myocardial infarction, unable to exercise, prior coronary revascularization of less than 3 months, left bundle branch block, diagnosed valvular heart disease, or idiopathic cardiomyopathy.

Study protocol

Figure 1 shows the flow diagram of the study protocol. Enrolled subjects were asked to have an overnight fast (>12 h). The imaging studies were arranged in the morning, and anti-angina medications were withheld for > 12 h before exercise testing. Patients first had their blood glucose levels measured using finger blood samples, and then were intravenously injected with ^{18}F-FDG (5–8 mCi) at rest. Thereafter, patients underwent two separate PET imaging sessions with a single dose of ^{18}F-FDG. This imaging protocol was named as dual-time-point imaging. Briefly, patients underwent the first ^{18}F-FDG imaging (rest) using PET/CT one hour after ^{18}F-FDG injection. After the first imaging session, they immediately underwent a symptom-limited exercise test using a bicycle ergometer with continuous electrocardiogram (ECG) and blood pressure monitoring. ^{99m}Tc-sestamibi (20–25 mCi) was intravenously injected at peak exercise. Approximately two hours after ^{18}F-FDG injection, the second ^{18}F-FDG imaging (exercise) was performed.

Exercise ^{99m}Tc-sestamibi myocardial perfusion imaging (MPI) was done after the second ^{18}F-FDG imaging using SPECT. Resting MPI was completed within 3 days of exercise imaging.

Image acquisition and reconstruction

^{18}F-FDG images were acquired, using a Biograph 64 PET/CT scanner (Siemens Medical Solutions, Knoxville, TN, USA) equipped with high-performance LSO PET crystals and a 64-slice CT. After a scout CT acquisition (120 kV, 10 mA), used for appropriate patient positioning, a CT transmission scan (140 kV, 35 mA) was performed for attenuation correction and anatomical localization. PET images were then acquired in list mode with a static 10-min frame. Raw images of ^{18}F-FDG were reconstructed by iterative ordered subset expectation maximization (OSEM) reconstructions (8 subsets, 4 iterations) and automatically corrected for photon attenuation using the CT scans.

Exercise ^{99m}Tc-sestamibi images were obtained as previously described using a dual-head, large-field-of-view SPECT (Infinia; GE Healthcare, Milwaukee, Wisconsin, USA), equipped with ultra-high-energy parallel-hole collimators [9, 11]. Resting ^{99m}Tc-sestamibi images were obtained using the same SPECT with ultra-high-energy parallel-hole collimators or low-energy high-resolution parallel-hole collimators. Thirty projection images were acquired over a 180° arc at 6° intervals. Perfusion images were reconstructed using standard filtered back projection.

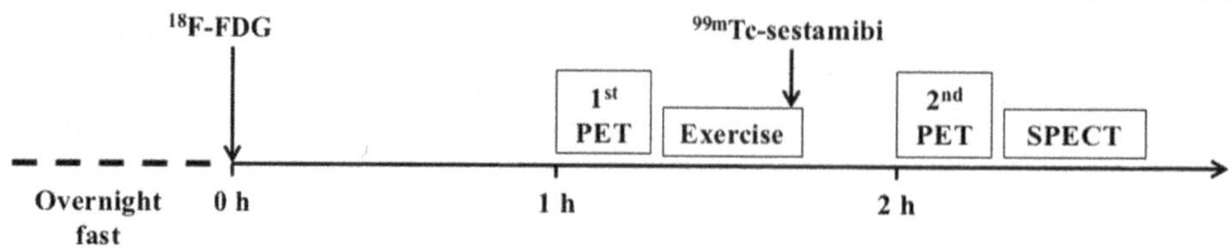

Fig. 1 Schematic of imaging protocols

Image analysis

^{18}F-FDG and ^{99m}Tc-sestamibi images were analyzed separately. Two experienced nuclear physicians interpreted the images independently, and disagreements were resolved by consensus.

^{18}F-FDG

^{18}F-FDG images were first semi-quantitatively analyzed using standard uptake value (SUV). The left ventricle was divided into 17 segments using the standard American Heart Association model, and each segment was further assigned to three major coronary territories. The maximal SUV of each segment (SUV_{myo}) was manually measured guided by CT and fusion images. The SUV of each coronary was represented by the highest segmental SUV_{myo} within its territory. Furthermore, a ROI of 3.0 cm^3 was placed over the LV chamber near the mitral valve plane to measure the SUV_{blood}. Each pair of ROIs on the rest and exercise images was carefully placed on the same region.

Thereafter, the myocardial^{18}F-FDG uptake of left ventricle as a whole was classified into four patterns, based on the results of semi-quantitative analysis as well as visual observation [11, 16, 17]: the 'none' pattern, indicated the SUV_{myo} in all segments was below or equal to the SUV_{blood}; the 'diffuse' pattern, indicated the SUV_{myo} in all segments was higher than the SUV_{blood}, nonetheless no significant difference existed among them (i.e., homogenous uptake); the 'focal' pattern, indicated that at least one segment had a SUV_{myo} higher than the SUV_{blood} and the SUV_{myo} in other segments was below or equal to the SUV_{blood}; and the 'focal on diffuse' pattern, indicated the SUV_{myo} in all segments was higher than the SUV_{blood}, and even higher uptake was identified in one or more segments. Finally, focal uptake in the 'focal' or 'focal on diffuse' pattern was defined as abnormal, except those on the basal segments and papillary muscle, which were considered normal [18]. Moreover, the changes of ^{18}F-FDG distribution pattern between exercise and resting images were analyzed.

^{99m}Tc-sestamibi

^{99m}Tc-sestamibi images were scored using the same 17-segment model, but with a 5-score scale (0 = normal uptake, 1 = mild, 2 = moderate and 3 = severe reduction in uptake, and 4 = no uptake). Exercise–rest perfusion defects were classified as fixed, reversible, or partially reversible. Abnormal ^{99m}Tc-sestamibi uptake was further assigned to three major coronary territories.

Coronary angiography

Coronary angiography within 3 months of scintigraphic imaging was analyzed. Angiographic results were reviewed for the presence, localization, and severity of coronary artery lesions. Luminal diameter narrowing of ≥ 50% in any of the major epicardial coronary arteries was considered significant and was defined as CAD.

Statistical analysis

Statistical analyses were performed using SPSS software (version 17.0, SPSS, Inc, Chicago, IL, USA). Continuous variables were described as means and standard deviations (SD) or medians and interquartile ranges, depending on the normality of distribution assessed using the Kolmogorov-Smirnoff test. Categorical variables were described as numbers and percentage. Paired *t* test or Wilcoxon rank test was used to compared the differences of SUVs between resting and exercise ^{18}F-FDG imaging, depending on the normality of the distribution. McNemar's test was used to compare the differences of the diagnostic performance between perfusion and ^{18}F-FDG imaging, and to compare the differences of the prevalence rate of ^{18}F-FDG abnormalities between resting and exercise imaging. The variables that potentially influenced the diagnostic sensitivity of ^{18}F-FDG imaging, were analyzed using χ^2 test. A P value of < 0.05 was considered statistically significant.

Results

Patient characteristics

Of 55 patients initially recruited, 3 cases without coronary angiography were excluded from the final analysis. The demographic, angiographic, and exercise testing data of the remaining 52 patients are listed in Table 1. Of them, 54% were men and the average age was 58 ± 8 years. Ten subjects (19%) had a history of percutaneous coronary intervention (>3 months). Coronary angiography showed significant coronary stenosis in 58 coronaries of 31 patients. Of them, 1-, 2- and 3-vessel disease was 42%, 29%, and 29%, respectively. The mean exercise time was 461 ± 169 s, and the rate-pressure product increased from (7.9 ± 1.9) x 10^3 at baseline to (22.0 ± 6.5) x 10^3 at peak exercise. During exercise, 32% of the patients had chest pain and 48% of the patients had ischemic ECG changes.

Myocardial perfusion imaging

In total, 20 CAD patients had perfusion abnormalities. Of them, 6 patients had partially reversible perfusion defects, and 14 had reversible perfusion defects. No patients without CAD showed perfusion abnormality. Therefore, the sensitivity and specificity of exercise MPI in the diagnosis of CAD was 64.5% and 100%, respectively. By vascular analysis, the sensitivity and specificity was 53.4% and 99.0%, respectively (Table 2).

Table 1 Patient characteristics

Characteristics	Results
Age (years)	58 ± 8
Male (%)	28 (54)
Diabetes mellitus (%)	22 (42)
Hypertension (%)	38 (73)
Hypercholesterolemia (%)	32 (62)
Smoker (%)	21 (40)
Family history of CAD	7 (14)
Previous PCI (%)	10 (19)
Blood glucose (mmol/L)	6.7 ± 1.5
Coronary angiography (%)	
One-vessel disease	13 (42)
Two-vessel disease	9 (29)
Three-vessel disease	9 (29)
Exercise test	
Exercise time (s)	461 ± 169
Baseline RPP	7900 ± 1900
Peak RPP	22000 ± 6500
Chest pain (%)	17 (32)
Positive ECG results (%)	25 (48)

CAD coronary artery disease, *PCI* percutaneous coronary intervention; and RPP, rate pressure product

^{18}F-FDG imaging

Changes of ^{18}F-FDG uptake on dual-time-point imaging

By semi-quantitative analysis, all coronary territories with abnormal ^{18}F-FDG uptake showed an increase in SUV_{myo} on exercise imaging, and that was only 44.6% in coronaries with normal ^{18}F-FDG uptake (Fig. 2a-c). Meanwhile, the SUV_{blood} was decreased on exercise imaging in all patients (Fig. 2d-f). Consequently, the SUV_{myo}/SUV_{blood} consistently increased from rest to exercise ^{18}F-FDG imaging in all coronaries, nevertheless, coronaries with abnormal ^{18}F-FDG uptake had a higher increment (Fig. 2g-i).

By qualitative analysis, 10 CAD patients had abnormal ^{18}F-FDG uptake on exercise imaging but normal uptake on resting imaging (Fig. 3a-b, Figs. 4 and 5). Fifteen patients had abnormal uptake on both imaging, but 7 of them had more myocardial segments involved on the exercise imaging (Fig. 6). Of the stenotic coronaries, 12 showed abnormal ^{18}F-FDG uptake exclusively on exercise imaging. Twenty-one stenotic coronaries showed abnormal uptake on both imaging, but 9 of them had more myocardial segments involved on the exercise imaging (Fig. 3c-d). In sum, 54.8% (17/31) of CAD patients and 36.2% (21/58) of stenotic coronaries exhibited exercise-induced ^{18}F-FDG changes.

Diagnostic performance of ^{18}F-FDG imaging

By patient analysis, abnormal ^{18}F-FDG uptake was present on exercise imaging in 26 patients (25 with CAD and 1 without CAD). The sensitivity and specificity of exercise ^{18}F-FDG imaging in the diagnosis of CAD was 80.6% (25/31) and 95.2% (20/21) (Table 2), respectively. Compared with MPI, ^{18}F-FDG imaging had a tendency to have higher sensitivity (80.6% vs 64.5%, P = 0.06), but similar specificity (95.2% vs 100%, P = 1.00).

By vascular analysis, abnormal ^{18}F-FDG uptake was present on exercise imaging in 35 coronary territories (33 with and 2 without significant stenosis). The sensitivity and specificity of exercise ^{18}F-FDG imaging in the detection of stenotic coronaries were 56.9% (33/58) and 98.0% (96/98) (Table 2), respectively. Both the sensitivity and specificity of exercise ^{18}F-FDG imaging were not significantly different from that of MPI (sensitivity: 56.9% vs 53.4%, P = 0.79; specificity: 98.0% vs 99.0%, P = 1.00).

Variables related to the diagnostic performance of ^{18}F-FDG imaging

The sensitivity of single-vessel and multi-vessel disease was comparable at both patient level (69.2% vs 94.1%, P = 0.14) and individual vessel level (69.2% vs 57.8%, P = 0.46) (Fig. 7a).

The sensitivity was not significantly different between patients with suspected stable angina and unstable angina both on patient and vascular level (Fig. 7b).

Diabetic patients had higher blood glucose than non-diabetes (7.6 ± 0.3 mmol/l vs 5.9 ± 0.1 mmol/l, $P < 0.0001$). Compared with normal subjects, diabetic patients had similar SUV_{blood} (1.66 ± 0.20 vs 1.70 ± 0.35, P = 0.59), but lower SUV_{myo} (1.62 ± 0.97 vs 2.78 ± 1.78, P = 0.0027) and SUV_{myo}/SUV_{blood} (1.19 ± 0.72 vs 1.99 ± 1.28, P = 0.0032) on resting imaging. ^{18}F-FDG imaging had a trend to have higher sensitivity for diabetic patients on the patient level (P = 0.07, Fig. 7c) but not on the vascular level (P = 0.57) (Fig. 7c).

Table 2 Diagnostic performance of exercise perfusion and ^{18}F-FDG imaging

	Patient analysis		Vascular analysis	
	Sensitivity	Specificity	Sensitivity	Specificity
^{99m}Tc-sestamibi	64.5% (20/31)	100% (21/21)	53.4% (31/58)	99.0% (97/98)
^{18}F-FDG	80.6% (25/31)	95.2% (20/21)	56.9% (33/58)	98.0% (96/98)
P value	0.06	1.00	0.79	1.00

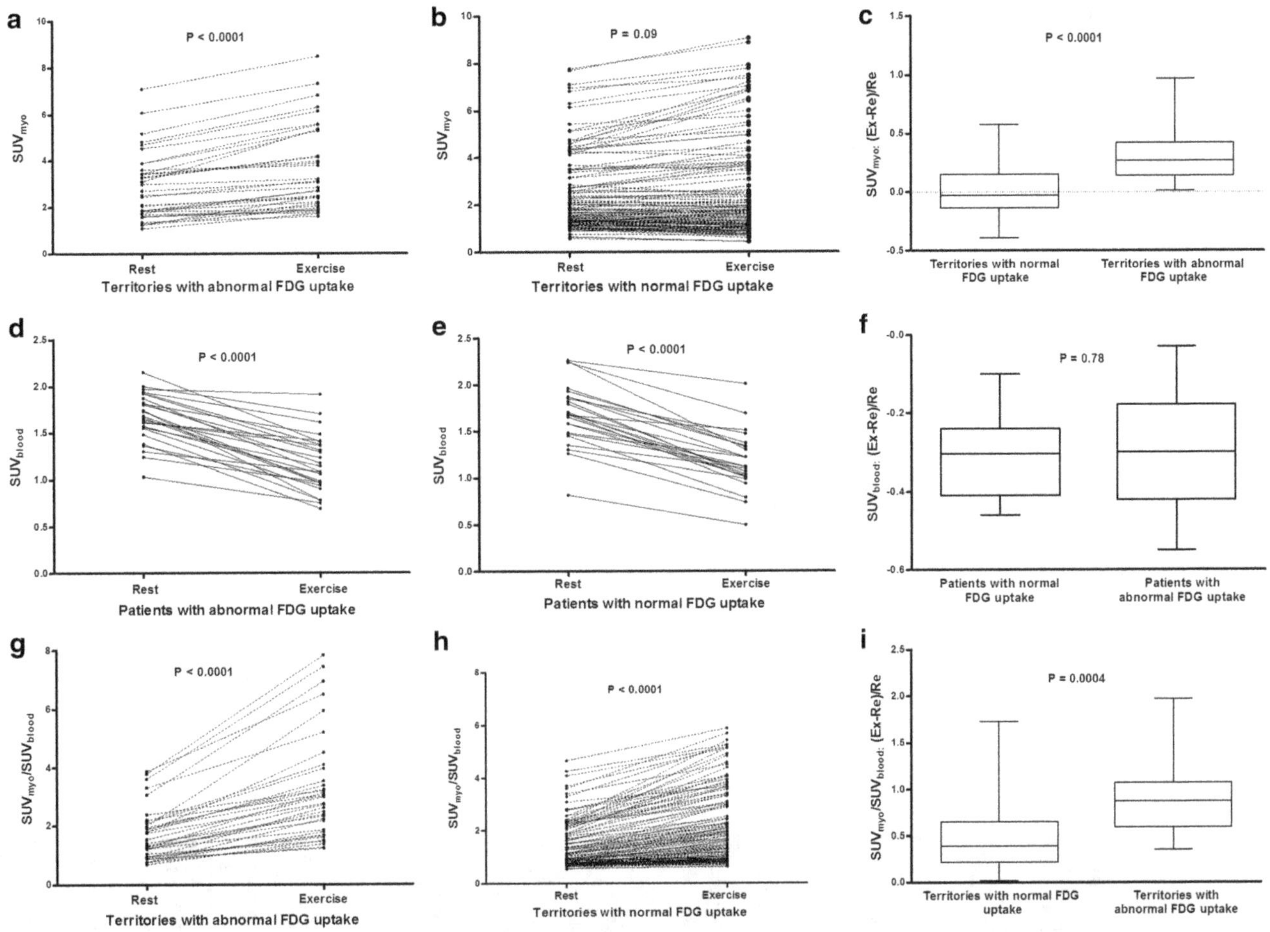

Fig. 2 SUV changes of ^{18}F-FDG uptake on dual-time-point imaging. All coronary territories with abnormal ^{18}F-FDG uptake show an increase in SUV_{myo} on exercise imaging (**a**). Contrarily, only 44.6% of coronaries with normal ^{18}F-FDG uptake show increased uptake (**b**). Therefore, the increment in territories with abnormal ^{18}F-FDG uptake is significant higher than that in normal territories (**c**). The SUV_{blood} consistently decreases from rest to exercise imaging in patients with abnormal (**d**) and normal ^{18}F-FDG uptake (**e**), and the reduction is similar between the two groups (**f**). As a result, although both abnormal and normal territories show an increase in SUV_{myo}/SUV_{blood} (**g, h**), the increment is higher in territories with abnormal ^{18}F-FDG uptake (**i**)

Discussion

By the direct comparison of the images obtained before and after an exercise test within two hours, the present study demonstrated a significant change of ^{18}F-FDG uptake in CAD patients and stenotic coronaries. Previous studies have reported enhanced ^{18}F-FDG uptake in patients with CAD under fasting conditions [3–11]. However, myocardial ^{18}F-FDG uptake is spatially heterogeneous even under strict dietary control [13–15]. Patients without documented CAD can also have regional or global myocardial uptake, which is known as 'non-specific' or 'physiological'. Physiological uptake is mostly localized on, but not confined to, the basal segments. Therefore, regional ^{18}F-FDG uptake, even in the territory supplied by the stenotic coronary, may only be physiological. As a result, although ^{18}F-FDG imaging had a relatively high sensitivity in the diagnosis of CAD, its specificity was rarely investigated and presumably poor [10]. To clarify the specificity of ^{18}F-FDG imaging, we had conducted exercise and resting ^{18}F-FDG imaging in CAD patients during two sequential days [9]. Resting imaging was 24 h after exercise imaging. We speculated that the ischemic uptake of ^{18}F-FDG on exercise imaging should decrease or disappear on resting imaging. In that study, 87% of the patients with increased ^{18}F-FDG uptake on exercise imaging showed decreased or no discernible uptake on resting imaging, which in part supported that ^{18}F-FDG uptake was a specific marker for myocardial ischemia. The other 13% patients had persistent uptake which was interpreted as ischemic memory. However, several studies have found that normal myocardium could also show a significant change in ^{18}F-FDG uptake among serial examinations [14, 15], which was considered as temporal heterogeneity. A number of known factors (hormones, dietary preparation, exercise, etc.) and unknown factors might

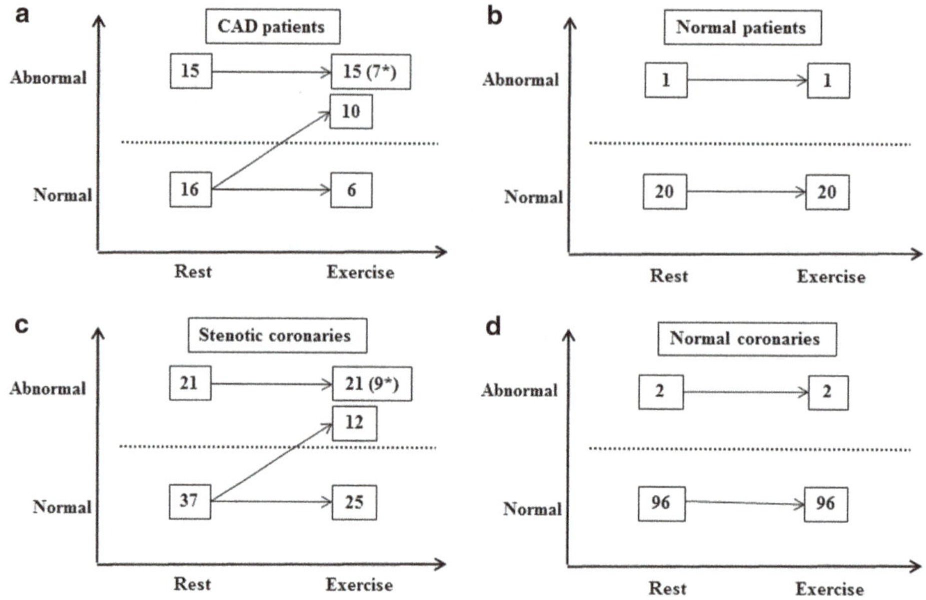

Fig. 3 Changes of ^{18}F-FDG distribution characteristics between resting and exercise imaging. By patientanalysis, the prevalence rate of ^{18}F-FDGabnormalities increases from 48.4% (15/31) on resting imaging to80.6% (25/31) (P = 0.004) on exercise imaging in CAD patient (**a**) nevertheless it does not significantly change in patients without CAD [4.8% (1/21) vs 4.8% (1/21) P = NS] (**b**) By vascular analysis, the prevalence rate of ^{18}F-FDG abnormalities on exercise imaging is significantly higher than that on resting imaging in stenotic coronaries [56.9% (33/58) vs 34.5% (21/58), P < 0.0001] (**c**) but not in normal coronaries [2.0% (2/98) vs 2.0% (2/98), P = NS] (**d**). (*)*Indicates the increased ^{18}F-FDG uptake is exclusively located on the basal segments or papillary muscle*

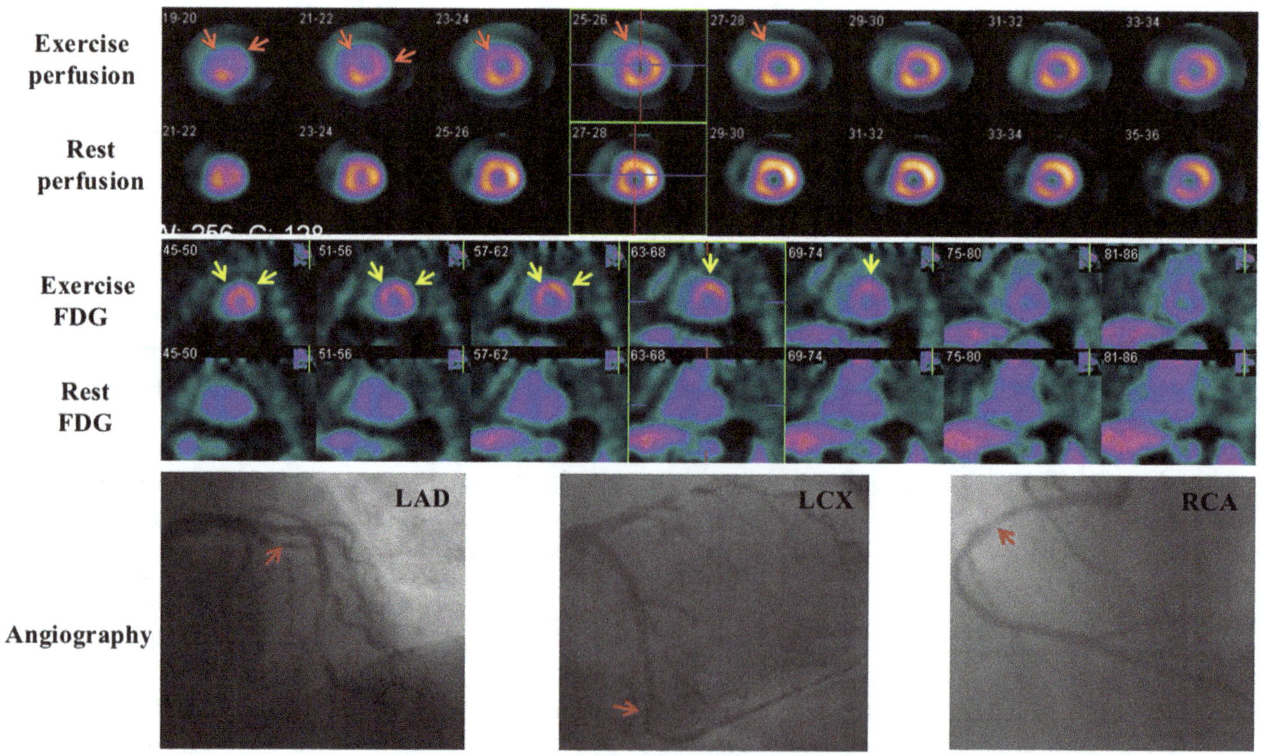

Fig. 4 Images of a 61-year-old woman. She had a 99% stenosis in the left anterior descending coronary (LAD), a 90% stenosis in the left circumflex coronary (LCX), and a 70% stenosis in the right coronary artery (RCA). Perfusion images show reversible defects in the anterior and lateral wall (*red arrows*). Resting ^{18}F-FDG images indicate only background uptake in the cardiac cavities and no visible uptake in the left ventricular wall ('none' pattern). Nevertheless, exercise ^{18}F-FDG images exhibit intense uptake in the anterior and lateral wall ('focal' pattern, *yellow arrows*) which is in accordance with exercise perfusion images

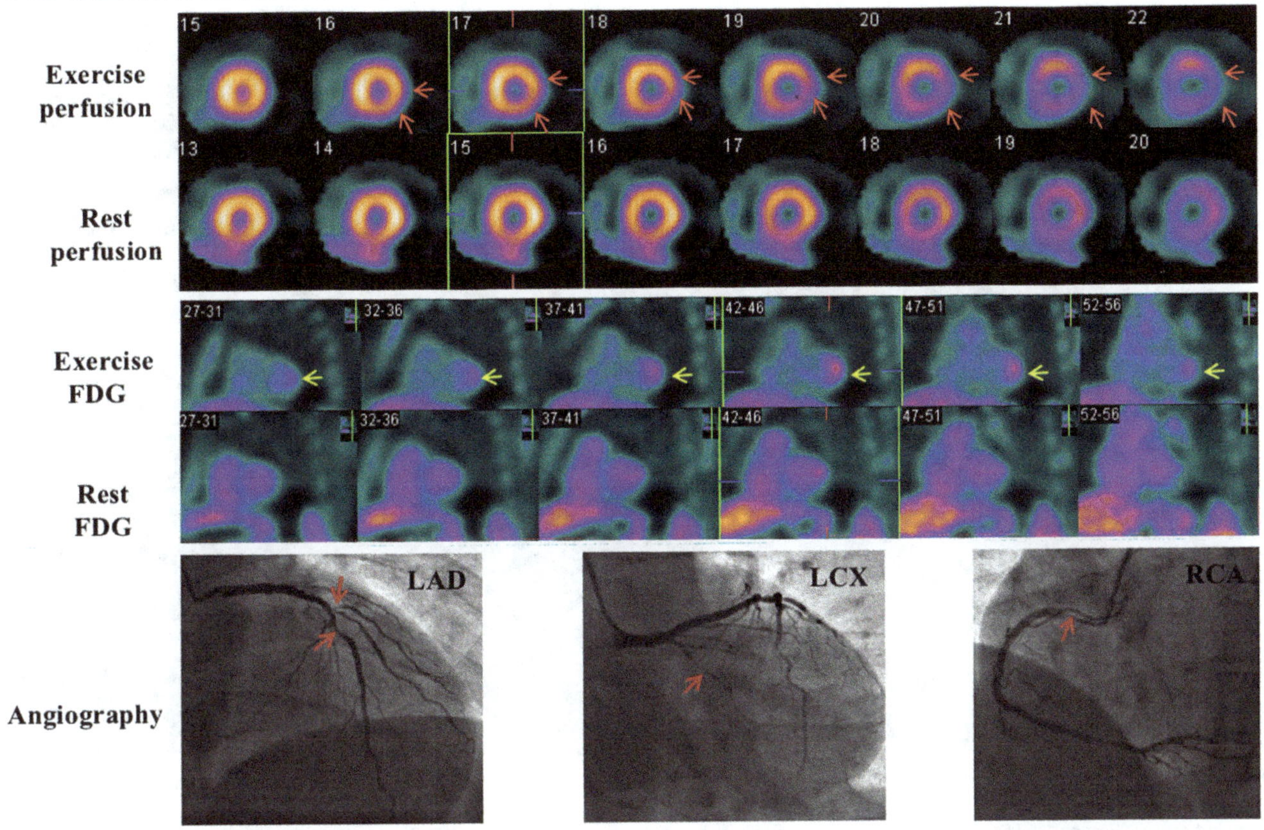

Fig. 5 Images of a 39-year-old man. He had a 70% stenosis in the LAD and a 90% stenosis in the diagonal branch, a 100% stenosis in the LCX, and a 90% stenosis in the proximal RCA. Perfusion images show reversible defects in the lateral wall (*red arrows*). Resting ^{18}F-FDG images indicate background uptake in the cardiac cavities and no visible uptake in the left ventricular wall ('none' pattern), exercise ^{18}F-FDG images exhibit intense uptake in the lateral wall ('focal' pattern, *yellow arrows*) which is in accordance with exercise perfusion images

influence myocardial ^{18}F-FDG uptake, and it was difficult to modulate these conditions to the same level on different days. Contrary to the prior studies [14, 15], the two ^{18}F-FDG imaging sessions in this study were performed within a very short interval of two hours, and only with a single administration of ^{18}F-FDG. This could, to the greatest extent, alleviate the differences of the aforementioned factors between exercise and resting imaging. Catecholamines released during exercise stress suppress exogenous glucose metabolism in normal myocardium but do not alter anaerobic glucose metabolism in ischemic myocardium [12, 19], but no study has reported that that effect was spatially heterogeneous. Hence, the regionally increased uptake on exercise imaging in CAD patients was most likely induced by myocardial ischemia. The significance of the present study was, for the first time, providing unequivocal evidence in support of that myocardial ischemia can induce ^{18}F-FDG uptake.

On the exercise imaging, the ^{18}F-FDG uptake in ischemic myocardium was consistently increased. Contrarily, non-ischemic myocardium showed variable changes of ^{18}F-FDG uptake and nearly half of them had decreased uptake. Moreover, the SUV_{blood} consistently decreased on the exercise imaging both in CAD and normal patients. Therefore, the ^{18}F-FDG distribution changes between resting and exercise imaging was due to the increased uptake ratio of ischemic to non-ischemic myocardium as well as the myocardium to background radioactivity.

Of note, some patients showed ischemic ^{18}F-FDG uptake on resting and nearly half (7/15) of them had more segments involved on exercise imaging. Abnormal ^{18}F-FDG uptake at rest may be induced by resting ischemia since 6 patients had perfusion abnormalities at rest in this study. Moreover, patients with unstable angina may have abnormal ^{18}F-FDG uptake at rest due to ischemic memory, even without perfusion abnormalities, which had been validated in prior studies [11, 20].

To determine the abnormality of ^{18}F-FDG uptake, we adopted the classification of ^{18}F-FDG distribution patterns and defined the uptake of basal segments and papillary muscle as normal, as recommended recently for the 'hot' spot imaging for the heart [18]. This study

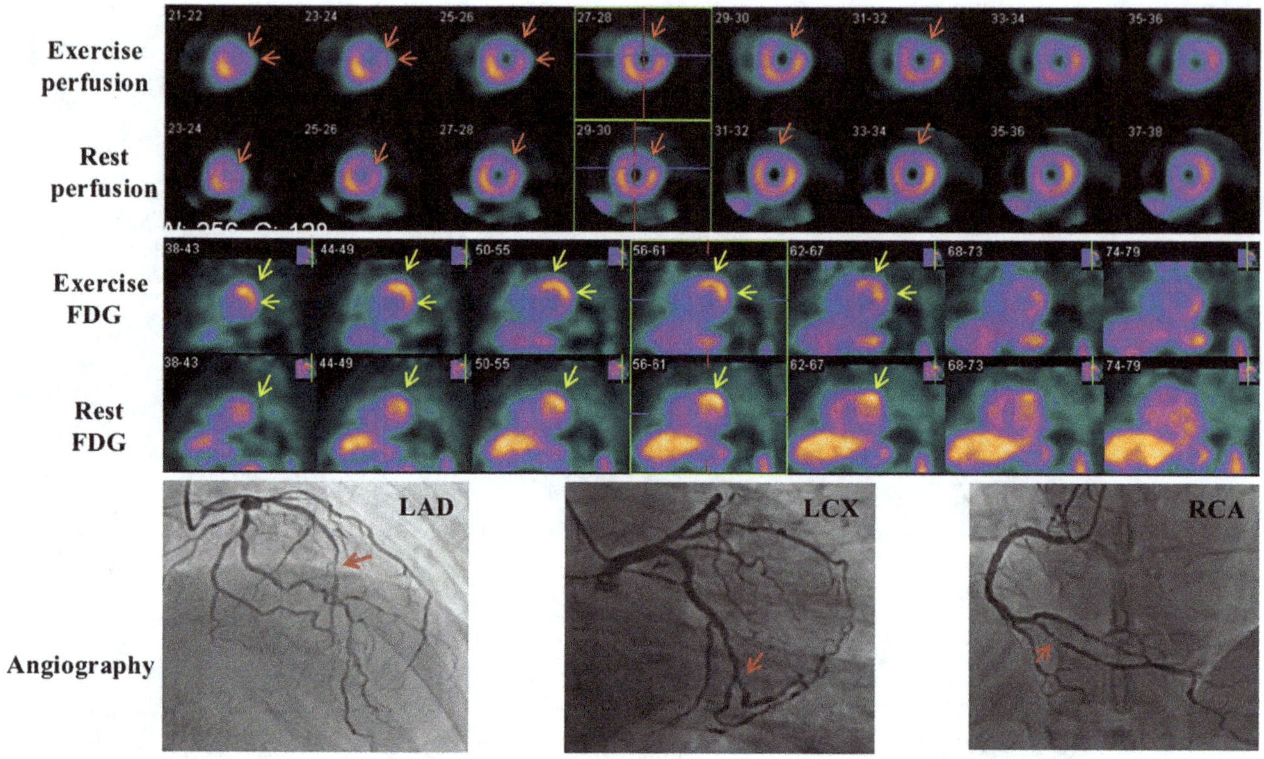

Fig. 6 Images of a 55-year-old woman. She had multiple lesions of > 90% stenosis in the LAD, multiple lesions of 60-80% stenosis in the LCX, and a distal lesion of 90% stenosis in the RCA. Perfusion images show partially reversible defects in the anterior and anterolateral wall ('focal' pattern, *red arrows*). Resting ^{18}F-FDG images show mild uptake in the anterior and anterolateral wall. On exercise images, ^{18}F-FDG uptake is further increased compared with resting images, and the involved area is enlarged as well ('focal' pattern, *yellow arrows*)

demonstrated this strategy was efficient for the detection of CAD. Overall, the diagnostic performance was comparable between ^{18}F-FDG imaging and MPI. Especially, a favorable specificity was obtained on both patient and vascular levels. In this study, all patients with perfusion abnormalities showed abnormal ^{18}F-FDG uptake on exercise imaging. Furthermore, 45.5% (5/11) of CAD patients with normal perfusion were detected by ^{18}F-FDG imaging as well. This implied that ^{18}F-FDG imaging may be more sensitive than MPI. It is important to note, the

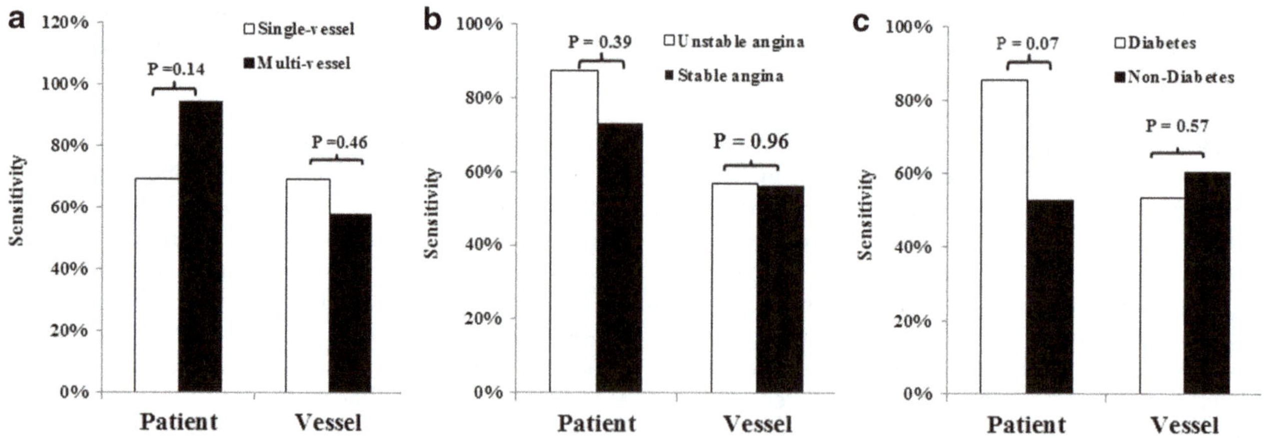

Fig. 7 Variables influence the diagnostic sensitivity of ^{18}F-FDG imaging. The sensitivity of single-vessel and multivessel disease was comparable at both patient level and individual vessel level (**a**) The difference of sensitivity is not significant between stable and unstable angina (**b**) and is borderline on the patient level but not on the vascular level between diabetic and non-diabetic patients (**c**)

difference of the sensitivity between ^{18}F-FDG imaging and MPI was merely borderline (P = 0.06) on the patient level. In contrast, previous studies have reported higher sensitivity of ^{18}F-FDG imaging over MPI [7, 10]. There were two major differences between the present and prior studies. First, ^{18}F-FDG was administered at peak exercise in previous studies. Contrarily, ^{18}F-FDG was injected one hour prior to exercise in the present study. Due to the extraction by myocardium and other tissues, and clearance from urinary and digestive system, ^{18}F-FDG in blood at the onset of exercise-induced ischemia was decreased. In addition, if physiological uptake of myocardium prior to exercise was too intense, new ischemic uptake might be masked. Second, only focally increased ^{18}F-FDG uptake was defined as abnormal in this study, whereas diffuse but homogeneous uptake and basal (including papillary muscle) uptake were also considered abnormal in prior studies [3–11]. The current definitions inevitably decreased the sensitivity, but rendered an improved specificity. Recent studies have demonstrated that most individuals without heart disease showed a 'none' or 'diffuse' pattern, 'focal' or 'focal on diffuse' uptake was mostly observed in unstable angina [11, 16]. These findings suggested that the pattern, rather than the extent, of ^{18}F-FDG uptake, is an indicator of myocardial involvement under fasting conditions. Therefore, we adopted these classifications in the present study. For the same reason, we did not consider quantitative evaluation of ^{18}F-FDG uptake as the diagnostic criteria.

The secretion of insulin is impaired and/or there is insulin resistance for diabetic patients. Therefore, the utilization of glucose is decreased in these subjects. However, recent studies have proposed that ischemia and insulin would trigger independent pathways of the translocation of glucose transporters (GLUTs) in the myocardium, to increase glucose transport to the myocyte: ischemia leads to GLUT-4 translocation via a phosphatidylinositol 3-kinase (PI3-kinase)-independent mechanism, and insulin via a PI3-kinase-mediated pathway [21, 22]. These differential regulations of GLUT-4 translocation suggest that even in diabetic patients who have myocardial insulin resistance, would have increased glucose uptake when triggered by ischemic events. Moreover, due to the lower ^{18}FDG uptake in non-ischemic myocardium demonstrated in this study, ^{18}FDG myocardial ischemic imaging may have a higher specificity in diabetic patients than that in non-diabetic patients.

There are some limitations in this study. This study included a subgroup of patients with suspected unstable angina, who had a higher incidence and more severity of perfusion abnormalities on both resting and exercise imaging. This may result in the overestimation of the sensitivity of ^{18}F-FDG imaging. However, we did not yet find significant differences in the diagnostic performance between stable and unstable angina (Fig. 7b). ^{18}F-FDG was only injected once and one hour prior to the exercise test in this study. This may, as discussed above, lower the sensitivity of ^{18}F-FDG imaging. Whether split dose (i.e., the ^{18}F-FDG was divided into 2 parts, and was administered separately at rest and exercise testing) or one injection after exercise followed by two imaging session, can improve the sensitivity needs to be further studied. We only examined the glucose level at the baseline and no other hormones were checked. The difference of these hormones between resting and exercise imaging, and their effects on the myocardial uptake of ^{18}F-FDG, could not be evaluated. Exercise perfusion images were acquired using SPECT equipped with ultra-high-energy collimators, which might have underestimated the sensitivity of MPI compared using SPECT equipped with low-energy collimators. Moreover, down-scatter of ^{18}F to the ^{99m}Tc window might bring quantitation error. The ratio of ^{99m}Tc to ^{18}F was more than 4–5 : 1 in this study, and the contribution of ^{18}F was estimated to be less than 5% of the total counts in the ^{99m}Tc window [23]. In addition to fasting, several other strategies have recently been developed to suppress the physiological uptake of ^{18}F-FDG in myocardium [24]. However, the application of these interventions in ischemic ^{18}F-FDG imaging was scarce and required further investigation [10]. Hence, we did not integrate them into our study protocol. We didn't integrate functional evaluation of wall motion into the study protocol, hence we couldn't correlate the metabolic abnormality with myocardial hypokinesis. Therefore, we couldn't decide in which patient myocardial stunning was the underlying mechanism of metabolic abnormality. Finally, since this was a small and exploratory study, larger studies are necessary.

Conclusion

The present study demonstrated that myocardial ischemia can induce ^{18}F-FDG uptake, and support the potential use of fasting ^{18}F-FDG imaging in detecting myocardial ischemia. As no satisfactory methods can completely suppress physiological uptake in non-ischemic myocardium so far, classification of the ^{18}F-FDG distribution pattern is an effective alternative in differentiating abnormal ^{18}F-FDG uptake.

Funding

This work was supported by the Beijing Municipal Science and Technology Commission (Z131107002213182), the Capital Health Research and Development of Special (SF2014-2-4033), and the National Natural Science Foundation of China (30970852, 81471694).

Authors' contributions

Study design: MY and KD. Data collection: XG, BX and YL. Data analysis: MY, ZH and KD. Manuscript writing: MY and KD. All authors read and approved the final manuscript.

Competing interests

The authors declare that they have no competing interests.

Author details

[1]State Key Laboratory of Cardiovascular Disease, Department of Cardiology, Cardiovascular Institute, Fuwai Hospital and National Center for Cardiovascular Diseases, Chinese Academy of Medical Sciences and Peking Union Medical College, Beijing, China. [2]National Center for Cardiovascular Diseases, Chinese Academy of Medical Sciences and Peking Union Medical College, A 167, Beilishi Road, Xicheng District, Beijing 100037, China. [3]Department of Cardiology, Beijing Chaoyang Hospital, Capital Medical University, Beijing, China. [4]Department of Nuclear Medicine, Cardiovascular Institute, Fuwai Hospital and National Center for Cardiovascular Diseases, Chinese Academy of Medical Sciences and Peking Union Medical College, Beijing, China. [5]Department of Nuclear Medicine, Beijing Chaoyang Hospital, Capital Medical University, 8th Gongtinanlu Rd, Chaoyang District, Beijing 100020, China.

References

1. Schwaiger M, Neese RA, Araujo L, Wyns W, Wisneski JA, Sochor H, et al. Sustained nonoxidative glucose utilization and depletion of glycogen in reperfused canine myocardium. J Am Coll Cardiol. 1989;13:745–54.
2. McNulty PH, Sinusas AJ, Shi CQ, Dione D, Young LH, Cline GC, et al. Glucose metabolism distal to a critical coronary stenosis in a canine model of low-flow myocardial ischemia. J Clin Invest. 1996;98:62–9.
3. Schelbert HR, Henze E, Phelps ME, Kuhl DE. Assessment of regional myocardial ischemia by positron-emission computed tomography. Am Heart J. 1982;103:588–97.
4. Camici P, Araujo LI, Spinks T, Lammertsma AA, Kaski JC, Shea MJ, et al. Increased uptake of ^{18}F-fluorodeoxyglucose in postischemic myocardium of patients with exercise-induced angina. Circulation. 1986;74:81–8.
5. Abramson BL, Ruddy TD, de Kemp RA, Laramee LA, Marquis JF, Beanlands RS. Stress perfusion/metabolic imaging: a pilot study for a potential new approach to the diagnosis of coronary artery disease in women. J Nucl Cardiol. 2000;7:205–12.
6. Araujo LI, McFalls EO, Lammertsma AA, Jones T, Maseri A. Dipyridamole-induced increased glucose uptake in patients with single-vessel coronary artery disease assessed with PET. J Nucl Cardiol. 2001;8:339–46.
7. He ZX, Shi RF, Wu YJ, Tian YQ, Liu XJ, Wang SW, et al. Direct imaging of exercise-induced myocardial ischemia with fluorine-18-labeled deoxyglucose and Tc-99 m-sestamibi in coronary artery disease. Circulation. 2003;108:1208–13.
8. Abbott BG, Liu YH, Arrighi JA. [18F]Fluorodeoxyglucose as a memory marker of transient myocardial ischaemia. Nucl Med Commun. 2007;28:89–94.
9. Dou KF, Yang MF, Yang YJ, Jain D, He ZX. Myocardial ^{18}F-FDG uptake after exercise-induced myocardial ischemia in patients with coronary artery disease. J Nucl Med. 2008;49:1986–91.
10. Arun S, Mittal BR, Bhattacharya A, Rohit MK. Comparison of Tc-99 m tetrofosmin myocardial perfusion scintigraphy and exercise F18-FDG imaging in detection of myocardial ischemia in patients with coronary artery disease. J Nucl Cardiol. 2015;22:98–110.
11. Dou KF, Xie BQ, Gao XJ, Li Y, Yang YJ, He ZX, et al. Use of resting myocardial 18 F-FDG imaging in the detection of unstable angina. Nucl Med Commun. 2015;36:999–1006.
12. Gould KL, Taegtmeyer H. Myocardial ischemia, fluorodeoxyglucose, and severity of coronary artery stenosis: The complexities of metabolic remodeling in hibernating myocardium. Circulation. 2004;109:e167–70.
13. Gropler RJ, Siegel BA, Lee KJ, Moerlein SM, Perry DJ, Bergmann SR, et al. Nonuniformity in myocardial accumulation of fluorine-18-fluorodeoxyglucose in normal fasted humans. J Nucl Med. 1990;31:1749–56.
14. Khandani AH, Isasi CR, Blaufox MD. Intra-individual variability of cardiac uptake on serial whole-body ^{18}F-FDG PET. Nucl Med Commun. 2005;26:787–91.
15. Inglese E, Leva L, Matheoud R, Sacchetti G, Secco C, Gandolfo P, et al. Spatial and temporal heterogeneity of regional myocardial uptake in patients without heart disease under fasting conditions on repeated whole-body 18 F-FDG PET/CT. J Nucl Med. 2007;48:1662–9.
16. Nose H, Otsuka H, Otomi Y, Terazawa K, Takao S, Iwamoto S, et al. The physiological uptake pattern of ^{18}F-FDG in the left ventricular myocardium of patients without heart disease. J Med Invest. 2014;61:53–8.
17. Ishimaru S, Tsujino I, Takei T, Tsukamoto E, Sakaue S, Kamigaki M, et al. Focal uptake on 18 F-fluoro-2-deoxyglucose positron emission tomography images indicates cardiac involvement of sarcoidosis. Eur Heart J. 2005;26:1538–43.
18. Dilsizian V, Bacharach SL, Beanlands RS, Bergmann SR, Delbeke D, Dorbala S. ASNC imaging guidelines/SNMMI procedure standard for positron emission tomography (PET) nuclear cardiology procedures. J Nucl Cardiol. 2016;23:1187–226.
19. Kemppainen J, Fujimoto T, Kalliokoski KK, Viljanen T, Nuutila P, Knuuti J. Myocardial and skeletal muscle glucose uptake during exercise in humans. J Physiol. 2002;542:403–12.
20. Araujo LI, Camici P, Spinks TJ, Jones T, Maseri A. Abnormalities in myocardial metabolism in patients with unstable angina as assessed by positron emission tomography. Cardiovasc Drugs Ther. 1988;2:41–6.
21. Davey KA, Garlick PB, Warley A, Southworth R. Immunogold labeling study of the distribution of GLUT-1 and GLUT-4 in cardiac tissue following stimulation by insulin or ischemia. Am J Physiol Heart Circ Physiol. 2007;292:H2009–19.
22. Bryant NJ, Govers R, James DE. Regulated transport of the glucose transporter GLUT4. Nat Rev Mol Cell Biol. 2002;3:267–77.
23. Sandler MP, Bax JJ, Patton JA, Visser FC, Martin WH, Wijns W. Fluorine-18-fluorodeoxyglucose cardiac imaging using a modified scintillation camera. J Nucl Med. 1998;39:2035–43.
24. Osborne MT, Hulten EA, Murthy VL, Skali H, Taqueti VR, Dorbala S, DiCarli MF, Blankstein R. Patient preparation for cardiac fluorine-18 fluorodeoxyglucose positron emission tomography imaging of inflammation. J Nucl Cardiol. 2017;24:86–99.

17

Prevalence and associated factors of ischemic heart disease (IHD) among patients with diabetes mellitus

Boonsub Sakboonyarat* and Ram Rangsin

Abstract

Background: Ischemic Heart Disease (IHD) is the first ranked among most common causes of death involving cardiovascular and other diseases. The information on the prevalence of IHD in Thailand is lacking especially among patients with diabetes mellitus. The objectives of this study were to determine the prevalence of IHD among patients with diabetes mellitus and to determine factors associated with IHD in a nation-wide survey.

Methods: A cross-sectional study to assess national outcomes among patients with diabetes who visited 831 public hospitals in Thailand was conducted in 2013 to evaluate status of care among patients with diabetes aged at least 18 years who received medical treatment in the target hospital for the last 12 months.

Results: A total of 25,902 patients with diabetes were included in this study. IHD was detected among 918 patients (3.54%; 95%CI 3.32–3.77). Multivariate analysis was conducted to determine which factors were most associated with IHD, and the results showed age (AORs 1.05; 95%CI 1.04–1.05), being male (AORs 1.78; 95%CI 1.53–2.07), hypertensive comorbidity (AORs 2.10; 95%CI 1.68–2.62), being in Health Region 4 (AORs 1.93; 95%CI 1.54–2.35), presenting hyperglycemic crisis (AORs 1.53; 95%CI 1.14–2.06) and insulin therapy (AORs 1.40; 95%CI 1.17–1.66) were the highest associated factors for IHD in this population.

Conclusion: Our data emphasized that IHD was a problem among patients with diabetes. Diabetic patients should be regularly assessed for IHD and their risk factors should be better controlled. Moreover, the Ministry of Public Health managers and clinicians should provide further preventative strategies to attenuate cardiovascular disease.

Keywords: Ischemic heart disease, Diabetes mellitus, Nation-wide survey, Prevalence, Associated factors

Background

Ischemic Heart Disease (IHD) is the first ranked and most common cause of death in cardiovascular and overall diseases [1]. The estimated prevalence of IHD among people aged ≥18 years in 2013 was 6.1, 6.4, 5.3 and 3.7% in Caucasian, African, Latino and Asian populations, respectively [1]. The prevalence increased with age and more prevalence was noted among males [2]. One recent study showed that the number of estimated deaths caused by IHD in Southeast Asia increased from 5.73 to 8.14 million from 1990 to 2013 [3]. Prevalence of IHD increased in patients with potential risk factors such as diabetes mellitus [4, 5]. Globally, adults with diabetes total 381 million. The estimated global prevalence of diabetes mellitus among adult populations was 8.3, 9.6, 5.7, 6.8, 8.6 and 6.4% in North American and Caribbean (NAC), African, European, Western Pacific and Thai populations [6]. Diabetes mellitus increases independent risk of IHD approximately 1.5 and 1.7 fold among males and females, respectively [7]. In 2007, a related study conducted among patients with diabetes reported that the age-standardized incidence rate (per 1000 person-years) of first coronary heart disease (CHD) events was 28.8 among males and 23.3 among females [8].

* Correspondence: Boonsub1991@pcm.ac.th
Department of Military and Community Medicine, Phramongkutklao College of Medicine, Bangkok 10400, Thailand

Epidemiological data of IHD in Asian populations has been studied in many countries. From 2007 to 2008, the prevalence of CHD in China was 0.63% [9]. In 2002, the overall prevalence of CHD in India was 8.2% [10]. However, limited information is available regarding the prevalence of IHD in the Thai general population in 1991 was 0.99% [11], especially among patients with major risk factors such as diabetes mellitus. We determined the prevalence of IHD among patients with diabetes mellitus using a nation-wide, cross-sectional survey among patients with diabetes mellitus. The secondary objective of this study was to determine factors associated with IHD.

Methods

Study designs

The data of this study were retrieved from database: An assessment in Quality of Care among Patients Diagnosed with Type2 Diabetes and Hypertension Visiting Ministry of Public Health and Bangkok Metropolitan Administration Hospital in Thailand (Thailand DM/HT) after the permission of the Medical Research Network of the Consortium of Thai Medical Schools (MedResNet).

The Thailand DM/HT evaluation survey was a nation-wide, cross-sectional study aiming to assess outcomes among patients with diabetes visiting public hospitals of the Ministry of Public Health (MoPH), Thailand and private hospitals and clinics in Bangkok was conducted from 2012 to 2013. The main objective of the Thailand DM/HT evaluation survey was to evaluate the status of care and was supported by the Thai National Health Security Office (NHSO).

Subjects

The healthcare system in Thailand can be categorized in two types comprising (1) healthcare under the MoPH and (2) private healthcare such as private clinics and hospitals. All Thais have healthcare coverage schemes such as the universal coverage scheme, social insurance scheme and government officer scheme. These healthcare schemes are supported by the NHSO. All of the hospitals under the MoPH at all levels, i.e., community (district), general (provincial) and regional nationwide and some private clinics in Bangkok were invited to participate in the study.

A stratified two-stage cluster sampling method proportional to the size was used to select national and provincial representative samples of patients with diabetes in Thailand. The stratified sample was drawn from a subset of all MoPH hospitals in Thailand. For Bangkok, the targeted institutes included all hospitals and clinics under the NHSO. The first level (province) comprised 77 strata while the second level constituted hospitals within each province. The second level was categorized in 5 strata by size, i.e., regional center hospital (> 500 beds), provincial general (middle) hospital (200–500 beds), first level one (F1) (90–120 beds), first level two (F2) hospital (60 beds) and first level three (F3) hospital (10–30 beds). All university medical centers were excluded from this study.

Inclusion criteria for this study comprised patients with diabetes aged at least 18 years receiving hospital medical treatment in hospital, drawn using the specified sampling method, during the previous 12 months. Any patient who had participated in a clinical trial was excluded. Those patients may have received trial medication or placebo, influencing the outcome of the study.

Data collection

A total of 833 hospitals under the MoPH were categorized as 33 regional hospitals, 83 general hospitals and 717 first level or community hospitals including the first level one (F1) 73 hospitals, the first level two (F2) 126 hospitals and the first level three (F3) 518 hospitals. All regional and general hospitals were selected, as well as 10% of F1 hospitals, 20% of F3 hospitals and 70% of F3 hospitals. This faction was based on the proportion of patient care provided at the various levels of hospitals. Patients with a diagnosis of diabetes mellitus were randomized and registered at each hospital. A standardized case report form was used to obtain the required information from medical records and was sent to the Thailand DM/HT study of the Medical Research Network of the Consortium of Thai Medical Schools (MedResNet) central data management unit in Nonthaburi. Data were retrieved from patient's medical records, status of diabetes complications and results of laboratory tests.

Measurements

Data collected included demographics, weight, height, body mass index (BMI), waist circumference, smoking behavior, systolic blood pressure (SBP), diastolic blood pressure (DBP), cardiovascular complications such as left ventricular hypertrophy (LVH), diabetic complications such as diabetic retinopathy (DR) and diabetic nephropathy (DN), blood chemistry data including fasting plasma glucose (FPG), hemoglobin A1c (HbA1c), hematocrit (Hct), hemoglobin (Hb), serum creatinine (Cr), uric acid, lipid profile including total cholesterol (TC), triglyceride (TG), high density lipoprotein cholesterol (HDL) and low density lipoprotein cholesterol (LDL), available electrocardiogram (ECG) data and results, history of anti-hyperglycemic and antiplatelet drug use and glomerular filtration rate (GFR) calculated using the epidemiology collaboration formula (EPI). Our study enrolled those patients with diabetes who were diagnosed and received ongoing medical care in a hospital. Hospitals in Thailand normally use the standard diagnosis and treatment following Thai clinical practice guidelines for diabetes and diagnosis and classification of diabetes mellitus using Diabetes Care, 2010. Diabetes mellitus was defined as FPG ≥126 mg/dl and confirmed by repeat testing at a second visit. Fasting is defined as no caloric intake for at least 8 h [12]. IHD was defined as myocardial infraction or history of coronary revascularization. Diagnosis of myocardial infraction was performed using standard criteria including stable angina and acute coronary syndrome, categorized as ST-T segment elevation myocardial infraction, nonST-T segment elevation myocardial infraction and unstable angina.

Statistical analysis

Data were coded and entered in the STATA/MP for Windows, Version 12 (Stata Corp LP, TX). Categorical data were presented as number and percentage. Continuous data were presented as mean and standard deviation (SD). Prevalence was analyzed using descriptive statistics and reported as percentage and 95% confident interval. The chi-square test was used to compare categorical data. Continuous data was compared using the *t*-test. Continuous data were grouped to analyze associated factor using odds ratio (OR). The magnitude of associations was presented as crude ORs with 95% confidence interval. The multivariate analysis was performed using logistic regression analysis and Forward Stepwise (LR) to adjust confounders. Stepwise *p*-value for entry was 0.05, and *p*-value for removal was set at 0.10. The Hosmer-Lemeshow goodness-of-fit of the logistic regression models was performed with $p\text{-value} = 0.494$. The complete case analysis and imputation method were used for any missing data. Missing values were imputed based on the means of the complete case. A *p*-value less than 0.05 was considered statistically significant.

Results

Demographic data

A total of 25,902 patients with diabetes mellitus were enrolled in this study from 2012 to 2013. Average age was 60.6 ± 10.5 years, 8076 (32.2%) were male and 17,836 (68.8%) were female. The average diabetes duration of patients was 7.1 ± 4.7 years while the average HbA1c level was 8.0 ± 2.2%. Baseline characteristics of this study are shown in Table 1. One third of participants lived in northeastern Thailand. In all, 62.5% subjects visited community or first level (F1, F2 and F3) hospitals. In this study, patients with hypertension totaled 29.1%. Prevalence of IHD among patients with diabetes was 3.54% (95%CI 3.32–3.77), increased with older age and was more common among males. Fig. 1 shows a bar graph representing IHD prevalence for every 10 years of age separated in male, female and overall.

Associated factors of IHD among patients with diabetes

Additional file 1 shows univariate analysis results regarding factors associated with IHD. Significant associated factors included older age, being male, health region, hospital level, insurance scheme, religion, occupation, GFR, HT co-morbidity, HT duration, LVH, LAE, AF, DM duration, DN, DR and insulin, sulfonylurea, thiazolidinedione and aspirin therapy. Because a number of patients had missing values for HbA1c, this may have decreased the statistical power of the complete cases analysis. As a result, we applied imputation to handle the missing value and the results of multivariate analysis after imputation showed similarity to the original independent associations with IHD. Multivariate analysis showed the risk factors of IHD included age, being male, being in Health Region 4, hypertensive comorbidity and insulin therapy (Table 2).

Discussion

Our present nation-wide survey showed the prevalence of IHD among Thai patients with diabetes mellitus was 3.54%. IHD was significantly associated with being male, age, being in Health Region 4, hypertensive comorbidity, presenting hyperglycemic crisis and insulin therapy. To our knowledge, this is the first report on the prevalence and risk factors of IHD among Thai patients with diabetes. The prevalence of IHD was 0.99% among the general population in Thailand reported in 1991 [11]. A related study in Sweden found a much higher prevalence of IHD (21.97%) among patients with diabetes including those aged from 45 to 74 years [13]. In contrast, our study enrolled all patients with diabetes aged from 35 to 97 years. However, when the same age groups as the Swedish study were analyzed, the prevalence of IHD was 2.75%. In the general population, the prevalence of IHD in Caucasian populations is normally higher than that among Asians [1, 7] and diabetes amplifies this morbidity. The present study enrolled patients with diabetes who received medical treatment in MoPH hospitals all over Thailand and public and private clinics in Bangkok under the NHSO. However, these populations did not include patients with diabetes who received medical treatment in health promoting hospitals (HPHs). These HPHs, primary care units of a community hospital, usually provide health care and medication for uncomplicated diabetes cases. The prevalence of IHD in this study may have been overestimated because the diabetic cases in HPHs were not included.

After adjusting for confounding factors by multivariate analysis, only older age, being male, being in Health Region 4, hypertensive comorbidity, presenting hyperglycemic crisis and insulin therapy remained significantly associated with IHD among patients with diabetes. Prevalence of IHD tended to be higher with older age similar to related studies in Sweden [13] and Finland

Table 1 Baseline characteristics of patients (total number of subjects =25,902)

Baseline Variables	*n*	Mean ± SD or number (%)
Gender	25,902	
Female		17,836 (68.8)
Male		8076 (32.2)
Age	25,902	60.6 ± 10.5
Hospital level	25,902	
Regional center		3096 (12)
General provincial		4911 (19)
Community		16,187 (62.5)
Bangkok metropolitan administration		1708 (6.5)
Diabetic duration	25,902	7.1 ± 4.7
Waist circumference	17,488	88.5 ± 10.4
Body mass index (kg/m^2)	24,643	25.5 ± 4.4
Fasting plasma glucose	23,048	154.7 ± 58.4
HbA1c level	20,481	8 ± 2.2
GFR_EPI	15,986	67.2 ± 31
LDL	15,544	108.6 ± 36.8
HDL	14,126	46.9 ± 13.8
Triglyceride	15,548	175.4 ± 110.9
Total cholesterol	14,775	187.7 ± 44.5
Uric acid	4553	6.1 ± 1.8
Smoking	23,806	
Never		21,249 (89.2)
Current Smoker		1036 (4.4)
Ex-smoker		1521 (6.4)
Hypertensive comorbidity	25,902	
No		7527 (29.1)
Yes		18,375 (70.9)

SD standard deviation, *HbA1c* hemoglobinA1c, *GFR_EPI* glomerular infiltration rate calculated by epidemiology collaboration formula, *LDL* low density lipoprotein cholesterol, *HDL* high density lipoprotein cholesterol

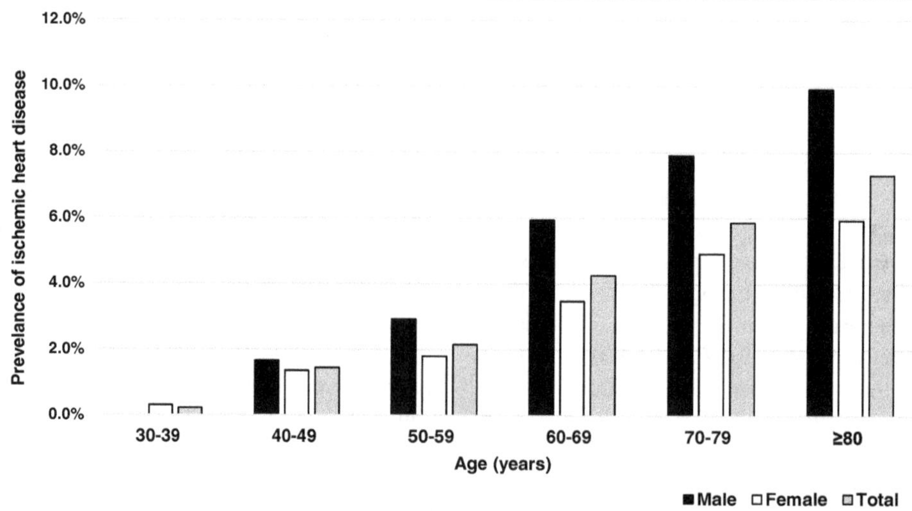

Fig. 1 Prevalence of ischemic heart disease in male and female at different age groups

Table 2 Multivariate logistic regression for factors associated with ischemic heart disease in diabetic patients. ($N = 25{,}902$)

Factors	IHD	No-IHD	AORs	95% CI
	n (%)	n (%)		
Age (years)	65.9 ± 9.5	60.4 ± 10.5	1.05[b]	(1.04–1.05)
Gender				
Female	523 (3)	17,303 (97)	1	
Male	395 (4.9)	7681 (95.1)	1.78[b]	(1.53–2.07)
Health regions				
Other health regions	774 (3.3)	22,877 (96.7)	1	
The 4th health region	144 (6.4)	2107 (93.6)	1.93[b]	(1.54–2.35)
Hypertensive Comorbidity				
No	129 (1.8)	7398 (98.2)	1	
Yes	789 (4.3)	17,586 (95.7)	2.10[b]	(1.68–2.62)
Hyperglycemic crisis				
No	846 (3.4)	23,680 (96.6)	1	
Yes	72 (5.2)	1304 (94.8)	1.53[a]	(1.14–2.06)
Insulin therapy				
No	659 (3.3)	19,685 (96.7)	1	
Yes	259 (4.7)	5299 (95.3)	1.40[b]	(1.17–1.66)

[a]$p < 0.01$, [b]$p < 0.001$

AORs Adjusted odds ratio for age, gender, health regions, hypertensive comorbidity, duration of diabetes mellitus, hyperglycemic crisis, insulin therapy and HbA1c level, *IHD* Ischemic heart disease, *CI* confidence interval

[14]. Among the elderly, changes occurring in endothelial function include loss of arterial elasticity and reduced arterial compliance, so more vascular aging and degenerative processes lead to atherosclerosis disease [15]. In addition, the endothelium experiences changed arterial function by decreased nitric oxide and increased endothelin causing a pro-coagulant state and promoting vascular smooth muscle growth and exaggerated increased risk of cardiovascular events [16]. Another reason is the elderly often have a low frequency of physical activity. A recent study showed that adults, who were physically active at least twice weekly, had decreased risk of CHD [17, 18].

The result of our study was similar to studies in the US and in western and Asian populations [2, 9, 19–21]. Most studies have found that IHD was more common among males than females [9, 11, 14, 19, 20, 22]. IHD being common among males was probably related to hormonal effects. In the premenopausal period, females' sex-hormones such as estrogen promote increased HDL and decreased LDL causing a cardio-protective effect [23, 24]. However, a related study in Pakistan showed that central adiposity is significantly higher among females compared with males regarding patients with type 2 diabetes mellitus [25]. Consequently, adiposity is positively related to IHD especially among females [26]. Patients presenting more adiposity may lead to IHD by adipocytokines by the inflammatory pathway causing vascular pathology and establishing atherothrombosis [27]. In addition, differing lifestyle or behavioral patterns between male and female indicate males present higher behavioral risks, e.g., from smoking, that predispose cardiovascular events [28].

However, several related studies have shown that higher BMI leads to risk for IHD [29–31]. The results of statistical analysis in this study found that a higher BMI exhibited a trend of dose response effect to IHD, but without significance. One result from the homogeneity in these diabetes populations is being categorized as overweight to obesity. In addition, patients, who have undergone a long duration with diabetes, may lead to presenting higher BMI. These diabetic populations are at greater risk for IHD; however, the duration of diabetes was not significant in the final model of this study.

The present study found that patients with diabetes, who present hypertensive comorbidity, are at increased risk for IHD. Hypertension is related to IHD and can be described by pathophysiology. The neuro-mediators of hypertension including angiotensin II can promote plasminogen activator inhibitor (PAI-1) expression and increased PAI-1 levels inhibiting the function of tissue plasminogen activator (tPA) resulting in increased myocardial infraction. In addition, the hypertensive stage adds extra pressure that can damage the arterial wall making it more vulnerable and building up plaque associated with atherosclerosis [32]. This study showed that hyperglycemic crisis was related to a high prevalence of IHD with an adjusted ORs of 1.53 (95% CI, 1.14–2.06). Acute hyperglycemia can attenuate endothelial function and reduce nitric oxide (NO) bioavailability [33, 34]. These actions promote monocyte and vascular smooth muscle cell migration into the intima and form macrophage foam cells, characterizing the initial morphological changes of atherosclerosis [35]. The study showed that insulin therapy was related to a high prevalence of IHD with an adjusted ORs of 1.40 (95% CI, 1.17–1.66). Insulin is more likely to be used among patients with more severe diabetes mellitus of longer duration and more complications such as chronic kidney disease. Therefore, these patients with insulin therapy have an increased number of cardiovascular events.

We have an explanation why IHD related to Health Region 4 in our study. The study showed this region had the highest prevalence of IHD at 6.4%. Health Region 4 is in central Thailand, a peripheral area near the Bangkok Metropolitan Area, where sufficient public health services are much more available. As a result, more patients can access services creating a higher load of reported cases. In addition, the area, which features several agriculture businesses, has more than enough dietary products combined with inappropriate patient dietary behaviors might have promoted a higher risk of cardiovascular disease. Consequently, the patients with diabetes in this area exhibited higher BMIs on average than others area, resulting in a higher risk for IHD [29, 30]. In addition, the patients with diabetic in Health Region 4 had higher age levels than the patients with diabetes in other areas. Although we adjusted age in the final model, the residual effect of age remained.

The study employed a cross-sectional design, and as such, the results could show only factors associated with IHD. The data presented in this study were obtained in the 2012–2013 Thailand DM/HT study of the NHSO from the Medical Research Network of the Consortium of Thai Medical Schools (MedResNet) central data management system. We were aware of missing data from this observational study. Even though this represented a relatively large sample size of the study population and some data were missing as from the nationwide observational (real life situation) study, the associations between factors and outcomes were able to be presented. In the study, we relied on evidence from medical records to identify ischemic heart disease; therefore, a small proportion of individuals with undiagnosed ischemic heart disease may have been misclassified non-differentially. The effect of misclassification decreases the observed effect size (odds ratio) of the associations (toward null). However, the officers who enter data in each hospital received proper training and verified reviewed medical records. The strength of this study was its nation-wide scope for IHD in a diabetic population. Thus, the finding of the study can be generalized and applied in others diabetic population.

Conclusion

The prevalence of IHD in a diabetic population in this study was 3.54%, higher than the prevalence of IHD in the general population in most related reports. Factors associated with IHD included age, being male, hypertensive comorbidity, being in Health Region 4, presenting hyperglycemic crisis and insulin therapy. Our data emphasized that IHD was a problem among patients with diabetes. Diabetic patients should be regularly assessed for IHD and their risk factors should be better controlled. Moreover, the Ministry of Public Health managers and clinicians should provide further preventative strategies to attenuate cardiovascular disease.

Abbreviations

BMI: body mass index; CI: confident interval; DBP: diastolic blood pressure; FPG: fasting plasma glucose; GFR_EPI: glomerular infiltration rate calculated by epidemiology collaboration formula; Hb: hemoglobin,;
HbA1c: hemoglobin A1c; Hct: hematocrit; HDL: high density lipoprotein cholesterol; HT: hypertension; IHD: ischemic heart disease; LDL: low density lipoprotein cholesterol; LVH: left ventricular hypertrophy; MoPH: Ministry of Public Health; NHSO: National Health Security Office ; SBP: systolic blood pressure; SD: standard deviation; TC: total cholesterol; TG: triglyceride

Acknowledgements

The authors wish to thank the entire staff members of the Department of Military and Community Medicine, Phramongkutklao College of Medicine, for their support in completing this study. The authors thank Professor Colonel Mathirut Mungthin for support and for proofreading this manuscript.

Funding

No funding was received.

Authors' contributions

B.S. and R.R. participated in conception, design and statistical analysis; B.S. drafted the manuscripts. Both authors read and approved the final manuscripts.

Competing interests

The authors declare that they have no competing interests.

References

1. Abubakar I, Tillmann T, Banerjee A. Global, regional, and national age-sex specific all-cause and cause-specific mortality for 240 causes of death, 1990–2013: a systematic analysis for the Global Burden of Disease Study 2013. Lancet (London, England). 2015;385(9963):117–71.
2. Mozaffarian D, Benjamin EJ, Go AS, Arnett DK, Blaha MJ, Cushman M, et al. Heart disease and stroke statistics--2015 update: a report from the American Heart Association. Circulation. 2015;131(4):e29–322.
3. Roth GA, Forouzanfar MH, Moran AE, Barber R, Nguyen G, Feigin VL, et al. Demographic and epidemiologic drivers of global cardiovascular mortality. N Engl J Med. 2015;372(14):1333–41.
4. Diabetes mellitus: a major risk factor for cardiovascular disease. A joint editorial statement by the American Diabetes Association; The National Heart, Lung, and Blood Institute; Th e Juvenile Diabetes Foundation International; The National Institute of Diabetes and Digestive and Kidney

Diseases; and The American Heart Association. Circulation 1999;100(10): 1132–1133.
5. Grundy SM, Benjamin IJ, Burke GL, Chait A, Eckel RH, Howard BV, et al. Diabetes and cardiovascular disease: a statement for healthcare professionals from the American Heart Association. Circulation. 1999; 100(10):1134–46.
6. Aguiree F, Brown A, Cho NH, Dahlquist G, Dodd S, Dunning T, et al. IDF diabetes atlas. 2013.
7. Wilson PW, D'Agostino RB, Levy D, Belanger AM, Silbershatz H, Kannel WB. Prediction of coronary heart disease using risk factor categories. Circulation. 1998;97(18):1837–47.
8. Avogaro A, Giorda C, Maggini M, Mannucci E, Raschetti R, Lombardo F, et al. Incidence of coronary heart disease in type 2 diabetic men and women: impact of microvascular complications, treatment, and geographic location. Diabetes Care. 2007;30(5):1241–7.
9. Yang ZJ, Liu J, Ge JP, Chen L, Zhao ZG, Yang WY. Prevalence of cardiovascular disease risk factor in the Chinese population: the 2007-2008 China National Diabetes and metabolic disorders study. Eur Heart J. 2012; 33(2):213–20.
10. Krishnan MN. Coronary heart disease and risk factors in India - on the brink of an epidemic? Indian Heart J. 2012;64(4):364–7.
11. Tatsanavivat P, Klungboonkrong V, Chirawatkul A, Bhuripanyo K, Manmontri A, Chitanondh H, et al. Prevalence of coronary heart disease and major cardiovascular risk factors in Thailand. Int J Epidemiol. 1998;27(3):405–9.
12. Diagnosis and classification of diabetes mellitus. Diabetes Care 2010;33 Suppl 1:S62–S69.
13. Wiréhn A-BE, Östgren CJ, Carstensen JM. Age and gender differences in the impact of diabetes on the prevalence of ischemic heart disease: a population-based register study. Diabetes Res Clin Pract. 2008;79(3):497–502.
14. Jousilahti P, Vartiainen E, Tuomilehto J, Puska P. Sex, age, cardiovascular risk factors, and coronary heart disease: a prospective follow-up study of 14 786 middle-aged men and women in Finland. Circulation. 1999;99(9):1165–72.
15. Jani B, Rajkumar C. Ageing and vascular ageing. Postgrad Med J. 2006; 82(968):357–62.
16. GE M, Allen PB, Morgan DR, Hanratty CG, Silke B. Nitric oxide modulation of blood vessel tone identified by arterial waveform analysis. Clin Sci. 2001; 100(4):387–93.
17. Sundquist K, Qvist J, Johansson S-E, Sundquist J. The long-term effect of physical activity on incidence of coronary heart disease: a 12-year follow-up study. Prev Med. 2005;41(1):219–25.
18. Oguma Y, Shinoda-Tagawa T. Physical activity decreases cardiovascular disease risk in women: review and meta-analysis. Am J Prev Med. 2004;26(5):407–18.
19. Ohira T, Iso H. Cardiovascular disease epidemiology in Asia: an overview. Circ J. 2013;77(7):1646–52.
20. Bhatnagar P, Wickramasinghe K, Williams J, Rayner M, Townsend N. The epidemiology of cardiovascular disease in the UK 2014. Heart. 2015; 101(15):1182–9.
21. Sanchis-Gomar F, Perez-Quilis C, Leischik R, Lucia A. Epidemiology of coronary heart disease and acute coronary syndrome. Ann Transl Med. 2016;4(13):256.
22. Ueshima H, Sekikawa A, Miura K, Turin TC, Takashima N, Kita Y, et al. Cardiovascular disease and risk factors in Asia: a selected review. Circulation. 2008;118(25):2702–9.
23. Shahar E, Folsom AR, Salomaa W, Stinson VL, McGovern PG, Shimakawa T, et al. Relation of hormone-replacement therapy to measures of plasma fibrinolytic activity. Atherosclerosis risk in communities (ARIC) study investigators. Circulation. 1996;93(11):1970–5.
24. Grady D, Rubin SM, Petitti DB, Fox CS, Black D, Ettinger B, et al. Hormone therapy to prevent disease and prolong life in postmenopausal women. Ann Intern Med. 1992;117(12):1016–37.
25. Akhter O, Fiazuddin F, Shaheryar A, Niaz W, Siddiqui D, Awan S, et al. Central adiposity is significantly higher in female compared to male in Pakistani type 2 diabetes mellitus patients. Indian J Endocrinol Metab. 2015;19(1):72.
26. Canoy D. Distribution of body fat and risk of coronary heart disease in men and women. Curr Opin Cardiol. 2008;23(6):591–8.
27. Golia E, Limongelli G, Natale F, Fimiani F, Maddaloni V, Russo PE, et al. Adipose tissue and vascular inflammation in coronary artery disease. World J Cardiol. 2014;6(7):539.
28. Mons U, Muezzinler A, Gellert C, Schottker B, Abnet CC, Bobak M, et al. Impact of smoking and smoking cessation on cardiovascular events and mortality among older adults: meta-analysis of individual participant data from prospective cohort studies of the CHANCES consortium. BMJ (Clinical research ed). 2015;350:h1551.
29. Flint AJ, Rexrode KM, Hu FB, Glynn RJ, Caspard H, Manson JE, et al. Body mass index, waist circumference, and risk of coronary heart disease: a prospective study among men and women. Obesity Res Clinical Practice. 2010;4(3):e171–e81.
30. Collaboration APCS. Body mass index and cardiovascular disease in the Asia-Pacific region: an overview of 33 cohorts involving 310 000 participants. Int J Epidemiol. 2004;33(4):751–8.
31. Joshy G, Korda R, Attia J, Liu B, Bauman A, Banks E. Body mass index and incident hospitalisation for cardiovascular disease in 158 546 participants from the 45 and up study. Int J Obes. 2014;38(6):848.
32. Libby P, Theroux P. Pathophysiology of coronary artery disease. Circulation. 2005;111(25):3481–8.
33. Williams SB, Goldfine AB, Timimi FK, Ting HH, Roddy MA, Simonson DC, et al. Acute hyperglycemia attenuates endothelium-dependent vasodilation in humans in vivo. Circulation. 1998;97(17):1695–701.
34. Low Wang CC, Hess CN, Hiatt WR, Clinical Update GAB. Cardiovascular disease in diabetes mellitus: atherosclerotic cardiovascular disease and heart failure in type 2 diabetes mellitus - mechanisms, management, and Clinical Considerations. Circulation. 2016;133(24):2459–502.
35. Perkins JM, Joy NG, Tate DB, Davis SN. Acute effects of hyperinsulinemia and hyperglycemia on vascular inflammatory biomarkers and endothelial function in overweight and obese humans. Am J Physiol Endocrinol Metab. 2015;309(2):E168–76.

18

Estimating the direct costs of ischemic heart disease: evidence from a teaching hospital

Rosane Paixão Schlatter[1,4,6*], Vânia Naomi Hirakata[5] and Carisi Anne Polanczyk[1,2,3,4]

Abstract

Background: Coronary artery disease is the most prevalent cardiovascular disease. In the United States, 7% of adults over 20 years of age are estimated to have coronary artery disease. In Brazil, a prevalence of 5 to 8% has been estimated in adults over 40 years of age, with an increased number of hospitalizations associated with both stable and acute clinical manifestations; and health care costs have quadrupled in the last decade. To estimate the direct costs of managing ischemic heart disease patient care in a teaching hospital in Brazil from the perspective of the service payer, the Brazilian Unified Health System.

Methods: This study was a retrospective cohort study for the identification and valuation of resources used at both the outpatient and in-hospital levels in a sample of 330 patients selected from the hospital's ischemic heart disease clinic. Data were collected from computerized hospital records and patients' hospital bills from January 2000 to October 2015. A bivariate analysis and binary logistic regression were performed with $p < 0.05$ considered statistically significant.

Results: The study population consisted of 330 patients with a mean age 61 ± 10 years and a follow-up period of 107 ± 2.6 months; of the patients, 55% were male, 89% had hypertension, 48% had diabetes, and 65% had acute myocardial infarction. The mean annual cost of outpatient management was US $1,521 per patient. The mean cost per hospitalization was US $1,976, and the expenses were higher in the first and last years of follow-up. Unstable angina, revascularization procedures, diabetes, hypertension and obesity were predictors of higher hospitalization costs ($p < 0.05$).

Conclusion: The cost estimates in this study indicate a high proportion of drug treatment costs in the treatment of ischemic heart disease. Treatment costs are higher in the first year and at the end of treatment, and some clinical factors are associated with greater hospital care costs. These results may serve as a basis for the evaluation of existing public policies and inputs for cost-effectiveness studies in coronary artery disease.

Keywords: Direct costs, Coronary artery disease, Disease cost study

* Correspondence: rschlatter@hcpa.edu.br
[1]Graduate Cardiology Program, Universidade Federal do Rio Grande do Sul (UFRGS), Porto Alegre, RS, Brazil
[4]National Health Technology Assessment Institute, CNPq, Porto Alegre, RS, Brazil
Full list of author information is available at the end of the article

Background

In 2012, cardiovascular disease accounted for 46.2% of non-communicable chronic disease deaths and 37% of deaths in people aged under 70 worldwide [1]. In Brazil, despite a reduction in the number of deaths since the 1990s, cardiovascular disease accounted for 28% of deaths in 2013 and incurred the highest spending in hospitalization in the Brazilian Unified Health System (SUS) in 2009 [2–4].

Coronary artery disease (CAD) is the most prevalent cardiovascular disease. In the United States, 7% of adults over 20 years of age are estimated to have a coronary artery disease diagnosis; by 2030, there will be an increase in this indicator [5]. In Brazil, a prevalence of 5 to 8% has been estimated in adults over 40 years of age [6], with an increased number of hospitalizations associated with both stable and acute clinical manifestations [6, 7].

Health costs have been increasing since the 1980s, mainly due to the incorporation of new technologies and demographic and epidemiological population transitions. In Brazil, health care costs have quadrupled in the last decade, reaching US $125 billion in 2013, of which 44% was paid by public health and 56% by the private sector [8].

The increase in spending on health, the need to balance public budgets and to seek efficiency in the allocation of resources, and the requirement of taking into account social demands in their entirety has led to a growing number of economic studies to aid in the decision-making process regarding the implementation of new public health policies.

Disease cost studies are important in Brazil because they provide a baseline for complete economic evaluations, such as cost-effectiveness studies. Identifying costs involves proper planning for data collection to enable the use of the generated information as an aid for future studies. In this context, this study aimed to estimate the direct costs associated with the treatment of ischemic heart disease at the outpatient and in-hospital levels in a public teaching hospital from the perspective of the main service public payer in Brazil, SUS.

Methods

This study was a retrospective cohort study to identify and value resource use in ischemic heart disease outpatients of the Hospital de Clínicas de Porto Alegre between January 2000 and October 2015. We used a bottom up microcosting methodology for 330 patients estimating direct costs during more than 10 years follow up. The inclusion criteria in this study were outpatients with follow-up of more than or equal to one year and a minimum of 3 consultations since January 2009. Of the 633 patients followed up in the ischemic heart disease clinic, 330 met the inclusion criteria and were included in the study.

Data collection

Forms were developed using REDCap [9] to collect retrospective data related to ambulatory care protocol clinical information. The information included CAD risk factors, medical history and current physical assessment, medication used, hospitalizations, procedures and tests performed during follow-up. Resource use for outpatient treatment and for hospitalization were analyzed separately.

Information relative to the following factors were recorded on the clinical assessment form: (A) Canadian Cardiovascular Society (CCS) functional class, (b) previous diagnosis of unstable angina, myocardial infarction, stroke, and congestive and valvular heart failure, (c) risk factors (diabetes mellitus, hypertension, dyslipidemia, and current and previous smoking), (d) medication use and (e) physical examination (weight, height, systolic and diastolic blood pressure, and heart rate).

Quantification of resources

The following factors were quantified during outpatient treatment: medical appointments, tests, outpatient catheterization procedures, medications in use, and transport of the patient to the hospital. Only medical consultations that took place in the ischemic heart disease clinic were considered. The number of consultations performed per patient was recorded.

The following drugs in use were considered in this study: acetylsalicylic acid, allopurinol, amiodarone, amlodipine, atenolol, atorvastatin, benazepril, captopril, clopidogrel, digoxin, diltiazem, enalapril, furosemide, hydrochlorothiazide, glibenclamide Isosorbide, losartan, lovastatin, metformin, metoprolol, nifedipine, omeprazole, paracetamol, pravastatin, propranolol, simvastatin, sustrate, warfarin, and verapamil. The list of drugs that were considered in this analysis is not exhaustive. The drugs included in the study were the ones prescribed by the cardiologists who tended to the patients while the study was ongoing as well as hypoglycemic drugs. All drugs were recorded in mg/day. We assumed that the drugs were purchased by the patients at pharmacies using their own resources without government subsidies and were taken with 100% treatment adherence.

The laboratory tests included alanine aminotransferase (ALT), albuminuria, aspartate aminotransferase (AST), total calcium, creatine kinase (CK and CK-MB), high density lipoprotein (HDL) cholesterol, low density lipoprotein (LDL) cholesterol, total cholesterol, creatinine, glycemic curve, qualitative urine test (QUT), urinary sediment test, phosphorus, glucose, glycated hemoglobin, potassium, C-reactive protein, thyrotropin, triglycerides, and urea.

Cardiac and imaging tests included were myocardial scintigraphy (stress and resting), echocardiography, stress echocardiography, resting electrocardiography, exercise test, Holter, ambulatory blood pressure monitoring (ABPM), chest X-ray, carotid and vertebral Doppler echocardiography, venous color Doppler echocardiography, and chest tomography.

The following factors were quantified in terms of hospital treatment: hospitalization days, intensive care unit (ICU) days, laboratory and diagnostic tests, angioplasty procedures with or without stent implantation, cardiac catheterization, and coronary artery bypass surgery performed during hospitalization.

Three pieces of information were evaluated for the hospitalizations (disease code, treatment code charged to the hospital account, and the specialty responsible for the hospitalization). The study included hospitalizations with International Classification of Diseases and Related Health Problems (ICD-10) relating to Chapter IX - Diseases of the Circulatory System (I00 to I99), Chapter XVIII - Symptoms, signs and abnormal clinical and laboratory findings, not classified elsewhere (R00, R07–4, R53, and R55), Septicemia, unspecified (A41.9), unspecified Diabetes Mellitus (E14), Transient cerebral ischemic attacks and related syndromes (G45), Prosthetic device, implant and cardiac and vascular graft complications (T82.0 to T82.9), Fitting and adjustment of other external prosthetic devices (Z44.8) and presence of implants and cardiac and vascular grafts (Z95.0 to Z95.9).

Death, hospitalization and coronary artery bypass surgery were defined as major events.

Resource valorization

The study used the SUS reimbursement system to estimate costs. The costs of consultations and tests were calculated by multiplying the quantity by the unit price of each resource used in the SUS table.

For pharmacological treatment, a survey of drug prices was performed in the same physical form across three pharmaceutical networks, and their mean prices were calculated. The average price of the medicines was calculated based on the generic version of the drug whenever it was available in Brazil. From the list of medications considered, only 2 drugs do not have the generic version available in Brazil: benazepril by the Novartis Laboratory and sublingual isosorbide-5 mononitrate by the Baldacci Laboratory. For patient transport costs, the price of public land transport in force in October of 2015 was used by assuming 2 journeys for residents in Porto Alegre and 4 journeys for residents in the metropolitan area, in the state interior, and in other states.

For hospitalization costs, the hospital bill amounts paid were used and adjusted for inflation by the National Consumer Price Index (Índice Nacional de Preços Amplo - IPCA) [10] considering the month of closure of the hospital bill as the initial date and October 2015 as the final date.

The total cost of each patient included outpatient care and hospitalization and was divided by the follow-up period to obtain the mean annual cost per individual. The costs were expressed as median values in Brazilian currency and converted to US dollars at an exchange rate of 1 Real = US \$3.60 (exchange rate of 10/2016). For the estimated annual hospitalization cost per patient, analyses were performed to identify potential clinical predictors of higher cost considering the following variables: gender, age, CCS functional class, stroke, unstable angina, myocardial revascularization surgery, myocardial infarction, diabetes mellitus, dyslipidemia, hypertension, body mass index, and active and prior smoking status.

Statistical analysis

Descriptive data are presented as absolute and relative frequencies for categorical variables and as means and standard deviations or medians and interquartile ranges (25th and 75th percentiles) for continuous variables. The Kolmogorov-Smirnov test was used to evaluate the data normality. The costs are presented as the mean and median. The cost variables were compared in relation to clinical predictors using the Mann-Whitney test for data with non-normal distributions after logarithmic transformation (bivariate analysis). A generalized linear model analysis (GLM) was performed to evaluate independent predictors of annual cost per patient. Binary logistic regression was performed to estimate the probabilities of major events and to establish a relationship with the estimated costs. A value of $p < 0.05$ was interpreted as statistically significant. To estimate the score, the cost ratio for significant risk factors was used and the individual probabilities of the presence of major events were calculated.

Results

A total of 633 patients were evaluated, of whom 330 met the inclusion criteria and constitute the study population. A total of 54.8% were male, and 51.8% lived in Porto Alegre. The mean age was 61 years, and the mean follow-up period in the ischemic heart disease clinic was 107.38 ± 2.62 months. Patients with CCS functional class I accounted for 73% of the sample, and patients with CCS class II accounted for 20.6%. There were 31 deaths (9.4%) during the follow-up period, of which 5 were related to concomitant malignancies. The baseline characteristics of the sample are presented in Table 1.

The use of outpatient resources in the follow-up period consisted of 9264 consultations, 71,114 laboratory tests, 5697 diagnostic tests and 416 outpatient catheterizations. On average, there were 28.1 consultations (median 28 and standard deviation 13.11) and 2 catheterizations

Table 1 Basic population characteristics (n = 330)

Characteristics	N (%)
Male gender	181 (54.8)
Mean age (years)*	61 ± 10.3
Acute myocardial infarction	204 (61.8)
Unstable angina	94 (28.5)
Coronary artery bypass surgery	102 (30.9)
Stroke	21 (6.4)
Heart failure	18 (5.5)
Angioplasty	169 (51.2)
Diabetes mellitus	115 (34.8)
Arterial hypertension	277 (83.9)
Dyslipidemia	185 (56.1)
Current smoking	53 (16.1)
Previous smoking	196 (59.4)
Obesity	86 (26.1)
Overweight	139 (42.1)
Regular physical activity	109 (33.0)
CCS class	
I	241 (73.0)
II	68 (20.6)
III	17 (5.2)
IV	4 (1.2)
Patient origin	
Porto Alegre	171 (51.8)
Metropolitan region	122 (37)
Interior	35 (10.6)
Other states	2 (0.6)
SBP*	138.7 (80–230)
DBP*	82.6 (50–160)
Follow-up time**	107.38 ± 2.62

*expressed as the mean and interquartile range. **expressed in months
CCS = Canadian functional class; SBP = Systolic blood pressure; DBP = Diastolic blood pressure

(median 2 and standard deviation 1.44) per patient. The patients' travel costs based on a return journey from their residence to the hospital totaled US $47,955 during the follow up. On average, the patients used 6 drugs per day, representing a mean cost of US $6174 (median US $5519) and a total of $2,037,298 during the period. Drug costs are shown in Table 2.

The total outpatient costs during the follow-up period were US $2,432,933 (Table 3), with a mean annual cost per patient of $854 (median US $765). The greatest drivers of the outpatient costs were pharmacological treatment (81%) and imaging tests (7%).

The mean estimated total hospitalization cost during the follow-up period was US $6104 (median US $4086), which generated a mean cost per hospitalization of US $1976 (median US $1710) (Table 4).

Regarding the total in-hospital procedures performed, catheterizations accounted for 33% (n = 186), angioplasties for 53% (n = 294) and coronary artery bypass surgery for 12% (n = 66). A total of 102 laboratory tests (median 52) and 11 imaging tests (median 7) were performed on average for each patient hospitalized during the follow-up period. In total, 26,092 laboratory tests and 2484 imaging tests were performed during the follow-up period.

Analysis of the total cost for the SUS showed that the highest costs occurred during the first year of follow-up; these costs average US $2865 per hospitalization, with a median of US $2799. The highest number of admissions also occurred during this period (Fig. 1).

Considering outpatient and hospitalization costs as a whole, the estimated total costs were US $3,965,228, with a mean annual cost per patient of US $1522 and median of US $1217 (Table 4). In this study, hospital costs accounted for 38.6% of the total cost of managing ischemic heart disease and outpatient costs accounted for 61.4%. The largest driver of costs was expenditure on drugs, followed by procedures during hospitalization (Fig. 2).

Significant factors that drove the greatest annual costs per patient in hospitalization included unstable angina, angioplasty, prior infarction bypass surgery, diabetes mellitus, hypertension, and obesity. Male gender and age were associated with greater hospitalization costs, but this result was not maintained after the multivariate adjustment (GLM) (Table 5).

Because this study involved a specialized outpatient clinic and a cohort with 10 years of follow-up, 76.7% of the patients had an event during this period. The estimated total cost for the SUS was assessed in relation to the likelihood of major events (hospitalization, death, and coronary artery bypass surgery) and the estimated annual cost per patient by considering the presence of significant risk factors in the bivariate analysis. The results are shown in Figs. 3 and 4.

Discussion

The results of this study offer up-to-date data regarding the outpatient and hospital management cost of patients undergoing clinical follow-up in an ischemic heart disease clinic in a public teaching hospital.

When estimating costs, some economic factors must be considered in the analysis, such as market prices, inflation, depreciation of goods, and opportunity cost [11]. Because this study involved a cohort with a ten-year follow-up, the amounts received in the years prior to the analysis were adjusted for inflation. The price tables used by the SUS were used to estimate the costs, with the

Table 2 Unit prices from the SUS table

Resources	US$ price
Consultations	2.10
Hospitalization days*	NA
ICU III days	141.29
Procedures**	
Coronary Angioplasty	712.25
Primary Coronary Angioplasty (including catheterization)	1303.28
Coronary Angioplasty with stent implantation	1277.39
Coronary Angioplasty with two stents implantation	2090.00
Cardiac catheterization	365.84
Myocardial Revascularization with extracorporeal use	3679.46
Diagnostic tests	
Myocardial scintigraphy with dipiridamol	113.48
Stress myocardial scintigraphy	113.48
Resting myocardial scintigraphy	106.41
Echocardiogram	11.09
Stress echocardiogram	45.83
Electrocardiogram	1.43
Exercise test	8.33
Holter	8.33
Ambulatory Blood Pressure Monitoring	2.80
BP Chest X-ray	1.81
Venous color Doppler ultrasound	11.00
Laboratory tests	
Calcium	0.51
CK	1.02
CK-MB	1.14
HDL and LDL cholesterol	0.98
Total cholesterol	0.51
Creatinine	0.51
Glycemic curve	1.01
Qualitative urinary test	1.03
Phosphorus	0.51
Glucose	0.51
Glycosylated hemoglobin	2.17
Potassium	0.51
C Reactive protein	0.79
Glutamic-oxaloacetic transaminase (GOT)	0.56
Glutamic-pyruvic transaminase (GPT)	0.56
Thyrotropin	2.49
Triglycerides	0.98
Troponin	2.50
Urea	0.51
Generic Drugs***	
Acetylsalicylic acid 100 mg	0.06
Allopurinol 100 mg	0.08
Amiodarone 200 mg	0.26
Amlodipine 5 mg	0.37
Atenolol 50 mg	0.22
Atorvastatin 20 mg	0.73
Captopril 12.5 mg	0.16
Captopril 25 mg	0.22
Captopril 50 mg	0.46
Clopidogrel 70 mg	1.45
Digoxin 0.25 mg	0.10
Diltiazem 60 mg	0.16
Enalapril 5 mg	0.24
Enalapril 10 mg	0.21
Enalapril 20 mg	0.36
Furosemide 40 mg	0.12
Hydrochlorothiazide 25 mg	0.20
Glibenclamide 5 mg	0.08
Isosorbide 10 mg	0.08
Losartan 50 mg	0.34
Lovastatin 20 mg	0.41
Metformin 850 mg	0.23
Metoprolol 100 mg	0.19
Nifedipine 10 mg	0.25
Omeprazole 20 mg	0.25
Paracetamol 500 mg	0.16
Pravastatin 10 mg	0.44
Propranolol 40 mg	0.06
Propranolol 80 mg	0.09
Simvastatin 10 mg	0.63
Simvastatin 40 mg	0.51
Sustrate 10 mg	0.13
Warfarin 5 mg	0.10
Verapamil 80 mg	0.20
Non-generic drugs***	
Benazepril 5 mg	0.54
Sublingual Isosorbide-5 mononitrate	0.11

*Inpatient stay in the SUS are included in the payment for the treatment performed. ** Includes normatives income. *** price for one tablet

exception of drug prices. The prices used by the SUS do not reflect the true costs of the intervention, rather reimbursement values, but represent the closest ones. They can be considered the opportunity cost of each system, which is considered by some authors to represent the real economic value of a resource used to perform an intervention [12, 13]. For the drugs price, we used the average price of the drugs; the estimates would

Table 3 Outpatient costs during the follow-up period in US$

	Consultations	Laboratory tests	Diagnostic tests	Drugs	Transport	Catheterization	Total outpatient cost
N	330	326	325	330	330	208	330
Mean	58.88	178.92	497.91	6.173.63	145.32	519.73	7372.53
Median	58.72	149.96	407.31	5.518.92	74.03	341.51	6539.51
Minimum	6.29	10.58	7.15	0.00	7.22	170.76	275.32
Maximum	159.39	913.76	1742.44	23,560.92	4613.83	2788.11	26,193.39
Total	19,428.67	58,328.71	161,819.60	2,037,297.67	47,954.91	108,104.27	243,293.83

be more accurate if it were possible to identify the amount paid by the government for the medication. However, in the Brazilian government's health database, called DATASUS, this information is not available.

In Brazil cost management accounting in the health area is a rather recent theme and institutions are still developing initiatives to know the real costs of patient care. In our hospital, there is no cost management system at the moment and thus, we cannot accurately state what percentage of the costs we find represents the real costs incurred. Since 2008, the readjustments of the Brazilian Health System reimbursements do not reflect Brazilian inflationary indices such as the National Broad Consumer Price Index (IPCA) and the National Consumer Price Index (NCPI). According to the Brazilian Federal Council of Medicine, in the performance of a coronary angioplasty with stent implantation this gap varies between 39% for the IPCA and 40% for the INPC.

Table 4 Hospitalization costs*

Mean cost per hospitalization	US$ value
N	251
Mean	1976.21
Median	1710.39
Standard deviation	1231.69
Minimum	103.82
Maximum	11,014.21
Cumulative cost of hospitalizations	
Mean	6104.76
Median	4086.02
Standard deviation	5843.72
Minimum	103.82
Maximum	38,890.29
Total	1,532,293.84
Costs per patient considering the outpatient and hospitalization basis	
Mean	12,015.84
Median	9726.93
Standard deviation	8134.67
Minimum	275.32
Maximum	59,437.76
Annual cost per patient	
Mean	1521.54
Median	1217.10
Standard deviation	1171.49
Minimum	237.79
Maximum	8171.83

*Includes tests, procedures, specialist materials, ICU days and fees when incurred

Although previous studies are scarce in the Brazilian literature, some have described the management costs of cardiovascular disease patients. Below, some of these studies are discussed, and the results prior to 2015 have been updated for inflation and are presented in this format for comparisons.

The mean annual cost per outpatient in the SUS was US $854 (median US $765); this finding was similar to the result reported by Ribeiro et al. [7] in a study conducted in 2002, which reported an annual per patient expenditure of US $779 (median US $760) with the same cohort of patients, and by Azambuja et al. [14], who estimated a mean annual cost of US $875 for cases of severe cardiovascular disease.

In terms of the composition of outpatient costs, spending on drug treatment was responsible for the highest expenditure. Regarding the mean annual cost of drugs, the studied sample showed values similar to US $830 found by Araújo et al. in heart failure patients [15]. This expenditure as a proportion of the total outpatient cost (81%) was higher than that found by Ribeiro et al. [7] (80%). This finding is consistent with the reality of Brazilian health care and may reflect the entry of new drugs with higher prices into the market, an increasing number of concomitant cardiovascular diseases, and cumulative price inflation. The cost results presented are similar to those of 10 years ago and we consider that this similarity can be partly explained by the gap in the correction of the Brazilian Health System reimbursements. For example, the value of the medical consultation for reimbursement is US $2.10 since 2005; similarly, several laboratory tests requested in the routine care of patients with ischemic heart disease remain unchanged at US $0.51. Another example, the value of stress scintigraphy

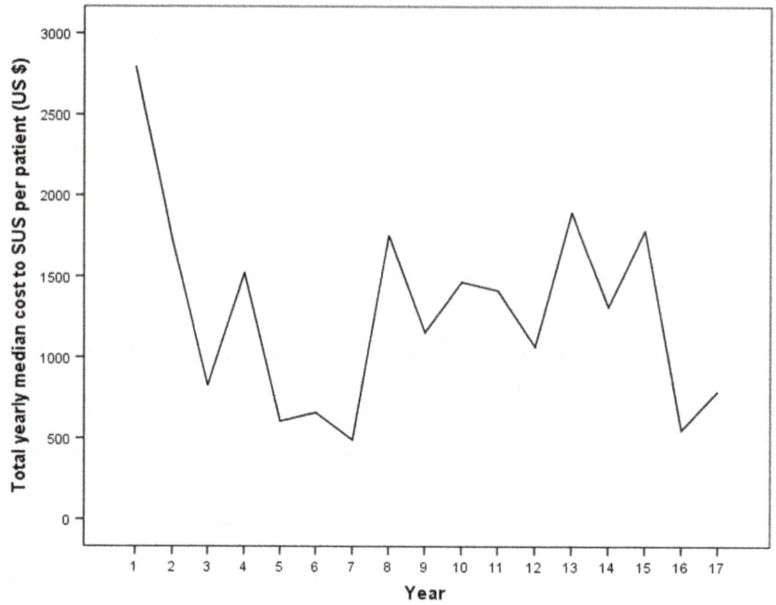

Fig. 1 Total cost to the SUS per year of follow-up (median)

found by Ribeiro was US $93.33; using by the IPCA index, it should be equivalent to US $167.63 (a variation of 79.61%) in this study. However, the reimbursement system only pays US $113.48 (a variation of 21.59%). This study considered that patients paid for 100% of the drugs and that there was 100% drug adherence, which might have led to overestimation of the total costs. Indeed, hypertension, diabetes, and dyslipidemia drugs are provided free in Primary Health Care Units (PHCUs) to public health system users, and there are government subsidies when these drugs are purchased by the private health system users as part of the National Pharmaceutical Assistance Policy [16]. Regardless, patient accessibility to this program was not ascertained in this study. In relation to treatment adherence in Brazil, Tavares et al. [17] found a high rate of adherence used to treat high blood pressure, ranging from 71% in the North to 84% in the South. Santos-Pinto et al. [18] analyzed the Popular Pharmacy Program aimed at private system users and estimated that approximately 70% of users in the North and Northeast who could obtain the drugs for free in the PHCUs acquired them from the Popular Pharmacy Program due to access problems in the PHCUs.

The mean cost to the SUS of each hospitalized patient of US $1976 was similar to the amount reported by Teich [4] (US $2005) in a study of acute coronary syndrome.

The analysis of the total cost to the SUS for each patient during the period suggests that the total costs were

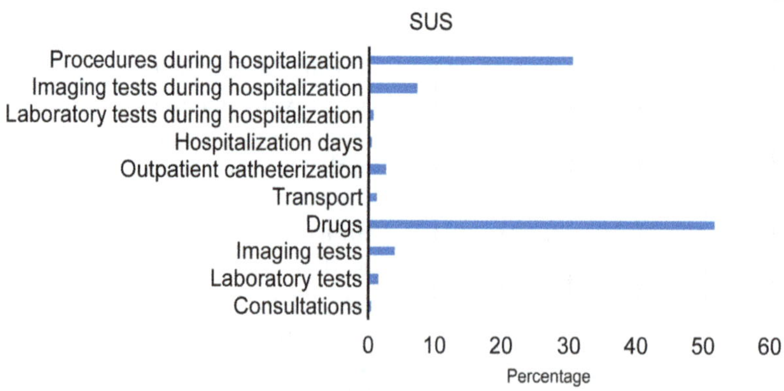

Fig. 2 Individual costs as a proportion of the total cost during follow-up

Table 5 Clinical predictors of the annual cost per patient

	Male		Female		P*
	Mean	Median	Mean	Median	
Annual cost per patient	1556.14	1171.74	1454.52	1298.85	0.884
	≤74 years		≥ 75 years		
	Mean	Median	Mean	Median	
Annual cost per patient	1508.29	1212.88	1649.38	1272.95	0.809
	Stroke		No Stroke		
	Mean	Median	Mean	Median	
Annual cost per patient	1727.86	1301.13	1507.52	1199.09	0.158
	Unstable angina		No Unstable angina		
	Mean	Median	Mean	Median	
Annual cost per patient	1742.73	1490.25	1433.45	1119.83	0.002
	CABS		No CABS		
	Mean	Median	Mean	Median	
Annual cost per patient	1649.55	1422.75	1464.28	1156.82	0.01
	AMI		No AMI		
	Mean	Median	Mean	Median	
Annual cost per patient	1578.52	1155.48	1429.29	1260.28	0.562
	Diabetes		No Diabetes		
	Mean	Median	Mean	Median	
Annual cost per patient	1781.96	1500.19	1382.25	1144.14	< 0.01
	Dyslipidemia		No Dyslipidemia		
	Mean	Median	Mean	Median	
Annual cost per patient	1475.45	1158.71	1580.36	1265.95	0.271
	Hypertension		No Hypertension		
	Mean	Median	Mean	Median	
Annual cost per patient	1568.30	1232.89	1277.17	1183.72	0.03
	BMI ≤ 29.9		BMI ≥ 30		
	Mean	Median	Mean	Median	
Annual cost per patient	1451.13	1145.89	1629.54	1498.74	0.011
	Current smoking		No Current smoking		
	Mean	Median	Mean	Median	
Annual cost per patient	1398.59	1059.38	1558.75	1179.43	0.838
	Previous smoking		No Previous smoking		
	Mean	Median	Mean	Median	
Annual cost per patient	1678.31	1059.38	1523.99	1177.12	0.545
	Heart failure		No Heart failure		
	Mean	Median	Mean	Median	
Annual cost per patient	2323.57	1.482.99	1475.28	1209.04	0.179
	Angioplasty		No Angioplasty		
	Mean	Median	Mean	Median	
Annual cost per patient	1832.63	1491.66	1195.00	976.29	< 0.01

*Mann-Whitney test

higher in the first year and at the end of follow-up, but it was not possible to establish an expenditure distribution pattern. When considering the major events in this cohort (n = 1021), the clinical variables that were predictive of increased costs were unstable angina, angioplasty, coronary artery bypass surgery, diabetes mellitus, obesity, and hypertension, with hospitalizations and readmissions responsible for 93% of all events. The higher number of hospitalizations during follow-up is consistent with literature, which shows re-hospitalization rates of over 30% during the first year of follow-up [16, 19]. As expected, the greater probability of events was associated with higher costs, which underscores the finding that the main drivers in this regard are related to the presence of severity markers, and consequent instability and need for hospitalization.

In this study, the outpatient costs were proportionately higher than the hospitalization costs in relation to the total cost primarily due to the drug expenditure. This result is different from the results found in the literature. The study with one year of follow-up conducted by Araujo [15] reported costs of 40% for hospitalization and 39% for medication. This difference may have been due to the data collection method used when quantifying drug use. In the study by Araújo, drug prices were calculated using the Brasíndice table in 2002. The Brasíndice table was a table published by a specialized company that had the price of drugs sold in Brazil, including the factory price and the maximum price to the consumer, plus taxes. Since May 2009, by resolution of the Regulation Chamber of the Brazilian Medicines Market, it is not allowed to divulge the maximum price of drugs to the consumer. We highlight that the Araújo study was carried out in 2002 with a cohort of 70 patients and used the methods of identifying the cost items and cost tables available at the time to estimate the actual costs of one year of treatment, including applying an overhead rate to the cost components. However, Araujo estimated the cost of hospitalization through the prospective analysis of 3 patients to identify the use of resources and establish the average cost of a day of hospital stay (top-down micro-costing). Today the methods used by Araujo could be considered a mix of the bottom-up and the top-down microcosting approaches. The top-down approach usually produces higher values than the bottom-up approach. Our study used the bottom-up micro-costing approach for identifying and quantifying all cost components. We believe that the differences found may also be influenced by the different methodological approaches used. In the United States, Sieck [20] estimated hospital costs as being responsible for 60% and drugs for 10% of direct costs in patients with congestive heart failure. Dunlay et al. [21] reported that 77% of

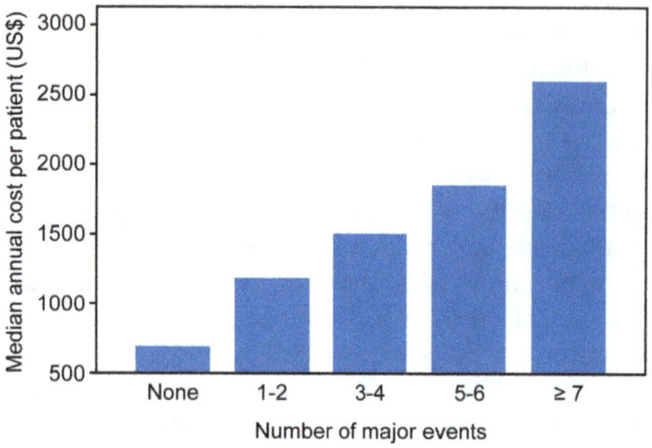

Fig. 3 Mean annual cost per patient considering the number of major events

costs in heart failure were incurred during hospitalization. The difference between our results and those of international studies may be that the hospitalization figures do not account for Brazilian inflation rates. Thus, the prices charged were below inflationary correction for the period. Another factor that may have contributed to this result was the reduction in the cost of orthotics and prostheses (stents) in recent years. In early 2000, the costs of these products were high, but the costs have subsequently reduced due to the entry of a wide range of products from the Indian and Chinese markets into the Brazilian market [22]. Moreover, in the past, stents were acquired by the hospitals with the insertion of a profit margin in the transfer to the hospital account but, currently, are acquired directly by the health plans, and the supplier is paid directly.

In the bivariate analysis, clinical factors such as heart failure, acute myocardial infarction, dyslipidemia, and stroke were not confirmed as major cost predictors. This finding confirmed the results of other studies [14, 23, 24]. Diabetes mellitus and unstable angina were the major cost drivers at both the outpatient and in-hospital levels. The association of the number of major events with costs can be explained by the long follow-up period of this cohort and the number of hospitalizations. A study of heart failure patients showed that 51.2% of the patients return to the emergency room between 1 and 12 times over a one-year period [25].

Considering the 2012 demographic census for the population over 18 years is 9,548,247 people and a prevalence of 7% for ischemic heart disease, the annual direct costs to the SUS for ischemic heart disease would be at least US $3.66 billion. This figure is similar to the figure reported by Teich [4].

Some limitations of this study should be mentioned. Costs related to drugs were assumed to be constant throughout the follow-up period, and the existence of subsidies from governmental pharmaceutical assistance programs and treatment adherence were not considered, which may have caused the share of these costs in the analysis to have been disproportionately high. Another limitation is that the costs in this study were calculated based on the value of the service provided and did not include institutional operating costs. This approach may have led to underestimation of the presented costs.

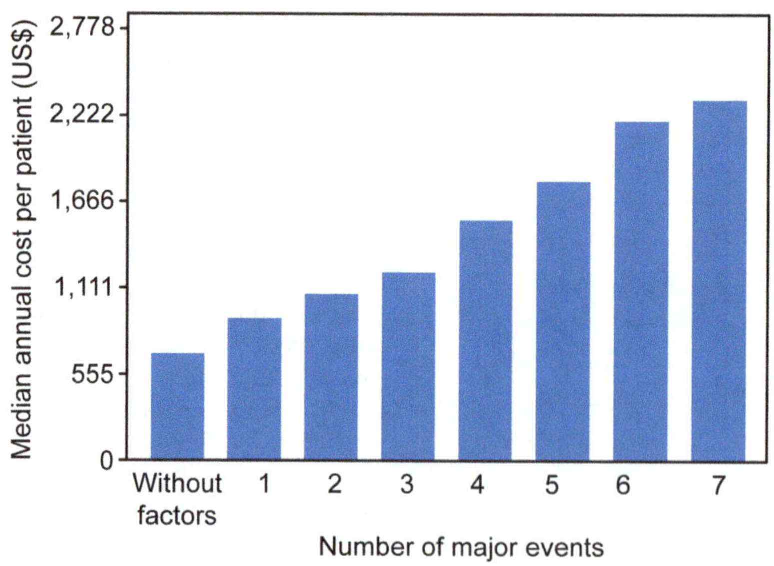

Fig. 4 Median annual cost per patient according to significant clinical predictors

Conclusion

This study showed that the direct costs of longitudinal ischemic heart disease treatment were high and were primarily driven by chronic pharmacological treatment and days of hospitalization; through out a 10-year period the costs were higher in the first year and the last years of follow-up.

In 2014, the per capita income of the Brazilian population was US $292. Thus, the cost of drugs in this study suggests the need to expand the National Pharmaceutical Assistance Policy to include drugs related to coronary heart disease and to review the drug distribution policy in the PHCUs to provide access to drugs and reduce morbidity and mortality.

Data from this study could help to define health care policies for ischemic heart disease patients in terms of the allocation of human resources (physicians and care staff), physical resources (admissions, tests, and drugs), and appropriate financial planning.

Abbreviations

ABPM: Ambulatory blood pressure monitoring; ALT: Alanine aminotransferase; AST: Aspartate aminotransferase; CAD: Coronary artery disease; CCS: Canadian Cardiovascular Society; CK: Creatinine kinase; GLM: Generalized linear model; HDL: High density lipoprotein; ICD: International Classification of Diseases and related Health Problems; ICU: Intensive care unit; IPCA: National Broad Price Index; LDL: Low density lipoprotein; PHCUs: Primary Health Care Units; QUT: Qualitative urine test; REDCap: Research electronic data capture; SUS: Unified Health System

Acknowledgements

The authors thank the Research Incentive Fund of the Clinical Hospital, Porto Alegre (Fundo de Incentivo à Pesquisa do Hospital de Clínicas de Porto Alegre) for its financial support.

Funding

This study was supported by the Research Incentive Fund of the Hospital de Clínicas de Porto Alegre (FIPE-HCPA).

Authors' contributions

RS and CP did the study design and wrote the article. RS made the collection of study data. VH contributes in the statistical analysis of the data. All authors read and approved the final manuscript.

Competing interests

The authors declare that they have no competing interests.

Author details

[1]Graduate Cardiology Program, Universidade Federal do Rio Grande do Sul (UFRGS), Porto Alegre, RS, Brazil. [2]Department of Cardiology, Hospital de Clinicas de Porto Alegre (HCPA), Porto Alegre, RS, Brazil. [3]Department of Cardiology, School of Medicine, UFRGS, Porto Alegre, RS, Brazil. [4]National Health Technology Assessment Institute, CNPq, Porto Alegre, RS, Brazil. [5]Research and Graduate Studies Department. Hospital de Clinicas de Porto Alegre HCPA, Porto Alegre, RS, Brazil. [6]Programa de Pós-graduação em Cardiologia, Hospital de Clínicas de Porto Alegre, Rua Ramiro Barcelos, 2350, CEP, Porto Alegre, RS 90035-903, Brazil.

References

1. WHO Library Cataloguing-In-Publication Data. Global status report on noncommunicable diseases 2010. http://www.who.int/nmh/publications/ncd_report2010/en/. Accessed 5 May 2014.
2. Duncan BB, Stevens A, Schmidt MI. Mortalidade por doenças crônicas no Brasil: situação em 2010 e tendências de 1991 a 2010. In: Saúde Brasil 2011: uma análise da situação de saúde e a vigilância da saúde da mulher. Saúde: Ministério da Saúde, Secretaria de Vigilância em Saúde, Departamento de Análise de Situação de Saúde; 2012. p. 93–104.
3. Brasil, Ministério da Saúde. Datasus. Sistema de informações de mortalidade. Óbitos por residência por ano do óbito segundo capítulo CID-10. Dados preliminares de mortalidade 2013.http://www.datasus.gov.br. Accessed 12 Jan 2016.
4. Teich V, Araujo DV. Estimativa do custo da síndrome coronariana aguda no Brasil. Rev Brascardiol. 2011;24:85–94.
5. Garko MG. Coronary heart disease - part I: the prevalence, incidence, mortality and pathogenesis of the leading cause of death in the United States. Health and Wellness Monthly. 2012; http://letstalknutrition.com/coronary-heart-disease-the-prevalence-incidence-mortality-and-pathogenesis-of-the-leading-cause-of-death-in-the-united-states-2/. Accessed 16 Jan 2016
6. Polanczyk CA, Ribeiro JP. Coronary artery disease in Brazil: contemporary management and future perspectives. Heart. 2009;95:870–6.
7. Ribeiro RA, Mello RGB, Melchior R, Dill JC, Hohmann CB, Lucchese AM, et al. Custo anual do manejo da cardiopatia isquêmica crônica no Brasil. Perspectiva pública e privada. Arq Bras Cardiol. 2005;85:3–8.
8. Brasil, Ministério da Saúde. Glossário temático: Economia da saúde. Série A: Normas e Manuais Técnicos. Ministério da Saúde: Saúde; 2006.
9. Harris PA, Taylor R, Thielke R, Payne J, Gonzalez N, Conde JG. Research electronic data capture (REDCap)–a metadata-driven methodology and workflow process for providing translational research informatics support. J Biomed Inform. 2009;42:377–81.
10. Instituto Brasileiro de Geografia e Estatística. Índice Nacional de Preços ao Consumidor Amplo - IPCA e Índice Nacional de Preços ao Consumidor – INPC. http://www.ibge.gov.br/home/estatistica/indicadores/precos/inpc_ipca/defaultinpc.shtm. Accessed 15 Aug 2015.
11. Brasil, Ministério da Saúde. Avaliação econômica em saúde: desafios para gestão no Sistema Único de Saúde. Série A: Normas e Manuais Técnicos. Saúde: Ministério da Saúde; 2008.
12. Stone DF. Clarifying (opportunity) costs. The American Economist: Forthcoming; 2014. http://papers.ssrn.com/sol3/papers.cfm?abstract_id=2321382 . Accessed 18 Jan 2016
13. Pinto MP, Ugá MAD. Os custos de doenças tabaco-relacionadas para o Sistema Único de Saúde. Cadernos de Saúde Pública. 2010;26:1234–45.
14. Azambuja MIR, Foppa M, Maranhão MFC, Achutti AC. Impacto econômico dos casos de doença cardiovascular grave no Brasil: uma estimativa baseada em dados secundários. Arq Bras Cardiol. 2008;91:163–71.
15. Araújo DV, Tavares LR, Veríssimo R, Ferraz MB, Mesquita ET. Cost of heart failure in the Unified Health System. Arq Bras Cardiol. 2005;84:422–7.
16. Brasil, Ministério da Saúde. Secretaria de Vigilância em Saúde, Departamento de Análise de Situação de Saúde. Plano de ações estratégicas para o enfrentamento das doenças crônicas não transmissíveis (DCNT) no Brasil: 2011–2022. Ministério da Saúde: Saúde; 2011.
17. Tavares NUL, Costa KS, Mengue SS, Vieira MLFP, Malta DC, Silva Júnior JB. Use of medication for treatment of noncommunicable chronic diseases in Brazil: results from the National Health Survey, 2013. Epidemiol Serv Saúde. 2015;24:315–23.
18. Santos-Pinto CDB, Costa NR, Osorio-de-Castro CGS. Quem acessa o Programa Farmácia Popular do Brasil? Aspectos do fornecimento público de medicamentos. Ciência Saúde Coletiva. 2011;16:2963–73.
19. Ambrosy AP, Fonarow GC, Butler J, Chioncel O, Greene SJ, Vaduganathan M, et al. The global health and economic burden of hospitalizations for heart failure: lessons learned from hospitalized heart failure registries. J Am Coll Cardiol. 2014;63:1123–33.
20. Sieck S. The Economics and Reimbursement of Congestive Heart Failure. In: Peacock WF, editor. Short stay management of acute heart failure. N Y; 2012. p. 9–32.
21. Dunlay SM, Shah ND, Shi Q, Morlan B, VanHouten H, Long KH, et al. Lifetime costs of medical care after heart failure diagnosis. Circ Cardiovasc Qual Outcomes. 2011;4:68–75.

19

The association of sleep disordered breathing with left ventricular remodeling in CAD patients

Audrius Alonderis*, Nijole Raskauskiene, Vaidute Gelziniene, Narseta Mickuviene and Julija Brozaitiene

Abstract

Background: There is still insufficient knowledge on the potential effect of mild to moderate sleep-disordered breathing (SDB) that is widely prevalent, often asymptomatic, and largely undiagnosed in patients with stable coronary artery disease (CAD). SDB affects 34% of men and 17% of women aged between 30 and 70. The objective of this study was to evaluate the association between SDB and left ventricular (LV) hypertrophy as well as structural remodeling in stable CAD patients.

Methods: The study was based on a cross-sectional design. Echocardiography and polysomnography was performed in 772 patients with CAD and with untreated sleep apnea. All study participants underwent testing by Epworth Sleepiness Scale questionnaire. Their mean age, NYHA and left ventricular ejection fraction were, respectively: 57 ± 9 years, 2.1 ± 0.5 and 51 ± 8%, and 76% were men. Sleep apnea (SA) was defined as an apnea-hypopnea-index (AHI) ≥5 events/h, and, non-SA, as an AHI <5.

Results: Sleep apnea was present in 39% of patients, and a large fraction of those patients had no complaints on excessive daytime sleepiness. The patients with SA were older, with higher body mass and higher prevalence of hypertension. LV hypertrophy (LVH), defined by allometrically corrected (LV mass/height$^{2.7}$) gender-independent criteria, was more common among the patients with SA than those without (86% vs. 74%, $p < 0.001$). The frequency of LVH by wall thickness criteria (interventricular septal thickness or posterior wall thickness ≥ 12 mm: 49% vs. 33%, $p < 0.001$) and concentric LVH (61% vs. 47%, $p = 0.001$) was higher in CAD patients with SA. The patients with SA had significantly higher values of both interventricular septal thickness and posterior wall thickness. Multiple logistic regression analysis showed that even mild sleep apnea was an independent predictor for LVH by wall thickness criteria and concentric LVH (OR = 1.5; 95% CI 1.04–2.2 and OR = 1.9; 1.3–2.9 respectively).

Conclusions: We concluded that unrecognized sleep apnea was highly prevalent among patients with stable CAD, and the majority of those patients did not report daytime sleepiness. Mild to moderate sleep apnea was associated with increased LV wall thickness, LV mass, and with higher prevalence of concentric LV hypertrophy independently of coexisting obesity, hypertension, diabetes mellitus or advancing age.

Keywords: Cad, Echocardiography, Hypertrophy, Left ventricular geometry, Polysomnography, Sleep apnea

* Correspondence: audrius.alonderis@lsmuni.lt
Behavioral Medicine Institute, Lithuanian University of Health Sciences, Vyduno 4, 00135 Palanga, Lithuania

Background

Coronary artery disease (CAD) is a major health issue in developed countries and constitutes a significant cause of death and disability. According to data from the Framingham Heart Study, a population-based longitudinal study, nearly one-half of males and one-third of females over 40 years of age will develop some manifestation of CAD [1]. Sleep-disordered breathing (SDB) and the related clinical syndrome, sleep apnea (SA), are highly prevalent in patients with ischemic heart disease and often remain undiagnosed, even after admission for myocardial infarction treatment [2, 3]. Sleep apnea is a condition in which breathing stops for more than ten seconds during sleep. Specific questions include whether SA is important in initiating the development of cardiac and vascular disease, whether SA in patients with established cardiovascular (CV) disease accelerates disease progression [4]. According to published data, atrial fibrillation, CAD, congestive heart failure, and arterial hypertension are clinical manifestations and are more common in patients with SA [2, 5–7]. SDB and nocturnal hypoxaemia are highly prevalent in stable heart failure with reduced left ventricular function and were identified as independent predictor of all-cause mortality in these patients [8]. Pathophysiology of acute coronary syndrome (ACS) deeply differs from stable angina, mainly due to peculiar features of plaque [9]. ACS, which is known to be characterized by a higher conventional CV risk, is caused by the loss of integrity of the protective covering of some atherosclerotic plaques, leading to thrombus formation and subsequent vessel obstruction [9, 10]. SA and sleep disruption have also been linked to an imbalance in circulatory thrombotic and anti-thrombotic activity [11]. Evidence linking SA and the severity of SDB to increased mortality and CV morbidity has been conflicting and inconclusive in both stable and unstable patients with established CAD [6, 12–17].

Abnormalities in left ventricular (LV) geometry, including LV hypertrophy (LVH), is both a target organ response to chronic arterial hypertension and other CV disorders; and LVH is an independent risk factor for coronary heart disease, heart failure, arrhythmias, including sudden cardiac death, stroke, and other major CV morbidity and mortality [16, 18–20]. Recurrent apneas during sleep lead to a sequence of events that, independently or in concert with other recognized risk factors, are likely to have harmful effects on CV structure and function. Several studies reported increased left-ventricular thickness or mass in association with SA but these relations were not significant after adjustment for body weight [21, 22].

Patients with SDB have a high prevalence of arterial hypertension and, more importantly, obesity, which represents the strongest predisposing factor for SDB [23–25]. Hypertrophy, defined as an increase in LV mass in relation to body size, is produced by an increase in chamber size, an increase in wall thickness, or both [26]. The relation between hypertension and obesity and its impact on LV geometry are known [27–33]. There is still insufficient knowledge on an impact of SA on LV geometry and on potential effect of mild to moderate sleep-disordered breathing, which is prevalent, often asymptomatic, and largely undiagnosed in stable CAD [12, 26].

The present study was performed to determine the association of SDB with LV geometry. We hypothesized, that in stable CAD patients even mild to moderate SA is an independent risk factor for: (1) a higher prevalence of LVH, by wall thickness criteria, with more pronounced both septal and posterior wall thickening; (2) a higher prevalence of concentric left ventricle than in patients without SA controlling for traditional recognized risk factors.

Methods

Design and setting

The study was a cross-sectional investigation of 1027 consecutive stable CAD patients attending the Clinic of Cardiovascular Rehabilitation, from October 2007 until December 2014 for routine cardiac rehabilitation program. Criterion for inclusion to the study are following: patients with CAD, men and women, from 18 years and older, consecutively referred to the rehabilitation clinic within two weeks after treatment for acute coronary syndromes (ACS), no current drug or mechanical treatment for SA. All patients were receiving standard treatment for secondary prevention of CAD and heart failure (HF) according to existing guidelines.

137 (13.3%) Of the patients were excluded from the study for meeting the criteria of being older than 80 years and having cognitive disorientation and communicative disabilities, having other severe diseases or has refused to participate in the program. In total, 887 (86.3%) Participants had successful echocardiographic data, 775 (75.4%) Participants had successful PSG of which 772 also had PSG data in conjunction with echocardiographic and ESS data (the other 115 with successful echocardiography data either elected not to undergo PSG or were ineligible due to medical reasons). Several echocardiograms and PSGs were technically inadequate (n = 6, 0.5%). Although the inclusion rate for eligible patients for study analysis was 772 (75%), the inclusion design was consecutive. Anthropometric and clinical profile of the patients not involved into the study did not differ significantly compared with the studied group. There were more cases of diabetes mellitus (23.5% Vs. 13.7%, $p < 0.001$) In studied patients than those in non-studied patients. The ratio of male patients was higher in not studied group (81.2% Vs. 73.6%, $p = 0.001$).

Ethic

The study and its consent procedures were approved by the Lithuanian Bioethics Committee (Certificate No. BE-2-21 issued at 2007–04-13) and conform to the ethical guidelines of the 2000 Declaration of Helsinki. Written informed consent was obtained from each study patient.

Patient assessment

All patients were evaluated for demographic characteristics (age, gender), CAD risk factors - diabetes mellitus, smoking, arterial hypertension, body mass index (BMI), and clinical characteristics, including New York Heart Association (NYHA) functional class, diabetes mellitus and use of medications. Hypertension was defined as a blood pressure > 140/90 mmHg measuring BP using sphygmomanometer or if the subject was receiving antihypertensive medications. All patients underwent overnight-polysomnography and were classified as sleep apneics or controls according to the apnea-hypopnea index.

Anthropometry

Weight and height for study subjects was measured in indoor clothing and without shoes. BMI was calculated as weight (in kg) divided by height (in m^2). Measured weight and height were used to calculate BMI, and categorized as follows: < 25, 25–29.9, and ≥30 kg/m^2, to represent normal, overweight, and obese (class I (30–34.9); class II (35–39.9), class III ≥40 kg/m^2) individuals for all analyses.

Polysomnography, classification of SA

Overnight fully attended polysomnography (PSG) monitoring was performed with the "Alice 4" Polysomnography System (Respironics Inc., USA) in the Sleep laboratory using standard recording techniques according to AASM (American Academy of Sleep Medicine) and precise protocol of PSG monitoring [34]. Surface electrodes were applied to perform electroencephalogram, chin electromyogram, electrocardiogram, and electrooculography. Airflow was monitored using a thermistor placed at the nose and mouth, and arterial oxygen saturation (SaO_2) was recorded continuously with a pulse oximeter. Apnea was defined as the disappearance of airflow for over 10 s; hypopnea was defined as a 50% or greater decrease in airflow lasting for more than 10 s associated with arousal or a 3% or greater decrease in arterial oxygen saturation from the baseline level. Physiological variables collected from the polysomnograms included the number of central apneas, obstructive or mixed apneas, mean oxygen saturation during sleep; and the max oxygen desaturation during sleep, oxygen desaturation index (ODI), respiration disturbance index (in total sleep time, AHI). The most common type of SA is obstructive sleep apnea (OSA), and much of the pathophysiologic understanding of SA relies on studies of OSA [4]. In our study the influence of central and obstructive events was not separately analysed.

The apnea-hypopnea index (AHI) was calculated as the total number of apnea and hypopnea episodes per hour of sleep [34]. According to the American Academy of Sleep Medicine criteria [34] SA was defined as five or more episodes of apnea and hypopnea per hour of sleep (AHI ≥ 5 n/h) and classified as mild (AHI 5–15), moderate (AHI 16–30), or severe (AHI > 30 n/h). Patients with AHI < 5 were classified as not having SA (non-SA group).

Epworth Sleepiness Scale (ESS) - was used for evaluation of the subjective excessive daytime sleepiness (EDS). Briefly, the patient rates the probability of dozing (0 to 3) in eight different situations. No specific time frame is specified. The ESS score represents the sum of individual items, and ranges from 0 to 24. A score 10 and more is considered as positive for the presence of excessive daytime sleepiness [35].

Echocardiography recording and analysis

Echocardiographic evaluation of the patients was blinded to the results of the PSG. Echocardiography studies were performed using Esaote echocardiography System (My Lab 50 Xvision, Italy). LV systolic function was assessed by LV ejection fraction (LVEF) using the modified biplane Simpson's method with apical two- and four-chamber views. It was defined as reduced LVEF while LVEF less than 45%. LV end-diastolic internal dimension (LVEDD), LV end-systolic internal dimension (LVESD), interventricular septal thickness (IVST), and LV posterior wall thickness (LVPWT) were determined from M-mode measurements according to the American Society of Echocardiography (ASE) guidelines [36]. The LV mass was calculated using the ASE convention [37, 38]:

$$\mathrm{LVM} = 0.8\left[1.04\left\{(\mathrm{IVST} + \mathrm{LVPWT} + \mathrm{LVEDD})^3 - \mathrm{LVEDD}^3\right\}\right] + 0.6$$

LVM was divided by $height^{2.7}$ and by body surface area (BSA) to obtain left ventricular mass index (LVMI). Because LVM was most strongly correlated with BMI and there is not a specific value adjusted for obesity, for this reason we adopted the most commonly used: LVM adjusted according to $height^{2.7}$ ($LVM/height^{2.7}$) [32] which is proposed to be similarly sensitive in detecting obesity-related and -unrelated LVH. The $height^{2.7}$ index was also important for the subcategorization of patients according to the presence of concentric or eccentric LVH because the prognostic value of such subcategorization was apparent only when the $height^{2.7}$-based criterion was applied [39].

LVH was defined as gender-neutral cutoff value for LVM indexed for height > 51 $g/m^{2.7}$ [40, 41]. Relative wall thickness (RWT) was computed by the ratio of sum of IVST and LVPWT to LVEDD. LV structure was categorized as normal (RWT ≤0.42 and no LVH), concentric remodeling (RWT >0.42 and no LVH), concentric hypertrophy (RWT >0.42 and LVH) and eccentric hypertrophy (RWT ≤0.42 and LVH) [36]. In addition, for the purposes of this study, we defined the prevalence of LVH on the basis of wall thickness criteria (IVST or LVPWT ≥12 mm) [22, 37].

Statistical analysis

Quantitative variables are expressed as means ± SD or medians (interquartile ranges [IQRs]) or in percentages, when appropriate. The Kolmogorov-Smirnov test was used to assess the normal distribution of continuous variables. To compare basic characteristics between non-SA and SA (AHI ≥ 5) groups the significance of differences was assessed using Mann–Whitney tests (or t tests, if data were normally distributed) or chi-squared tests, respectively. Analysis of variance (ANOVA) was used to determine whether there are any statistically significant differences between the means of three (non-SA group excluded) or four independent SA severity (coded as 1 = non-SA, 2 = mild, 3 = moderate, 4 = severe) groups. For the linear trend the *p* value for F-ratio was presented. A Bonferroni correction was applied to post hoc pairwise comparisons of means.

To further substantiate the notion that mild-severe SA was an independent determinant of LVH by wall thickness criteria or concentric LV geometry (dependent variable coded 0 = absent/1 = present), bivariate analysis and multiple logistic regression analyses were performed. In the multiple logistic regression analysis, statistically significant variables in the bivariate analysis, as well as the non-significant variables with suggested clinical relevance, were included. The candidate explanatory (independent) variables for entering in the multiple regression model were hypoxemia during sleep SaO_2 and age, AHI (4 categories), BMI (4 categories), age over 60, sex, hypertension, diabetes mellitus, NYHA class, current smoking, history of MI as well as LVEF lower than 45%, excessive daytime sleepiness (ESS ≥ 10). Because daytime sleepiness is common in patients with SA, this factor was taken into account as potential confounding factor. The goodness of fit and Nagelkerke R^2 for these models presented. Forward stepwise selection was then performed to identify factors independently associated with LVH. Data were analyzed with SPSS 17.0 statistical software (SPSS Inc., Chicago, Illinois, USA). A *p*-value <0.05 was considered significant.

Results

Clinical characteristics

Patients were predominantly male (76%), mean age was 57 ± 9 years (ranged from 32 to 81 years). The median value of the AHI in the sample was 3.4 and the interquartile range (25th percentile to 75th percentile) was 1 to 9. Sleep apnea defined as five or more episodes of apnea and hypopnea per hour of sleep (AHI ≥ 5 n/h) was present in 300 (39%) of patients and 175 (22.7%) of patients had LVEF ≤ 45%.

General characteristics comparison according to SA status

Compared to non-SA patients, individuals with SA were on average older (SA: 59 ± 9 years vs. non-SA: 56 ± 9 years, $p < 0.001$), more frequently male (83% vs. 72%; $p = 0.004$), and had a higher prevalence of traditional CV risk factors such as obesity and hypertension (53% vs. 43% and 91% vs. 78%, respectively; both $p < 0.01$). Current smoking was more common in the non-SA patients than that in patients with SA. Almost equal proportions were in NYHA classes ($\chi^2 = 4.8$ $p = 0.09$) (Table 1). We also estimated that 42% of men and 28% of women had an AHI ≥5 ($\chi^2 = 12.3, p < 0.001$).

ESS ranged from 0 to 18 with a median of 6 (interquartile range 4–9). The patients with SA had higher scores on the ESS than those non-SA patients ($p = 0.006$). No statistically significant between-group differences were found for frequency of excessive daytime sleepiness (ESS ≥ 10) (respectively 16% and 19%; $p = 0.14$) (Table 1). The mean ESS score was within the normal range in both groups (6.0 ± 3.5 vs. 6.7 ± 3.5). ACE inhibitors/angiotensin II receptor blockers and beta-blockers were prescribed to 81% and 89% of study patients, respectively. Antihypertensive and antiagregant drugs were used by larger number of patients with SA than non-SA patients ($p = 0.012$ and $p = 0.003$, respectively; data not shown).

Clinical, polysomnographic and echocardiographic characteristics according to SA severity

There were no statistically significant differences in their mean age and sex in SA patients groups according to severity of SA. Prevalence of NYHA class, percentage of hypertension and LVEF ≤ 45%, as well as diabetes mellitus, history of MI, smoking history did not differ between mild, moderate and severe SA patients groups. However, BMI was higher in the severe SA patients than that in patients with moderate ($p = 0.025$) and mild ($p = 0.002$) SA (Table 2).

There was (as expected) a gradual increase in mean AHI and ODI with increase in SA severity (p for trend < 0.001). Patients with severe SA had both the lowest average SaO_2 and highest maximal oxygen desaturation ($p < 0.001$). Severity of SA did not manifest by sleepiness (p for trend = 0.062). Even in the most severe apnea category (AHI ≥ 30) the mean ESS score statistically significant differ from that in non-SA patients (being within the normal range 7.6 ± 3.8) (Table 3).

Table 1 Univariate analysis of demographic, clinical characteristics and comorbidities of the CAD patients according to SA status

Characteristic	Total sample *N* = 772	Non-SA AHI: <5 *n* = 472	SA AHI: ≥5 *n* = 300	p
Age, years	57 ± 9	56 ± 9	59 ± 9	<0.001
Age over 60 years, n (%)	344 (47)	191 (40)	153 (50)	χ^2 = 8.2 p = 0.004
Male gender, n (%)	586 (76)	338 (72)	248 (83)	0.001
BMI, kg/m^2	30.0 ± 4.8	29.4 ± 4.6	31.0 ± 5.0	<0.001
BMI, n (%):				χ^2 = 11.8 p = 0.003
Normal (<25 kg/m^2)	104 (13.5)	78 (16.5)	26 (8.7)	
Overweight (25–24.9 kg/m^2)	305 (39.5)	189 (40.0)	116 (38.7)	
Obese (≥30 kg/m^2)	363 (47.0)	205 (43.4)	158 (52.7)	
Coronary artery disease (CAD), n (%):				χ^2 = 3.8 *p* = 0.43
Stable angina pectoris	230 (29.8)	140 (29.7)	90 (30.0)	
First myocardial infarction	729 (94.4)	278 (58.8)	173 (57.7)	
Previous myocardial infarction	91 (11.7)	54 (11.5)	37 (12.3)	
NYHA class, n (%):				χ^2 = 4.8 p = 0.09
I	65 (8.4)	48 (10.2)	17 (5.7)	
II	598 (77.5)	359 (76.4)	239 (79.9)	
III	106 (13.7)	63 (13.4)	43 (14.4)	
LVEF ≤45%, n (%)	175 (22.7)	95 (20.1)	80 (26.7)	χ^2 = 4.5 p = 0.034
Hypertension n (%)	641 (83.0)	369 (78.2)	272 (90.7)	χ^2 = 20 p < 0.001
Diabetes mellitus, n (%)	165 (21.4)	102 (21.6)	63 (21.0)	χ^2 = 0.04 *p* = 0.84
History of smoking, n (%)	97 (12.6)	67 (14.3)	30 (10.0)	χ^2 = 2.9 *p* = 0.08
Median (IQR) Epworth Sleepiness Scale, score	6 (4–9)	6 (3–8)	6 (4–9)	0.006[a]
Excessive day time sleepiness ESS > 10, n (%)	131 (17)	74 (15.7)	57 (19.0)	χ^2 = 1.4 p = 0.14

Values are mean ± standard deviation, or number of patients (%) unless stated otherwise
BMI body mass index, *ESS* Epworth Sleepiness Scale, *LVEF* left ventricular ejection fraction, *IRQ* interquartile range, *SA* sleep apnea, *AHI* apnea-hypopnea index, *NYHA* New York Heart Association
[a]Mann-Whitney U test

We found no statistically significant differences in a frequency of EDS among patients without (15.7%) and with SA despite the severity (17.7% to 24.5%, p = 0.556) (Table 3).

Reduced LVEF (≤45%) was more frequent in the patients with SA than those in non-SA patients (26.7% and 20.1% respectively, p = 0.034) (Table 1). There were no significant differences in LVEF (mean ejection fraction) of patients included in any of the groups of SA severity ($p_{\text{for trend}}$ = 0.38), suggesting that SA severity was not affecting changes in their LV systolic function. Post hoc analysis (data not shown) demonstrated that only the LVEDD was marginally significantly higher in severe SA patients than those in mild SA patients (mild-SA vs. severe-SA p = 0.044 (not shown), model F = 3.03 $p_{\text{for trend}}$ = 0.05) (Table 4).

There were not found statistically significant differences in left atrium diameter, in thickness of IVST and LVPWT, in value of LVM and LVMI (g/m^{-2} and g/m$^{2.7}$) of patients included in any of the groups of SA severity. This suggests that SA severity according to AHI categories was not inducing changes in their LV thickness and mass (ANOVA for SA severity groups all $p_{\text{for trend}}$ > 0.05, Table 4).

Left ventricular hypertrophy

In univariate analysis the CAD patients with SA had a 1.9-fold higher prevalence of LVH on the basis of wall thickness criteria (IVST or LVPWT ≥12 mm) compared to non-SA patients (49.3 vs. 33.4%; odds ratio, OR = 1.9; 95% confidence interval (CI), 1.4–2.6; p < 0.001) (Table 4, Fig. 1).

Left atrium diameter, IVST and LVPWT was significantly higher in patients with SA, than those in non-SA patients (all p < 0.001). However, no between-group differences were found for RWT (Table 4).

LVH defined by allometrically corrected (LV mass/height$^{2.7}$) gender-independent criteria was present in 86% of the SA patients compared to 74% in non-SA patients group (p < 0.001).

Table 2 Basic characteristics of the CAD patients with SA according to SA severity

Variable	SA severity group			p for trend[a]
	Mild AHI: 5–14.9 n = 192	Moderate AHI: 15–29.9 n = 59	Severe AHI: ≥30 n = 49	
	1	2	3	
Age, years	59.1 ± 8.7	59.7 ± 9.3	60.9 ± 7.3	0.401
Age over 60 years, n (%)	88 (47)	32 (54)	33 (67)	0.037
Male, n (%)	148 (79.1)	52 (88.1)	44 (89.8)	0.087
BMI, kg/m^2	30.5 ± 4.9	30.7 ± 4.5	33.2 ± 5.5[b]	0.003
Hypertension, n (%)	171 (91.4)	53 (89.8)	45 (91.8)	0.965
Diabetes mellitus, n (%)	38 (20.3)	9 (15.3)	15 (30.6)	0.139
NYHA class, mean	2.05 ± 0.43	2.14 ± 0.47	2.16 ± 0.47	0.203
Myocardial infarction, n (%)	133 (71)	39 (66)	16.9 (71)	0.746
LVEF ≤ 45%, n (%)	53 (28.3)	13 (22.0)	13 (26.5)	0.600
Smoking history, n (%)	19 (10.2)	7 (11.9)	3 (6.1)	0.588

Values are mean ± standard deviation, or number of patients (%)
SA sleep apnea, *AHI* apnea-hypopnea index, *BMI* body mass index, *LVEF* left ventricular ejection fraction, *NYHA* New York Heart Association
[a]ANOVA or χ^2 (differences between different SA severity groups)
[b]p < 0.002 severe SA vs. mild SA and p = 0.025 severe SA vs. moderate SA

Distribution of LV geometrical pattern

Some form of LV geometric remodeling was present in 92% of patients, with concentric LVH as the most common geometric abnormality. Eccentric LVH occurred in 26.3% (n = 192), concentric LVH in 52.4% (n = 382) of patients, concentric LV remodeling in 13.4% (n = 98). Eccentric LVH is much less prevalent than concentric hypertrophy.

The frequency distribution of the LV geometric groups indicated significant differences between SA and non-SA patients (χ^2 = 18.9; p < 0.001) (Fig. 2). Percentage of concentric hypertrophy defined as the combination of an increased RWT and an increased LVMI (LVM/height$^{2.7}$) was 60.9% in CAD patients with SA compared to 47.1% (p < 0.001) in non-SA patients (Fig. 2).

LVH (high LVMI) is traditionally two right panels designate subjects with increased LVMI (Fig. 2). As it described in Table 4 pattern of concentric remodeling – comprising high RWT without an absolute increase in mass index, pattern of concentric hypertrophy depend on increased LV wall thickness and chamber dilation is present.

Table 3 Polysomnography characteristics of the CAD patients according to SA severity

Variable	non-SA AHI < 5 n = 472	SA severity group			p for trend[c]
		Mild AHI: 5–14.9 n = 192	Moderate AHI: 15–29.9 n = 59	Severe AHI: ≥30 n = 49	
		1	2	3	
AHI, n/h	1.7 ± 1.5[a]	9.0 ± 2.9	21.7 ± 4.5	44.3 ± 10.8	<0.001
ODI, %	2.6 ± 7.7[a]	8.1 ± 12.4[23]	14.0 ± 17.4[13]	35.1 ± 25.1[12]	<0.001
Average SaO_2, %	94.5 ± 1.7[a]	93.9 ± 1.8[3]	93.4 ± 2.8[3]	91.9 ± 4.9[12]	0.001
$DeSaO_2$ max, %	6.7 ± 8.3[a]	12.0 ± 8.0[3].	15.2 ± 10.5[3]	24.6 ± 17.5[12]	<0.001
ESS score	6.0 ± 3.5[b]	6.7 ± 3.5	6.0 ± 3.2	7.6 ± 3.8	0.062
ESS > 10, n (%)	74 (15.7)	34 (17.7)	11 (18.6)	12 (24.5)	0.556

Data are presented as mean ± SD or number of patients (%)
SA sleep apnea, *AHI* apnea-hypopnea index, events per hour, *ODI* oxygen desaturation index, *SaO_2* saturation of nocturnal arterial oxygen, *$DeSaO_2max$* maximal oxygen desaturation, *ESS* Epworth sleepiness scale
[a]p < 0.01 between non-SA and every SA groups
[b]p < 0.05 between non-SA and Sever SA (ANOVA for all four groups, post hoc with Bonferroni correction)
[c]ANOVA or χ^2 test for SA severity groups, non-SA group was excluded from this analysis
[123]the number in superscript indicates the SA severity groups, with significant differences p < 0.05 (ANOVA for three SA severity groups, post hoc with Bonferroni correction)

Table 4 Basic echocardiographic measurements of the left ventricle in SA and non-SA patients

Variable	Non-SA AHI: <5 n = 472	SA AHI: ≥5 n = 300	t test, Mann–Whitney or χ^2 test	p for trend[a]
Thickness and diameters				
Left atrium, cm	3.8 ± 0.5	4.1 ± 2.2	<0.001	0.110
LVPWT, mm	11.1 ± 1.1	11.6 ± 1.1	<0.001	0.904
IVST, mm	11.2 ± 1.6	11.8 ± 1.7	<0.001	0.829
LVEDD, mm	50.3 ± 5.1	51.6 ± 5.6	0.003	0050
LVESD, mm	33.8 ± 6.1	34.7 ± 5.7	0.013	0.052
LVWT, mm	22.3 ± 2.4	23.4 ± 2.4	<0.001	0.829
RWT	0.45 ± 0.06	0.45 ± 0.06	0.149	0.232
LVH by wall thickness criteria, n (%)	151 (33.4)	138 (49.3)	<0.001	0.268
IVST ≥ 12 mm	126 (27.9)	118 (42.1)	<0.001	0.381
LVPWT ≥ 12 mm	79 (17.5)	89 (31.7)	<0.001	0.593
LV mass index ≥51 g/m$^{2.7}$, n (%)	333 (74.0)	241 (86.4)	<0.001	0.348
RWT > 42, n (%)	285 (63.3)	195 (69.9)	0.077	0.348
Concentric LVH, n (%)	214 (47.1)	168 (60.9)	0.001	0.438
Left ventricular mass				
LVM g	256.4 ± 63.4	285.9 ± 68.5	<0.001	0.210
LVMI g/m^2	128.7 ± 26.9	139.5 ± 29.4	<0.001	0.765
LVMI g/m$^{2.7}$	59.7 ± 13.9	66.1 ± 15.4	<0.001	0.550
LVEF, %	52.1 ± 8.4	50.4 ± 8.7	0.007	0.380
LVEF ≤ 45%, n (%)	95 (20.1)	80 (26.7)	0.034	0.135

Data are presented as mean ± SD or number of patients (%)
SD indicates standard deviation, *SA* sleep apnea, *AHI* apnea-hypopnea index, *IVST* interventricular septum thickness in diastole, *LVPWT* left ventricular posterior wall thickness in diastole, *LVEDD* left ventricular end-diastolic diameter, *LVESD* left ventricular end-systolic diameter, *LVWT* left ventricular wall thickness, *RWT* relative wall thickness, *LVH* left ventricular hypertrophy, *LVM* left ventricular mass, *LVMI* left ventricular mass index, *LVEF* LV ejection fraction
[a]ANOVA or χ^2 for SA severity groups, data not shown, non- SA patients were excluded from this analysis

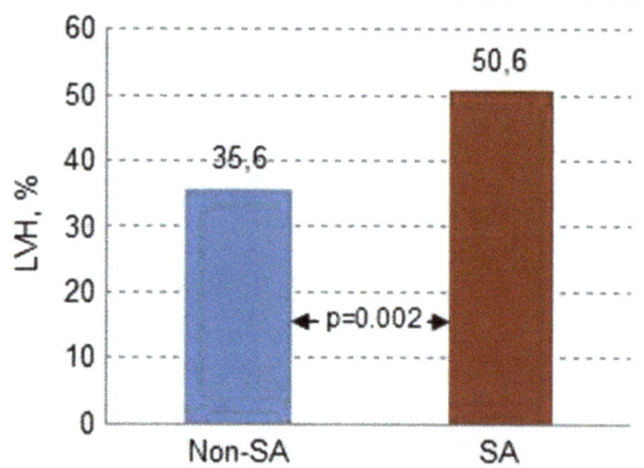

Fig. 1 Prevalence of left ventricular hypertrophy on the basis of wall thickness criteria (interventricular septal thickness or posteriorwall thickness ≥ 12 mm). LVH = left ventricular hypertrophy; SA = sleep apnea

Determinants of LV hypertrophy in the CAD patients

Predictors of LVH on the basis of wall thickness criteria

Multiple logistic regression analysis highlighted cross sectional predictors of LVH on the basis of wall thickness criteria (interventricular septal thickness or posterior wall thickness ≥ 12 mm) such as male sex (OR = 2.6) $p < 0.001$), hypertension (OR = 1.8 $p = 0.016$), age over 60 years (OR = 1.7 $p = 0.002$), LVEF ≤45% (OR = 0.7 p < 0.001) and AHI (for trend $p = 0.029$): mild SA versus non-SA (OR = 1.5; $p = 0.030$), moderate SA versus non-SA (OR = 2.1; $p = 0.012$) (Fig. 3).

The prevalence of LVH on the basis of wall thickness criteria was lower in patients with LVEF ≤ 45% and did not differ significantly between the patients with severe SA (AHI ≥ 30) and non-SA (OR = 0.96; $p = 0.91$). Furthermore, the risk progressively increased with higher BMI values (p for trend <0.001) but this increase slowed down in patients with BMI ≥ 40 versus normal (OR = 3.5 95% CI, 1.3–9.6; p < 0.001) (Fig. 3).

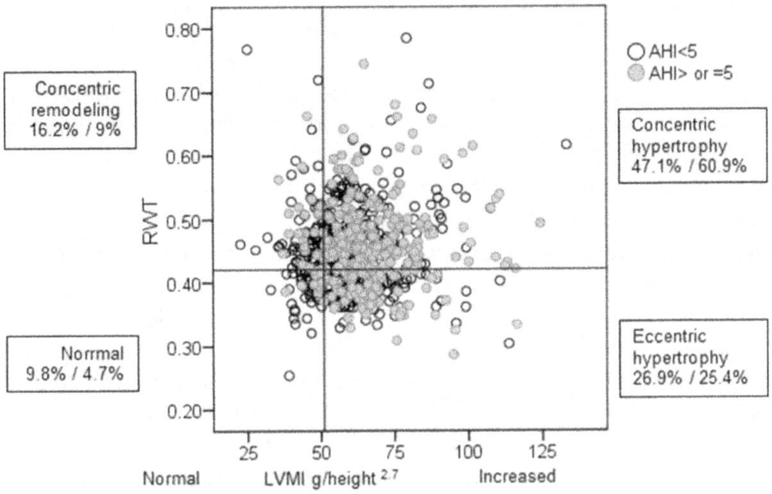

Fig. 2 Frequency distribution of the four different LV–geometrical patterns in patients with vs without sleep apnea. The spreadsheet showed the distribution of LV mass index versus relative wall thickness (RWT). Apnea-hypopnea index (AHI) ≥5 n/h = sleep apnea. Left ventricular geometry, including concentric remodeling as well as eccentric and concentric hypertrophy based on normal/high RWT and left ventricular hypertrophy (LVH) based on left ventricular mass index (LVMI g/height $^{2.7}$) criteria. The reference lines indicate the gender-independent LVH cut-off, (51 g/m $^{2.7}$, vertical line), and the upper limit of RWT (0.42, horizontal line). In boxes: geometric pattern, percentage: without sleep apnea/with sleep apnea; χ^2-test df = 3 $p < 0.001$

Predictors of concentric LVH

Mild SA (AHI = 5–14.9 /h), performing multiple logistic regression analysis, was found as a strong independent cross sectional predictor *of concentric LVH* in the CAD patients (OR = 1.9). The risk of concentric hypertrophy did not increase with the greater level of SA severity.

For BMI increase every 5 kg/m^2 (e.g., moving from normal weight to overweight, or from overweight to mild obesity), the risk of concentric LVH also increased

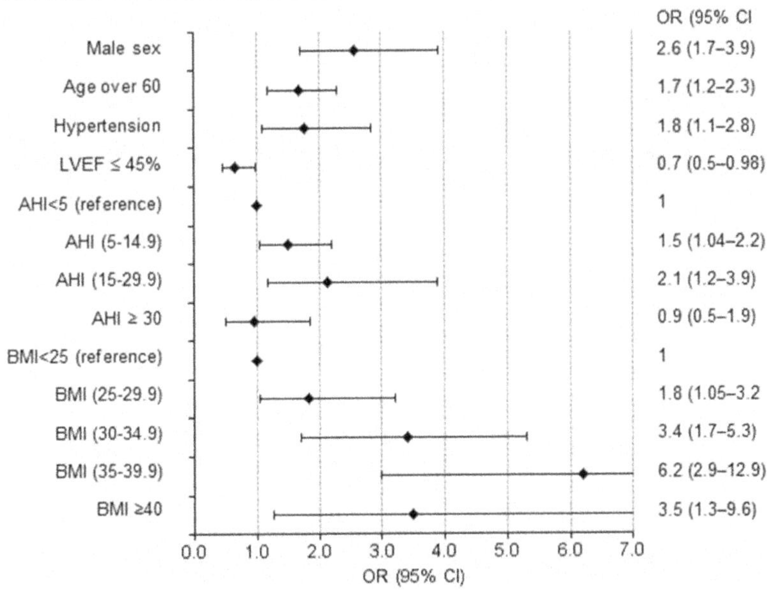

Fig. 3 Cross sectional predictors of left ventricular hypertrophy on the basis of wall thickness criteria (interventricular septal thickness or posterior wall thickness ≥ 12 mm). The independent variables entered in the multiple regression model were: age, sex, ESS score, hypoxemia during sleep SaO_2, age over 60, AHI (4 categories), BMI (4 categories), NYHA class, hypertension, diabetes mellitus, current smoking, history of MI as well as LVEF lower than 45% and excessive daytime sleepiness (ESS ≥ 10). Model: Hosmer & Lemeshow test $\chi^2 = 8.9$ df = 8 $p = 0.349$; Nagelkerke $R^2 = 0.213$. Abbreviations: ESS = Epworth sleepiness scale, LVEF = left ventricular ejection fraction; AHI = apnea-hypopnea index; BMI = body mass index; OR = odds ratio; CI = confidence interval

by 50% (OR = 1.5). Such factors as gender, history of smoking, diabetes mellitus were not statistically significant (Fig. 4).

Discussion

Summary of findings

Previous studies, that often lacked adjustment for important cardiovascular risk factors suggested that SDB was associated with changes in heart structure, including LV hypertrophy. The present study was performed in a large sample of consecutive *stable CAD patients* characterized by a relatively high degree of comorbidity. This study extends these results with the novel finding that *even mild level* of SDB is strongly associated with LVH, with increase LV wall thickness (both interventricular septum and posterior wall) and concentric LVH, independently of coexisting traditionally recognized risk factors. The risk of concentric hypertrophy did not increase with greater levels of SDB severity.

These results could suggest that the effect of SA on LVH risk is fully realized at certain SA severity level. As hypothesized, there was almost 2-fold increase in risk of having LVH on the basis of wall thickness criteria, and 1.5-fold higher risk of concentric hypertrophy, adjusted for the traditionally recognized risk indicators in CAD patients with the disordered breathing.

Although patients with SA had a higher mean value of the ESS than non-SA patients, this value was lower than the reference value for excessive sleepiness (ESS ≥10). Therefore, this value did not seem to be a determining factor in the diagnosis of SA in these patients. The limitations of ESS are known in cardiovascular patients and the existence of patients with severe SA without excessive sleepiness is controversial [41, 42].

Though we do not claim any causal relation our results could suggest that even mild SA had additive effect in changes to the heart shape, similar to the effects of both hypertension and obesity. This effect includes increased mass and thickening of the heart wall. As patients with stable CAD and with SA often do not show typical SA symptoms, the presence of one or more established predictors of LVH *on the basis of wall thickness criteria or concentric LVH,* such as male sex, older age, higher BMI, ejection fraction >45%, or SA may *constitute independent risk factors* for adverse long-term outcomes. The increase recognition of SA as an independent, additive or even synergistic risk factor for CAD brings a growing need for early identification of high-risk individuals and a consensus regarding well defined treatment strategies in such patients.

The prevalence of SA in CAD patients

The data in our cross-sectional study indicates that undiagnosed SA was highly prevalent (39%) among patients with CAD. The prevalence of SA in patients with CAD was higher than in normal population, as stated by numerous studies, and was in range or higher than in our study. The studies reported a wide range of prevalence, ranging from 26% to 66%, partially explained by the

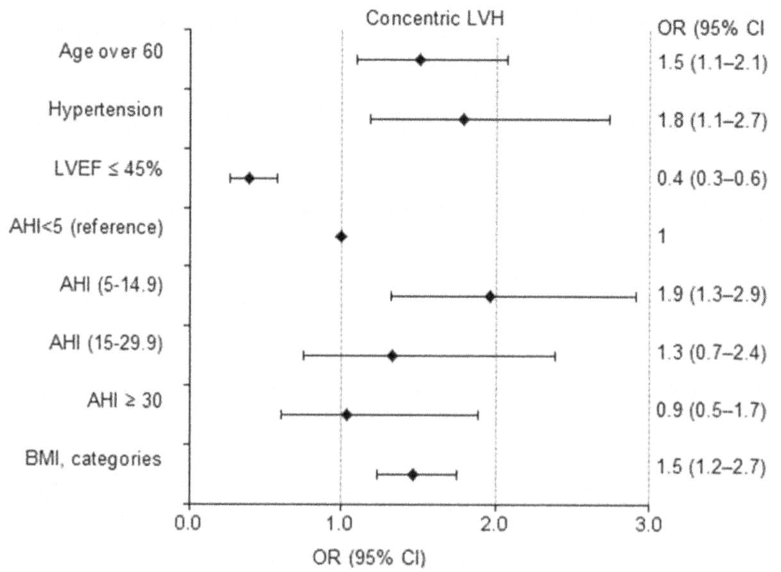

Fig. 4 Cross sectional predictors of concentric left ventricular hypertrophy. The independent variables entered in the multiple regression model were: age, sex, ESS score, hypoxemia during sleep SaO_2, age over 60, AHI (4 categories), BMI (ORs per 5 kg/m^2 higher BMI above 25 kg/m^2), NYHA class, hypertension, diabetes mellitus, current smoking, history of MI as well as LVEF lower than 45% and excessive daytime sleepiness (ESS ≥ 10). Model: Hosmer & Lemeshow test $\chi^2 = 5.1$ df = 8 $p = 0.746$; Nagelkerke $R^2 = 0.132$. Abbreviations: ESS = Epworth sleepiness scale; LVEF; left ventricular ejection fraction; AHI = apnea-hypopnea index; BMI = body mass index; OR = odds ratio; CI = confidence interval

different value of AHI used to establish the diagnosis of SA in the different studies [3, 5, 41].

There is some evidence suggesting that the prevalence and the severity of SA are modified along the CAD evolution. Mooe et al. reported that clinically significant sleep apnea (AHI >10) was documented in 37% of investigated 142 patients with stable angina pectoris and angiographically confirmed CAD [43]. Peker et al. reported 30% prevalence of SA in patients admitted with an acute coronary syndrome, while Areias et al. claimed SA to be present in 43% of the study patients [12, 17, 41]. In CAD patients immediately after an acute myocardial infarction and after clinical stabilization of unstable angina pectoris Moruzzi et al. observed a significantly higher AHI compared to stable angina pectoris patients [12, 44]. In the study conducted in Greece, the authors concluded that there was a high prevalence of SA during the acute phase of coronary syndrome ACS (54%); this prevalence decreased 6 months after ACS and persisted in 21% of the patients, which indicates that this abnormality may be transient [41, 45]. Recently, Fox et al. (2016) investigating the prevalence of SDB in cardiac rehabilitation patients, reported a prevalence of SDB (AHI ≥ 15) by different cardiac condition. They found that patients who had undergone coronary artery bypass graft (CABG) had a higher prevalence of SDB and more severe SDB compared to patients with stable CAD or ACS (prevalence of 53%, 46% and 45% respectively) [46]. As noted, patients with heart failure and SA (in particular CSA) do not generally present with symptoms that distinguish them from heart failure patients without SA. Arzt et al. (2016) reported a prevalence of 46% in a large representative population of patients with stable chronic HF receiving optimized medical treatment [47].

In general, there is a stronger relationship between SDB and CAD in clinical cohorts than in the general population because clinical cohort studies are particularly influenced by comorbidity and confounding factors, including obesity, hypertension, smoking, and hyperlipidemia. This circumstance may also suggest that SDB constitutes an additive or synergistic risk factor for development of CAD [14, 16].

Cardiac remodeling in hypertension and obesity

Despite the high prevalence of SA reported in patients with CAD, it is frequently underdiagnosed [12]. In addition, comorbidities such as obesity and hypertension that coexist with the majority of SA patients make it more difficult to assess the independent risk of SA on vascular disease. *Both hypertension and obesity* strongly affect cardiovascular structure and function. Since obesity and hypertension are closely linked and often coexist, while obesity is an independent risk factor for arterial hypertension these two disorders often exert a dual burden on the left ventricle, leading to both dilatation and hypertrophy [30] as well as markedly increasing the premature risk of CV disease [19]. The presence of hypertension in patients with SA likely contributes to the association with LVH or increased wall thickness [48]. Data supporting a possible cause and effect relationship between SA and LVH were published by Cloward et al., who found that 6 months of nocturnal positive airway pressure administration to patients with severe OSA was associated with a significant reduction in LV wall thickness [49].

Many studies have shown that obesity is associated with LVH, a potential contributor to heart failure [29]. It is unclear to what extent LVH results directly from obesity or from associated conditions, such as hypertension, impaired glucose homeostasis, or obstructive sleep apnea [23]. Early studies from Ochsner demonstrated that the cardiac adaptation to these two disorders differed considerably [19]. Hypertension causes fundamental response to an isolated increase in pressure load or afterload such as an increase in LV wall thickening without chamber dilatation. On the other hand, obesity leads to LV chamber dilatation with only minimal increases in LV wall thickness. Cardiac remodeling in obesity is characterized by concentric geometry at least as often as eccentric geometry [33]. However, some investigators have found evidence of eccentric LVH (an increase in cavity volume that is greater than the increase in wall thickness) in obese subjects [30, 31, 48].

In fact, LVH in SDB is as closely related to the severity of the sleep disturbances as it is to the levels of blood pressure and BMI [23]. Our study findings also confirm the strong independent association between concentric LVH and obesity at any value of BMI. It helps to dispel the notion that LVH in this condition is exclusively eccentric. When obesity and hypertension coexist, there is a substantial increase in the prevalence of LVH at any value of BMI confirmed in many studies [23, 33, 49]. However, the increase in LV mass/height$^{2.7}$ is more pronounced in patients with hypertension than in those without [33]. MacMahon and colleagues demonstrated that weight loss in hypertensive subjects with overweight reduced LVM and posterior wall thickness [50]. In contrast, Niroumand et al. concluded that SA is not associated with increased LVM independently from obesity, hypertension or advancing age [21].

LV geometry

We found that male sex, age 60+, hypertension, higher BMI, higher than 45% LVEF and SA were independent predictors of LVH *on the basis of wall thickness criteria and predictors of concentric LVH (w*ith the exception of sex). These indicators showed additive effects of SA and are consistent with those of other studies. Drager et al. (2007) looked at arterial stiffness by measuring pulse wave velocity and heart structure in OSA patients with and without hypertension. They demonstrated that patients with untreated OSA had increased left atrial diameter, septal wall thickness, LV posterior wall thickness, LV mass index, and LVH, even controlling for cardiovascular risk factors [51]. These indicators showed additive effects of hypertension and OSA.

SDB produces a series of mechanical, hemodynamic, chemical, neural, and inflammatory responses (i.e. intermittent apnea-induced hypoxia, hypercapnia, increases in sympathetic drive and LV myocardial afterload, daytime hypertension, loss of vagal heart rate regulation and systemic vasculature remodeling) [23, 26, 49]. These strongly impact the CV system, being all potent stimuli to myocyte necrosis and apoptosis, myocardial ischemia, and finally, predict development of concentric LV geometry [26].

The associations between SDB and LV geometry have been previously investigated in a lot of studies conducted on patients with obesity and hypertension, yet the results are irreconcilable [21, 23, 26, 29, 31]. Both overweight and increased blood pressure determine a state of chronic myocardial LV overload and represent two of the main predisposing factors for LVH and systolic dysfunction. In theory, the two conditions are hemodynamically different and should lead to different LV geometry adaptations [30]. In clinical practice, such dichotomy is less evident because obesity and hypertension lead to heterogenic and unpredictable changes in LV geometry [18, 19, 23].

Although less well established than for hypertension, there is growing evidence that SA is a risk factor for incident diabetes [52]. In addition, some reports have demonstrated metabolic syndrome independent association of SA with LV structure [53, 54]. The relative absence of effects of diabetes mellitus on LVM in our study could be explained by relatively low prevalence of this CAD risk factor in our patient population, and the fact that this prevalence was similar in patients with SA and non-SA (21%). The impact of diabetes mellitus on LVM is predominantly through an interaction with obesity and age rather than a direct and independent effect. After adjusting for confounding factors there was no difference between diabetic and non-diabetic participants with regard to apnea-hypopnea events [14, 52].

Despite significant scientific evidence pointing to SA as an emerging CV risk factor, SA is still underdiagnosed in several cardiology subspecialties (hypertension, coronary, arrhythmia, heart failure, valvular heart disease) and consequently undertreated [55]. On account of the high prevalence of SA in the general population, the sleep medicine field is confronted by a demanding challenge to provide sufficient resources for the management of this disorder. In spite of the differences in the diagnostic procedures as well as different AHI cut-off values for definitions of SA, there seems to be enough evidence to warrant overnight sleep screening in individuals with CAD, given that concomitant SA may worsen long-term outcomes. Furthermore, several subsequent studies have demonstrated that patients with untreated severe SA exhibit an increased incidence of fatal and nonfatal cardiovascular events (including MI and ACS) compared with those without SA or even with those with untreated mild to moderate SA [6, 14, 16]. In a longitudinal study of 408 patients with CAD, Mooe and co-workers (2001) noted that SA independently increased the risk for incident cerebrovascular events [13]. Yet such an association suggests but does not demonstrate a causal relationship, and the role of treating SA to prevent CV diseases remains unclear [6]. SA is prevalent in our study population, especially *in its mild form*. Although severe SA is associated with adverse health consequences, the association with mild disease is unclear. Reports differ regarding the clinical relevance of mild SA. Improved diagnostic techniques and evidence based approaches to management in mild SA require further research. Exploring potential causes and improving recognition as well as SA treatment in cardiology might have benefits in the reduction of CV morbidity and mortality [56].

Limitation and strength of the study

We acknowledge a few *limitations* of this study. First, the cross-sectional design does not permit us to evaluate the longitudinal impact of SA on cardiac structure, as the real duration of the SA is not known. A potential limitation is that our study was performed in a clinic-based sample. Second, in our study we do not separately analyze the influence of central and obstructive events. The causative mechanisms of obstructive and central type sleep apnea differ, but the physiological and hence cardiovascular sequelae can be considered in unison [4, 5, 7].

The strengths of this study include relatively large sample size. First, by including a large sample of patients and numerous confounding covariates, our study has overcome many of methodological limitations and provides strong support for an independent cross-sectional association between SA and LV. Second, adjustments of echocardiographic parameters to BMI and hypertension have been successfully implemented. Third, all of our subjects had comprehensive overnight standardized polysomnography data.

Conclusion

We concluded that among patients with stable CAD, unrecognized SA was highly prevalent, and the majority of these patients did not report excessive daytime sleepiness. Mild to moderate SA was associated with increased LV wall thickness, LV mass, and was associated with higher prevalence of concentric LV geometry independently of coexisting obesity, hypertension, diabetes mellitus or advancing age.

Abbreviations

ACS: Acute coronary syndromes; AHI: Apnea-hypopnea index; ASE: American Society of Echocardiography; BMI: Body mass index; CV: Cardiovascular; HF: Heart failure; IVST: Interventricular septal thickness; *LV*: Left ventricular or left ventricle; LVEDD: Left ventricular end-diastolic diameter; LVEF: LV ejection fraction; LVESD: LV end-systolic diameter; LVH: LV hypertrophy; LVM: LV mass; LVMI: LV mass index; LVPWT: LV posterior wall thickness; LVWT: LV wall thickness; MI: Myocardial infarction; NYHA: New York Heart Association; ODI: Oxygen desaturation index; OSA: Obstructive sleep apnea; RWT: Relative wall thickness; SA: Sleep apnea; SDB: Sleep disordered breathing.

Acknowledgements

Not applicable.

Funding

This research did not receive any specific grant from funding agencies in the public, commercial, or not-for-profit sectors.

Authors' contributions

AA first author of this work participated in the polysomnographic measurement, involved in the early conception of the idea, proposal development data analysis, manuscript writing and submitting to the publishing journal. NR gave guidance on writing this paper and contributed to the statistical analysis. VG was the focal person responsible for doing echocardiograms and participated in the study design. JB participated in an assessment clinical state of patients, lead the interpretation of research findings. NM and JB revised the manuscript critically for important intellectual content. All authors have read and approved the final manuscript.

Competing interests

The authors declare that they have no competing interests.

References

1. Lloyd-Jones DM, Larson MG, Beiser A, Levy D. Lifetime risk of developing coronary heart disease. Lancet. 1999;353(9147):89–92.
2. De Torres-Alba F, Gemma D, Armada-Romero E, Rey-Blas JR, López-de-Sá E, López-Sendon JL. Obstructive sleep apnea and coronary artery disease: from pathophysiology to clinical implications. Pulmonary Medicine. 2013;2013: 768064. https://doi.org/10.1155/2013/768064.
3. Konecny T, Kuniyoshi FH, Orban M, Pressman GS, Kara T, Gami A, et al. Under-diagnosis of sleep apnea in patients after acute myocardial infarction. J Am Coll Cardiol. 2010;56(9):742–3.
4. Somers VK, White DP, Amin R. Sleep apnea and cardiovascular disease: an American Heart Association/American College of Cardiology Foundation scientific statement from the American Heart Association Council for high blood pressure research professional education committee, council on clinical cardiology, stroke council, and council on cardiovascular nursing. Circulation. 2008;118:1080–1111.
5. Bradley TD, Floras JS. Obstructive sleep apnoea and its cardiovascular consequences. Lancet. 2009;373(9657):82–93. doi:10.1016/S0140-6736(08)61622-0.
6. Kasai T, Floras JS, Bradley TD. Sleep apnea and cardiovascular disease: a bidirectional relationship. Circulation. 2012;126(12):1495–510.
7. Stopford E, Ravi K, Nayar V. The association of sleep disordered breathing with heart failure and other cardiovascular conditions. Cardiol Res Pract. 2013;2013:356280, 9 pages. https://doi.org/10.1155/2013/356280.
8. Oldenburg O, Wellmann B, Buchholz A, Bitter T, Fox H, Thiem U, Horstkotte D, Wegscheider K. Nocturnal hypoxaemia is associated with increased mortality in stable heart failure patients. Eur Heart J. 2016 Jun 1;37(21):1695–703.
9. Iannaccone M, Quadri G, Taha S, D'Ascenzo F, Montefusco A, Omede P, et al. Prevalence and predictors of culprit plaque rupture at OCT in patients with coronary artery disease: a meta-analysis. Eur Heart J Cardiovasc Imaging. 2015;17:1128–37.
10. Libby P. Current concepts of the pathogenesis of the acute coronary syndromes. Circulation. 2001;104(3):365–72.
11. Terada S, Koyama T, Watanabe H, Makabe S, Igarashi G, Seki K, et al. Abnormal coagulation and platelet profile in patients with obstructive sleep apnea syndrome. Int J Cardiol. 2011;146:423–5. https://doi.org/10.1016/j.ijcard.2010.10.095.
12. Carpio C, Álvarez-Sala R, García-Río F. Epidemiological and pathogenic relationship between sleep apnea and ischemic heart disease. Pulmonary Medicine. 2013;2013:405827. https://doi.org/10.1155/2013/405827.
13. Mooe T, Franklin KA, Holmström K, Rabben T, Wiklund U. Sleep-disordered breathing and coronary artery disease, long-term prognosis. Am J Respir Crit Care Med. 2001;164(10):1910–3. https://doi.org/10.1164/ajrccm.164.10.2101072.
14. Gottlieb D, Yenokyan G, Newman A, O'Connor G, Punjabi N, Quan S, et al. Prospective study of obstructive sleep apnea and incident coronary heart disease and heart failure: the sleep hearth health study. Circulation. 2010;122:352–60.
15. Hagenah GC, Gueven E, Andreas S. Influence of obstructive sleep apnoea in coronary artery disease: a 10-year follow-up. Respir Med. 2006;100(1):180–2.
16. Hedner J, Grote L, Bonsignore M, McNicholas W, Lavie P, Parati G, et al. The European sleep Apnoea database (ESADA): report from 22 European sleep laboratories. Eur Respir J. 2011;38:635–42.
17. Peker Y, Kraiczi H, Hedner J, Loth S, Johansson A, Bende M. An independent association between obstructive sleep apnoea and coronary artery disease. Eur Respir J. 1999;14:179–84.
18. Artham SM, Lavie CJ, Milani RV, Patel DA, Verma A, Ventura HO. Clinical impact of left ventricular hypertrophy and implications for regression. Prog Cardiovasc Dis. 2009;52:153–67.
19. Lavie CJ, Milani RV, Shah SB, Gilliland Y, Bernal JA, et al. Impact of left ventricular geometry on prognosis—a review of Ochsner studies. Ochsner J. 2008;8:11–7.
20. Lavie CJ, Patel DA, Milani RV, Ventura HO, Shah S, Gilliland Y. Impact of echocardiographic left ventricular geometry on clinical prognosis. Prog Cardiovasc Dis. 2014;57(1):3–9.
21. Niroumand M, Kuperstein R, Sasson Z, Hanly PJ. Impact of obstructive sleep apnea on left ventricular mass and diastolic function. Am J Respir Crit Care Med. 2001;163:1632–6.
22. Noda A, Okada T, Yasuma F, Nakashima N, Yokota M. Cardiac hypertrophy in obstructive sleep apnea syndrome. Chest. 1995;107:1538–44.
23. Avelar E, Cloward TV, Walker JM, Farney RJ, Strong M, Pendleton RC, et al. Left ventricular hypertrophy in severe obesity: interaction among blood pressure, nocturnal hypoxemia and body mass. Hypertension. 2007;49:34–9.
24. Peppard PE, Young T, Palta M, Skatrud J. Prospective study of the association between sleep-disordered breathing and hypertension. N EnglJ Med. 2000;342:1378–84.
25. Peppard PE, Young T, Barnet JH, Palta M, Hagen EW, Hla KM. Increased prevalence of sleep-disordered breathing in adults. Am J Epidemiol Oxford University Press. 2013 May 1;177(9):1006–14.
26. Cioffi G, Russo TE, Stefenelli C, Selmi A, Furlanello F, Cramariuc D, Gerdts E, de Simone G. Severe obstructive sleep apnea elicits concentric left ventricular geometry. J Hypertens. 2010 May;28(5):1074–82.
27. Ganau A, Devereux RB, Roman MJ, de Simone G, Pickering TG, Saba PS, et al. Patterns of left ventricular hypertrophy and geometric remodeling in essential hypertension. J Am Coll Cardiol. 1992;19:1559–60.
28. Silangei LK, Maro VP, Diefethal H, Kapanda G, Dewhurst M, Mwandolela H, Hame B. Assessment of left ventricular geometrical patterns and function among

hypertensive patients at a tertiary hospital. Northern Tanzania BMC Cardiovascular Disorders. 2012;12:109. https://doi.org/10.1186/1471-2261-12-109.
29. Lauer MS, Anderson KM, Kannel WB, Levy D. The impact of obesity on left ventricular mass and geometry. The Framingham Heart Study JAMA. 1991;266:231–6.
30. Messerli FH, Sundgaard-Riise K, Reisin ED, Dreslinski GR, Ventura HO, Oigman W, Frohlich ED, Dunn FG. Dimorphic cardiac adaptation to obesity and arterial hypertension. Ann Intern Med. 1983;99:757–61.
31. de Simone G, Devereux RB, Roman MJ, Alderman MH, Laragh JH. Relation of obesity and gender to left ventricular hypertrophy in normotensive and hypertensive adults. Hypertension. 1994;23:600–6.
32. de Simone G, Izzo R, De Luca N, Gerdts E. Left ventricular geometry in obesity: is it what we expect? Nutr Metab Cardiovasc Dis. 2013;23(10):905–12.
33. Aurigemma GP, de Simone G, Fitzgibbons TP. Cardiac remodeling in obesity. Circ Cardiovasc Imaging. 2013 Jan 1;6(1):142–52.
34. Iber C, Ancoli-Israel S, Chesson A, Quan SF. The AASM manual for the scoring of sleep and associated events: rules, terminology and technical specifications. 1st ed. American Academy of Sleep Medicine: Westchester, Illinois; 2007.
35. Johns MW. Daytime sleepiness, snoring and obstructive sleep apnea: the Epworth sleepiness scale. Chest. 1993;103:30–6.
36. Schiller NB, Shah PM, Crawford M, DeMaria A, Devereux R, Feigenbaum H, Gutgesell H, Reichek N, Sahn D, Schnittger I. Recommendations for quantitation of the left ventricle by two-dimensional echocardiography, American Society of Echocardiography Committee on Standards, Subcommittee on quantitation of two-dimensional echocardiograms. J Am Soc Echocardiogr. 1989;2:358–67.
37. Devereux RB, Alonso DR, Lutas EM, Gottlieb GJ, Campo E, Sachs I, Reichek N. Echocardiographic assessment of left ventricular hypertrophy: comparison to necropsy findings. Am J Cardiol. 1986;57:450–8.
38. Foppa M, Duncan BB, Rohde LE. Echocardiography-based left ventricular mass estimation. How should we define hypertrophy? Cardiovascular Ultrasound. 2005;3:17. https://doi.org/10.1186/1476–7120–3-17.
39. Cuspidi C, Meani S, Negri F, Giudici V, Valerio C, Sala C, et al. Indexation of left ventricular mass to body surface area and height to allometric power of 2.7: Is the difference limited to obese hypertensives? J Hum Hypertens. 2009;23:728–734.
40. Lang RM, Bierig M, Devereux RB, Flachskampf FA, Foster E, Pellikka PA, et al. Recommendations for chamber quantification: a report from the American Society of Echocardiography's guidelines and standards committee and the chamber quantification writing group, developed in conjunction with the European Association of Echocardiography, a branch of the European Society of Cardiology. J Am Soc Echocardiogr. 2005;18:1440–63.
41. Areias V, Romero J, Cunha K, Faria R, Mimoso J, Gomes V, et al. Sleep apnea-hypopnea syndrome and acute coronary syndrome an association not to forget. *Rev Port Pneumol.* 2012;18(1):22–8.
42. Somnologie. 2017;20(2):97–180. doi:https://doi.org/10.1007/s11818-016-0093-1.
43. Mooe T, Rabben T, Wiklund U, Franklin KA, Eriksson P. Sleep-disordered breathing in women: occurrence and association with coronary artery disease. Am J Med. 1996;101:251–6.
44. Moruzzi P, Sarzi-Braga S, Rossi M, Contini M. Sleep apnoea in ischaemic heart disease: differences between acute and chronic coronary syndromes. Heart. 1999;82(3):343–7.
45. Bouloukaki I, Simantirakis E, Mermigis C, Arfanakis D, Chrysos-tomakis S, Kallergis E, et al. Sleep-disordered breathingin patients with acute coronary syndrome. J Sleep Res. 2010;19:296–7.
46. Fox H, Purucker HC, Holzhacker I, Tebtmann U, Bitter T, Horstkotte D, Graml A, Woehrle H, Oldenburg O. Prevalence of sleep-disordered breathing and patient characteristics in a coronary artery disease cohort undergoing cardiovascular rehabilitation. J Cardiopulm Rehabil Prev. 2016 Nov/Dec;36(6): 421–429.
47. Arzt M, Woehrle H, Oldenburg O, Graml A, Suling A, Erdmann E, Teschler H, Wegscheider K. SchlaHF investigators. Prevalence and predictors of sleep-disordered breathing in patients with stable chronic heart failure: the SchlaHF registry. JACC Heart Fail. 2016 Feb;4(2):116–25.
48. Kraiczi H, Peker Y, Caidahl K, Samuelsson A, Hedner J. Blood pressure, cardiac structure and severity of obstructive sleep apnea in a sleep clinic population. J Hypertens. 2001;19:2071–8.
49. Cloward TV, Walker JM, Farney RJ, Anderson JL. Left ventricular hypertrophy is a common echocardiographic abnormality in severe obstructive sleep apnea and reverses with nasal continuous positive airway pressure. Chest. 2003;124:594–601.
50. MacMahon SW, Wilcken DE, Macdonald GJ. The effect of weight reduction on left ventricular mass: a randomized controlled trial in young, overweight hypertensive patients. N Engl J Med. 1986;314:334–9.
51. Drager LF, Bortolotto LA, Figueiredo AC, Figueiredo AC, Silva BC, Krieger EM, Lorenzi-Filho G. Obstructive sleep apnea, hypertension, and their interaction on arterial stiffness and heart remodeling. Chest. 2007;131:1379–86.
52. Marshall NS, Wong KKH, Phillips CL, Liu PY, Knuiman MW, Grunstein RR. Is sleep apnea an independent risk factor for prevalent and incident diabetes in the Busselton health study? J Clin Sleep Med. 2009;5:15–20.
53. Usui Y, Takata Y, Inoue Y, Katsunori S, Hirofumi T, et al. Coexistense of obstructive sleep apnoea and metabolic syndrome is independently associated with left ventricular hypertrophy and diastolic dysfunction. Sleep Breath. 2012;16(3):677–84.
54. Drager LF, Togeiro SM, Polotsky VY, Lorenzi-Filho G. Obstructive sleep apnoea: a cardiometabolic risk in obesity and the metabolic syndrome. J Am Coll Cardiol. 2013;62:569–76.
55. Costa LE, Uchôa CH, Harmon RR, Bortolotto LA, Lorenzi-Filho G, Drager LF. Potential underdiagnosis of obstructive sleep apnoea in the cardiology outpatient setting. Heart. 2015;101:1288–92.
56. Fietze I, Penzel T, Alonderis A, Barbe F, Bonsignore MR, Carverly P, et al. Management of obstructive sleep apnea in Europe. Sleep Med. 2011;12:190–7.

20

Burden of Ischaemic heart disease and attributable risk factors in China from 1990 to 2015: findings from the global burden of disease 2015 study

Ganshen Zhang[1], Chuanhua Yu[1*], Maigeng Zhou[2], Lu Wang[1], Yunquan Zhang[1] and Lisha Luo[1]

Abstract

Background: Ischaemic heart disease (IHD) is a major barrier to sustainable human development, but its health burden and geographic distribution among provinces of China remain unclear. This study aimed to estimate IHD burden in provinces of China, and attributable to risk factors from 1990 to 2015.

Methods: Data were collected from the Global Burden of Disease 2015 Study, which evaluated IHD burden and attributable risk factors using deaths and disability-adjusted life years (DALYs). Statistical models including cause of death ensemble modelling, Bayesian meta-regression analysis, and comparative risk assessment approaches were applied to reduce bias and produce comprehensive results of IHD deaths, DALYs and attributable risks. The 95% uncertainty intervals (UIs) were calculated and reported for mortality and DALYs.

Results: The age-standardised death rate per 100,000 people increased by 13.3% from 101.3 (95%UI: 95.3–107.5) to 114.8 (95%UI: 109.8–120.1) from 1990 to 2015 in China, whereas the age-standardised DALY rate declined 3.9% to 1760.2 per 100,000 people (95%UI: 1671.6–1864.3). In 2015, the age-standardised death rate per 100,000 people was the highest in Heilongjiang (187.4, 95%UI: 161.6–217.5) and the lowest in Shanghai (44.2, 95%UI: 37.0–53.1), and the age-standardised DALY rate per 100,000 people was the highest in Xinjiang (3040.8, 95%UI: 2488.8–3735.4) and the lowest in Shanghai (524.4, 95%UI: 434.7–638.4). Geographically, the age-standardised death and DALY rates for southern provinces were lower than northern provinces, especially in southeastern coastal provinces. 95.3% of the IHD burden in China was attributable to environmental, behavioural and metabolic risk factors. The five leading IHD risks in 2015 were high systolic blood pressure, high total cholesterol, diet high in sodium, diet low in whole grains, and smoking.

Conclusions: Population growth and ageing has led to a steady increase in the IHD burden. Regional disparities in IHD burden were observed in provinces of China. The distribution characteristics of IHD burden provide guidance for decision makers to formulate targeted preventive policies and interventions.

Keywords: Ischaemic heart disease, Mortality, Disability-adjusted life years, Risk factors

* Correspondence: YuCHua@whu.edu.cn
[1]Department of Epidemiology and Biostatistics, School of Health Sciences, Wuhan University, #185 Donghu Road, Wuhan, Hubei 430071, China
Full list of author information is available at the end of the article

Background

Cardiovascular diseases (CVDs), which accounted for one-third of global deaths in 2015, are recognised as a major barrier to sustainable human development [1, 2]. Of all CVDs, ischaemic heart disease (IHD) is one of the leading causes of mortality and disease burden worldwide [3], resulting in approximately 8.9 million deaths and 164.0 million disability-adjusted life years (DALYs) globally in 2015 [4–6]. A number of risk factors have been found to be associated with IHD such as hypertension, high total cholesterol, diet high in sodium, and smoking [7–9]. Additionally, mortality from IHD has decreased in developed countries in the past three decades [10] but has increased continuously in many low- and middle- income countries [11–14].

China, one of the largest developing countries in the world, has undergone rapid health transition in the past decades under the background of economic growth and social change. The prevalence and mortality of non-communicable diseases (NCDs), including IHD, has been rising rapidly in China [15]. Therefore, the Chinese Government has implemented the Plan of Healthy China 2030 in response to the Sustainable Development Goals (target 3.4.1) by the United Nations to reduce premature mortality from major NCDs [16, 17]. Furthermore, IHD is one of the major health threats to Chinese people and was the second leading causes of mortality next to stroke in 2013 [18]. However, IHD burden and its geographic distribution among provinces of China remain unclear due to the lack of comparable data. The Global Burden of Diseases, Injuries, and Risk Factors 2015 Study (GBD 2015) estimated health lost from fatal and non-fatal outcomes by integrating all available data on incidence, prevalence, and mortality to produce accurate, consistent, transparent, and up-to-date estimates for global, regions, nations, and subnational regions for some countries [2, 19]. In this study, we aimed to estimate the disease burden of IHD on mortality and DALYs in various provinces of China, as well as DALYs attributed to IHD risk factors, by using the data from the GBD 2015 study.

Methods

Data sources

Data for this study were obtained from the GBD 2015 study, which estimated the burden of 315 diseases and injuries, 2619 unique sequelae, and 79 risk factors in 195 countries worldwide from 1990 to 2015 [4–7]. Original data from three main data sources including the Disease Surveillance Points (DSPs), the Maternal and Child Surveillance System, and the Chinese Center for Disease Control and Prevention (CDC) Cause of Death Reporting System were adapted by the GBD 2015 collaborators to estimate outcomes of IHD in China. IHD cases were identified using the World Health Organization clinical criteria and the 10th revision of the International Classification of Diseases and Injuries (ICD-10) discharge diagnosis codes (codes I20-I25).

Mortality, disability-adjusted life years and risk factors

The general methodological approaches of GBD 2015 and the specific methodology used to study IHD in China have been described elsewhere [4–7]. We used mortality and DALYs to measure the burden caused by IHD. DALYs from IHD consisted of two parts, years of life lost (YLLs) that quantifies life loss caused by premature mortality from fatal IHD and years lived with disability (YLDs) that evaluates health loss from living with non-fatal IHD sequelae such as non-fatal myocardial infarction, angina, and ischaemic heart failure [6, 20]. Cause of Death Ensemble modelling (CODEm) was the principal method adapted to estimate fatal IHD mortality and YLLs [4]. Prevalence for non-fatal IHD sequelae was estimated using Bayesian meta-regression analysis using the DisMod-MR 2.1 software, and its disability weight was evaluated by population-based health surveys and an open web-based survey [5, 21]. We computed DALYs via the summation of YLLs and YLDs [5]. Comparative risk assessment (CRA) approaches were used to evaluate the number of excess DALYs from IHD observed in a given year that can be attributed to past exposure to a risk factor [7]. We used the revised GBD 2015 global population age standard to determine all the age-standardised death and DALY rates.

Uncertainty interval

For each estimated rate and number of deaths and DALYs, we reported its 95% uncertainty interval (UI), which was estimated by taking 1000 samples from the posterior distribution of each quantity and using the 25th and 975th-ordered draws of the uncertainty distribution [4–7].

Results

Mortality

The IHD death rate per 100,000 people in China increased significantly from 52.2 (95%UI: 49.2–55.6) in 1990 to 105.6 (95%UI: 101.0–110.8) in 2015. A total of 1461.2 thousand IHD deaths (95%UI: 1396.8–1532.9) occurred in 2015 in China compared to 6,03.1 thousand in 1990. IHD deaths accounted for 15.5% of all deaths in 2015, ranking only next to stroke (20.1%), with a sharp increase from 6.8% in 1990. Nevertheless, the age-standardised death rate only increased slightly in both males (19.5%) and females (4.5%) from 1990 to 2015. Of all IHD deaths in 2015, 58.0% were in males and 66.4% were in those aged 70+ years.

Table 1 provides the number of deaths and age-standardised death rates from IHD in various provinces

Table 1 Number of deaths and age-standardised death rates from ischaemic heart disease with percent change, 1990–2015, in provinces of China

Locations	Number of deaths (thousand)			Age-standardized death rate per 100,000 people		
	1990	2015	% change	1990	2015	% change
China	603.1 (568.0–642.2)	1461.2 (1396.8–1532.9)	142.3	101.3 (95.3–107.5)	114.8 (109.8–120.1)	13.3
Anhui	22.8 (18.4–28.7)	65.2 (55.3–76.8)	186.0	86.6 (69.9–106.1)	107.8 (91.7–126.1)	24.4
Beijing	7.5 (6.0–9.2)	16.9 (14.6–19.7)	125.7	116.7 (94.9–141.2)	86.5 (74.7–100.6)	−25.9
Chongqing	6.5 (5.2–8.1)	28.3 (22.0–34.7)	332.3	73.2 (58.9–89.8)	87.3 (69.1–105.8)	19.3
Fujian	11.0 (8.9–13.6)	22.7 (18.5–27.1)	105.9	78.0 (64.0–94.8)	70.7 (57.7–84.1)	−9.4
Gansu	7.8 (6.2–9.6)	23.3 (19.0–27.9)	197.0	87.8 (71.3–105.5)	117.3 (97.6–138.2)	33.6
Guangdong	30.4 (24.1–37.5)	79.7 (69.2–92.2)	162.3	94.9 (75.8–116.1)	97.7 (85.0–112.7)	2.9
Guangxi	21.7 (17.5–26.9)	61.1 (50.6–72.8)	181.6	98.6 (79.4–121.7)	136.3 (113.4–161.7)	38.3
Guizhou	12.7 (10.1–16.0)	34.5 (27.1–43.7)	172.1	87.7 (70.3–109.8)	114.6 (91.0–143.0)	30.7
Hainan	4.0 (3.2–4.9)	7.5 (6.0–9.3)	88.2	120.2 (98.6–145.4)	91.5 (72.7–113.2)	−23.9
Hebei	38.4 (30.0–48.5)	92.7 (77.1–111.7)	141.6	114.3 (90.3–141.6)	143.5 (120.8–169.7)	25.5
Heilongjiang	28.2 (21.9–35.3)	66.7 (56.3–78.7)	136.4	198.0 (158.3–242.3)	187.4 (161.6–217.5)	−5.4
Henan	55.1 (44.0–67.2)	121.7 (101.2–146.6)	120.8	119.8 (96.2–144.7)	152.4 (127.7–181.4)	27.2
Hong Kong Special Administrative Region of China	4.2 (3.9–4.7)	7.4 (6.6–8.7)	78.6	91.7 (85.5–103.6)	58.3 (52.1–67.7)	−36.4
Hubei	27.5 (22.1–33.9)	58.4 (49.1–69.1)	112.5	106.5 (86.8–129.6)	111.4 (94.8–131.3)	4.6
Hunan	31.1 (24.6–38.6)	93.5 (79.5–110.2)	201.0	99.4 (79.8–121.7)	139.2 (118.1–163.3)	40.0
Inner Mongolia	13.7 (10.8–17.4)	32.3 (26.7–38.5)	136.5	157.0 (127.8–193.9)	158.7 (134.1–184.1)	1.1
Jiangsu	23.5 (18.5–29.7)	55.7 (47.1–65.2)	137.0	59.5 (47.3–74.7)	63.4 (53.8–74.2)	6.5
Jiangxi	17.1 (13.6–21.3)	38.2 (31.8–45.3)	123.4	101.6 (81.5–124.5)	106.4 (89.3–124.9)	4.8
Jilin	22.3 (17.7–28.0)	45.4 (36.5–56.8)	103.3	201.9 (165.0–248.9)	182.0 (148.4–223.1)	−9.9
Liaoning	28.1 (22.3–34.6)	66.0 (56.7–77.2)	134.8	129.6 (104.3–156.8)	135.7 (117.6–157.1)	4.7
Macao Special Administrative Region of China	0.41 (0.36–0.46)	0.43 (0.34–0.54)	6.0	174.0 (153.2–194.4)	83.1 (64.7–103.2)	−52.3
Ningxia	2.0 (1.5–2.4)	7.2 (5.6–9.1)	266.0	122.0 (97.7–148.7)	166.8 (133.8–206.2)	36.7
Qinghai	1.8 (1.4–2.2)	6.6 (5.1–8.5)	278.8	114.6 (91.5–141.6)	176.5 (140.2–218.6)	54.0
Shaanxi	17.1 (13.7–21.2)	47.3 (36.0–58.8)	177.5	113.0 (91.8–138.0)	151.9 (119.6–184.4)	34.5
Shandong	50.3 (41.0–61.2)	146.4 (123.6–171.5)	191.0	103.8 (84.0–125.1)	145.9 (123.6–170.4)	40.6

Table 1 Number of deaths and age-standardised death rates from ischaemic heart disease with percent change, 1990–2015, in provinces of China *(Continued)*

Locations	Number of deaths (thousand)			Age-standardized death rate per 100,000 people		
	1990	2015	% change	1990	2015	% change
Shanghai	5.9 (4.7–7.1)	13.1 (11.0–15.7)	123.2	57.6 (46.3–69.2)	44.2 (37.0–53.1)	−23.3
Shanxi	16.6 (13.2–20.8)	41.0 (31.4–51.5)	146.5	114.9 (92.9–141.9)	137.4 (108.5–168.8)	19.6
Sichuan	47.7 (38.6–59.5)	65.4 (51.9–80.8)	37.0	88.1 (72.2–108.4)	75.4 (60.3–92.4)	−14.4
Tianjin	6.8 (5.5–8.5)	16.8 (14.2–19.6)	145.5	126.4 (103.3–153.2)	134.8 (115.6–155.4)	6.7
Tibet	1.4 (1.1–1.9)	2.3 (1.8–2.8)	61.0	138.6 (107.7–185.2)	135.6 (110.3–168.7)	−2.1
Xinjiang	10.9 (8.6–13.8)	27.1 (22.2–33.2)	148.0	169.5 (137.3–211.1)	178.4 (148.5–214.2)	5.2
Yunnan	14.7 (11.7–18.5)	44.6 (37.1–54.3)	202.9	86.0 (68.6–107.2)	118.2 (99.2–142.2)	37.4
Zhejiang	14.0 (11.3–17.1)	26.0 (21.3–31.2)	85.6	57.1 (46.5–68.9)	45.0 (37.0–53.8)	−21.2

of China from 1990 to 2015. In 2015, Shandong had the greatest number of IHD deaths at 146.4 thousand (95%UI: 123.6–171.5), and Heilongjiang had the highest age-standardised death rate at 187.4 per 100,000 people (95%UI: 161.6–217.5) followed by Jilin and Xinjiang. The lowest age-standardised death rate occurred in Shanghai with 44.2 per 100,000 people (95%UI: 37.0–53.1) followed by Zhejiang and Hong Kong. Age-standardised death rates for southern provinces were lower than northern provinces, especially in southeastern coastal provinces such as Shanghai, Zhejiang, Hong Kong, Jiangsu, and Fujian (Fig. 1a). Age-standardised death rates for 22 provinces increased while the remaining 11 provinces decreased between 1990 and 2015; the highest increases occurred in Qinghai (54.0%), Shandong, and Hunan, and the largest declines were observed in Macao (− 52.3%), Hong Kong, and Beijing.

YLLs and YLDs

In 2015, YLLs from IHD was 24,407.2 thousand person years (95%UI: 23,041.1–25,809.1), which increased by 84.6% from 13,221.8 thousand (95%UI: 12,382.0–14,098.7) in 1990. However, the age-standardised YLL rate per 100,000 people decreased 4.3% from 1761.1 (95%UI: 1656.4–1877.2) in 1990 to 1671.9 (95%UI: 1585.1–1763.4) in 2015 (Table 2). Among all provinces, Xinjiang had the highest age-standardised YLL rate at 2956.7 (95%UI: 2403.7–3659.6) in 2015, and the lowest occurred in Shanghai at 427.6 (95%UI: 346.8–536.0). Age-standardised YLL rates for 20 provinces decreased whereas the remaining 13 provinces increased from 1990 to 2015; Macao showed the most rapid decline while Qinghai experienced the most rapid increase.

IHD caused an estimated 1358.0 thousand YLDs (95%UI: 915.7–1870.3) in China in 2015, which was 2.5 times higher than the YLDs in 1990 at 524.6 thousand (95%UI: 352.5–720.2). The age-standardised YLD rate per 100,000 people rose 23.8% from 71.3 (95%UI: 47.9–97.7) to 88.3 (95%UI: 59.4–120.9) (Table 2). All provinces experienced increases in age-standardised YLD rates between 1990 and 2015. In 2015, the highest age-standardised YLD rate appeared in Tianjin, followed by Beijing and Macao, whereas the lowest YLD rate occurred in Tibet.

For IHD, YLLs was much higher than YLDs, as the YLLs/YLDs ratio for IHD was 25.2 in 1990 and reduced to 18.0 in 2015. Although the ratios decreased for all provinces during 1990 to 2015, they remained greater than 10 for most provinces.

DALYs

IHD caused a total of 2576.5 thousand DALYs (95%UI: 2439.1–2737.4) in China in 2015, accounting for 7.5% of total DALYs from all causes, ranking only second to stroke (10.1%). The IHD DALY rate per 100,000 people increased from 1190.7 (95%UI: 1120.9–1268.9) in 1990 to 1862.4 (95%UI: 1763.1–1978.6) in 2015. However, the age-standardised DALY rate showed a 3.9% reduction to 1760.2 (95%UI: 1671.6–1864.3) in 2015.

Table 3 shows the number of DALYs and age-standardised IHD DALY rates for various provinces of China in 1990 and 2015. IHD DALYs for all provinces increased except in Macao. Xinjiang had the highest age-standardised DALY rate at 3040.8 per 100,000 people (95%UI: 2488.8–3735.4) in 2015, followed by Qinghai and Heilongjiang, while Shanghai, Zhejiang and Hong Kong had the lowest rates. Age-standardised

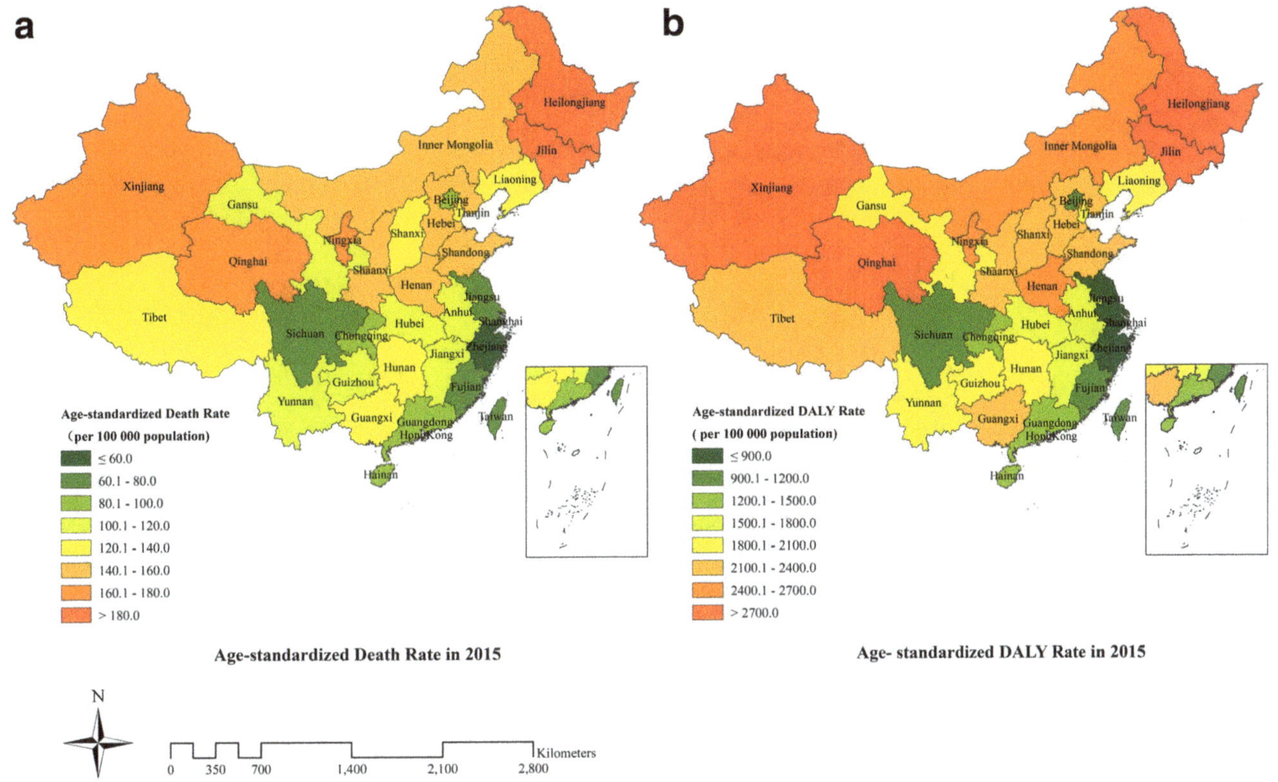

Fig. 1 Age-standardised death rate (**a**) and age-standardised DALY rate (**b**) from ischaemic heart disease for both sexes combined in 2015 in China. DALYs = disability-adjusted life years

DALY rates for southern provinces were lower than northern provinces, especially in southeastern coastal provinces (Fig. 1b). Nineteen provinces showed a downward trend for age-standardised DALY rates with the most rapid decline observed in Macao, Hong Kong, and Beijing. The remaining 14 provinces showed an upward trend, where Qinghai, Guangxi and Yunnan had the fastest growth rate. Before 2005, the age-standardised DALY rates for most provinces increased except in ten provinces including Macao, Hong Kong, Hainan, Shanghai, Sichuan, Zhejiang, Beijing, Hubei, Jilin and Heilongjiang. However, after 2005, the age-standardised DALY rates for the majority of provinces declined except in Guangxi, Qinghai, and Guizhou (Fig. 2and Additional file 1).

Risk factors

In China, 95.3% of IHD DALYs (24,561.9 thousand, 95%UI: 23,193.9–26,122.8) were attributable to metabolic, environmental, and behavioural risks and their overlaps in 2015 compared to 91.4% of IHD DALYs (12,560.7 thousand, 95%UI: 11,813.6–13,405.6) in 1990. From 1990 to 2015, the proportion of the three metabolic-related risks and overlaps increased while other clusters decreased, including metabolic risks alone, interaction of behavioural and metabolic risks, and interaction of metabolic and environmental risks (Fig. 3). A substantial portion of IHD DALYs was attributable to behavioural-related risks, including behavioural risks alone (7.8%), interaction of behavioural and metabolic risks (51.1%), and interaction of behavioural and metabolic and environmental risks (25.3%).

Figure 4 shows the changes to the 22 leading risk factors for IHD DALYs between 1990 and 2015 in China. In 2015, the five leading IHD risk factors and their DALY rates per 100,000 people were high systolic blood pressure (1080.1, 95%UI: 922.5–1226.9), high total cholesterol (839.4, 95%UI: 685.0–1004.8), diet high in sodium (825.2, 95%UI: 586.6–1081.7), diet low in whole grain (487.3, 95%UI: 302.0–682.2), and smoking (487.0, 95%UI: 395.6–581.0). DALY rates for all risk factors increased between 1990 and 2015 except for household air pollution from solid fuels. The largest increase in the DALY rate occurred for diet low in polyunsaturated fatty acids (283.5%), followed by high body mass index (160.6%) and high systolic blood pressure (128.4%). However, only seven risk factors increased in age-standardised IHD DALY rates, while the remaining 15 risk factors declined. The age-standardised IHD DALY rate for household air pollution from solid fuels showed the greatest decline (50.3%). Six risk factors, including high systolic blood pressure (2nd to 1st), diet low in whole grains (5th to 4th), ambient particulate matter

Table 2 Age-standardised YLL and YLD rates and YLLs/YLDs ratios for ischaemic heart disease in 1990 and 2015 in provinces of China

Province	Age-standardized YLL rate per 100,000 people			Age-standardized YLD rate per 100,000 people			YLL/YLD ratio 1990	YLL/YLD ratio 2015
	1990	2015	% change	1990	2015	% change		
China	1761.1 (1656.4–1877.2)	1671.9 (1585.1–1763.4)	−4.3	71.3 (47.9–97.7)	88.3 (59.4–120.9)	23.8	25.2	18.0
Anhui	1426.7 (1137.0–1795.5)	1505.4 (1249.9–1812.1)	5.5	70.9 (48.1–97.7)	87.5 (58.4–120.7)	23.5	19.8	16.4
Beijing	1849.3 (1477.0–2306.9)	1040.6 (873.1–1251.1)	−43.7	90.4 (61.4–124.2)	111.3 (76.0–153.9)	23.0	20.3	8.9
Chongqing	1216.8 (968.3–1527.6)	1215.7 (925.1–1533.8)	−0.1	63.7 (42.3–88.3)	79.2 (52.9–110.1)	24.4	18.7	14.5
Fujian	1307.5 (1054.8–1636.3)	925.6 (738.6–1128.8)	− 29.2	68.6 (46.4–94.4)	84.2 (56.7–115.8)	22.8	19.0	10.3
Gansu	1565.7 (1239.1–1908.2)	1755.2 (1422.3–2120.7)	12.1	64.7 (43.4–88.8)	80.4 (54.3–110.5)	24.3	24.6	20.3
Guangdong	1611.02 (1259.93–2005.35)	1272.8 (1087.1–1502.2)	−21.0	74.2 (50.4–102.4)	91.3 (61.7–125.6)	23.2	22.1	13.2
Guangxi	1719.6 (1377.1–2179.6)	2152.1 (1748.0–2640.7)	25.2	68.2 (46.0–94.0)	83.9 (56.8–115.8)	23.1	25.5	25.1
Guizhou	1510.6 (1197.1–1917.9)	1845.2 (1434.4–2379.7)	22.2	61.7 (41.3–85.7)	76.9 (51.3–106.5)	24.6	24.2	23.0
Hainan	1957.9 (1559.9–2444.0)	1315.4 (1006.4–1708.9)	−32.8	67.3 (45.2–93.1)	83.1 (56.2–114.9)	23.4	28.6	15.5
Hebei	2065.0 (1598.0–2632.7)	2255.2 (1846.2–2780.1)	9.2	73.2 (49.8–100.8)	90.0 (60.4–124.5)	22.9	29.4	23.9
Heilongjiang	3606.6 (2791.8–4496.9)	2761.8 (2291.2–3302.4)	−23.4	80.2 (54.6–109.3)	98.2 (67.1–133.4)	22.4	49.7	26.1
Henan	2173.8 (1734.0–2676.7)	2324.5 (1903.3–2855.6)	6.9	75.6 (50.8–104.0)	93.1 (63.6–127.8)	23.1	30.2	24.0
Hong Kong Special Administrative Region of China	1298.6 (1228.1–1434.1)	699.7 (624.8–794.3)	−46.1	71.2 (48.1–99.1)	86.3 (57.2–119.3)	21.2	17.7	8.5
Hubei	1840.91 (1471.74–2290.86)	1577.4 (1308.6–1890.7)	−14.3	68.7 (46.3–94.5)	84.6 (57.0–116.4)	23.1	26.9	17.1
Hunan	1733.0 (1364.6–2157.8)	2004.2 (1664.3–2402.9)	15.7	65.3 (43.5–89.9)	80.2 (53.7–112.1)	22.9	26.6	23.8
Inner Mongolia	2829.3 (2252.6–3587.8)	2371.5 (1935.4–2863.1)	−16.2	78.7 (53.5–108.4)	96.3 (64.9–132.2)	22.2	38.6	23.3
Jiangsu	928.2 (724.2–1179.2)	787.0 (653.1–944.7)	− 15.2	71.8 (47.8–98.3)	88.3 (59.7–121.3)	23.0	12.6	8.3
Jiangxi	1703.8 (1351.9–2135.7)	1482.1 (1206.5–1773.0)	−13.0	67.5 (45.4–92.5)	82.8 (55.9–113.3)	22.8	25.0	16.5
Jilin	3586.3 (2839.1–4495.1)	2654.5 (2088.9–3408.8)	− 26.0	80.4 (54.4–110.8)	97.9 (67.1–135.1)	21.8	47.4	25.0
Liaoning	2236.8 (1763.7–2773.4)	1875.8 (1578.9–2236.1)	−16.1	84.9 (57.9–115.7)	103.8 (70.2–142.9)	22.2	27.6	16.7
Macao Special Administrative Region of China	2589.3 (2267.0–2883.6)	988.1 (763.2–1240.8)	−61.8	90.3 (61.2–124.2)	110.1 (74.7–151.8)	21.9	28.6	8.2
Ningxia	2085.0 (1626.4–2558.8)	2552.9 (1963.4–3248.2)	22.4	78.5 (53.0–108.3)	96.5 (65.4–132.3)	22.9	27.7	25.3
Qinghai	2092.9 (1642.2–2671.4)	2793.5 (2127.3–3591.7)	33.5	63.3 (42.0–87.5)	79.0 (53.2–109.8)	24.8	34.6	33.3
Shaanxi	1993.6 (1603.5–2489.0)	2216.3 (1659.0–2795.6)	11.2	72.2 (49.0–99.3)	89.8 (60.3–124.4)	24.3	28.6	22.8
Shandong	1808.6 (1466.0–2224.1)	2043.7 (1698.1–2462.8)	13.0	77.0 (52.2–106.2)	95.0 (64.8–130.1)	23.4	24.1	20.3

Table 2 Age-standardised YLL and YLD rates and YLLs/YLDs ratios for ischaemic heart disease in 1990 and 2015 in provinces of China *(Continued)*

Province	Age-standardized YLL rate per 100,000 people			Age-standardized YLD rate per 100,000 people			YLL/YLD ratio 1990	YLL/YLD ratio 2015
	1990	2015	% change	1990	2015	% change		
Shanghai	802.7 (640.8–982.9)	427.6 (346.8–536.0)	−46.7	78.5 (53.2–108.0)	96.8 (65.7–133.2)	23.3	9.7	4.1
Shanxi	2092.7 (1651.9–2621.9)	2117.0 (1592.1–2701.9)	1.2	75.3 (51.1–104.3)	92.8 (63.2–126.9)	23.2	29.2	21.9
Sichuan	1468.84 (1184.9–1844.6)	1092.6 (841.8–1371.1)	− 25.6	60.6 (40.1–83.0)	75.0 (49.9–103.5)	23.7	23.4	13.7
Tianjin	2205.8 (1759.3–2747.8)	1780.0 (1492.3–2154.6)	−18.4	90.8 (62.2–125.1)	112.2 (77.7–153.3)	23.6	25.5	15.1
Tibet	2682.3 (2055.1–3581.9)	2257.6 (1809.1–2847.6)	−15.8	57.0 (38.1–79.9)	71.2 (47.2–98.9)	24.9	49.3	31.8
Xinjiang	3177.8 (2481.1–4037.5)	2956.7 (2403.7–3659.6)	− 7.0	68.0 (45.9–93.0)	84.0 (56.0–115.7)	23.5	50.0	35.0
Yunnan	1526.2 (1205.6–1927.2)	1884.4 (1537.7–2325.8)	23.5	63.2 (42.4–87.7)	78.3 (52.4–109.8)	23.8	24.3	23.4
Zhejiang	864.4 (685.2–1069.9)	552.3 (446.4–673.8)	− 36.1	68.4 (45.9–94.7)	83.7 (55.8–114.3)	22.4	12.1	6.2

YLLs = years of life lost, YLDs = years lived with disability

pollution (8th to 7th), high fasting plasma glucose (11th to 8th), high body-mass index (14th to 11th), and diet low in polyunsaturated fatty acids (20th to 19th), increased in rank between 1990 and 2015.

Discussion

Main findings

In this study, we found that the number of deaths and DALYs from IHD have increased significantly in China since 1990, but age-adjusted DALY rate has declined. The IHD burden increased in most provinces before 2005 but declined after 2005. Geographically, the IHD burden in southern provinces were lower than northern provinces, especially in southeastern coastal provinces. Furthermore, 95.3% of the IHD burden in China was attributable to environmental, behavioural and metabolic risk factors. The top five IHD risks were high systolic blood pressure, high total cholesterol, diet high in sodium, diet low in whole grains, and smoking.

Mortality and disability-adjusted life years

IHD was the second leading cause of disease burden in China only after stroke. IHD deaths and DALYs have greatly increased for both sexes since 1990. Moreover, China made the second greatest contribution to global IHD burden after India, accounting for 15.7% of total global IHD DALYs in 2015 [5]. These findings call for comprehensive approaches to prevent and reduce the IHD burden in China.

The IHD death rate and the DALY rate increased greatly, but the age-adjusted death rate and DALY rate showed no obvious increases between 1990 and 2015. These findings were mainly caused by population growth and ageing during this period. YLLs were the main component of IHD burden in China with over 90% of DALYs attributed to YLLs. A global level assessment has shown that YLL rates for CVDs increased with the Socio-demographic Index for countries and regions in the middle of the socio-demographic rankings [4]. Most provinces in China remain in the middle of the socio-demographic rankings despite experiencing an increase in the Socio-demographic Index since 1990 [4]. Evidence has also shown that IHD patients in low- and middle-income countries have less access to affordable and high quality CVD medications [22]. All of these findings imply that, in most provinces of China, economic growth and social development have led to an increase in the life expectancy to allow individuals to survive long enough to develop IHD; however, many of them are not able to access to optimal medical or surgical treatments for IHD. Therefore, both the YLL rate and YLD rate from IHD in China have increased significantly since 1990. However, age-standardised YLL and DALY rates have declined, implying improvements in medical care and social security in China that provided more available and affordable treatments for IHD patients.

Differences in the burden of IHD existed between sexes, time periods, and provinces in China. With respect to gender, the IHD burden was higher and increased more rapidly among males than females. Because females are more sensitive to heath information, females are more likely to seek healthcare and have better access to primary prevention compared to males [23]. Regarding time period, the IHD burden in most

Table 3 Number of DALYs and age-standardised DALY rates from ischaemic heart disease with percent change, 1990–2015, in provinces of China

Province	Number of DALY (thousand)			Age-standardized DALY rate per 100,000 people		
	1990	2015	% change	1990	2015	% change
China	1374.6 (1294.0–1464.9)	2576.5 (2439.1–2737.4)	87.4	1832.4 (1728.7–1948.7)	1760.2 (1671.6–1864.3)	−3.9
Anhui	520.8 (411.4–661.6)	1057.5 (878.0–1264.8)	103.0	1497.6 (1207.2–1870.7)	1592.9 (1331.6–1895.2)	6.4
Beijing	159.0 (126.7–201.3)	266.1 (224.9–320.0)	67.3	1939.7 (1566.7–2398.3)	1151.9 (982.1–1369.1)	− 40.6
Chongqing	143.8 (113.5–181.0)	462.3 (356.0–581.1)	221.5	1280.5 (1027.7–1588.0)	1294.9 (1002.3–1615.8)	1.1
Fujian	244.5 (195.9–308.2)	362.5 (292.0–435.5)	48.3	1376.1 (1116.7–1710.6)	1009.8 (818.3–1206.1)	−26.6
Gansu	205.5 (160.8–252.1)	466.1 (375.0–567.3)	126.8	1630.4 (1309.0–1969.3)	1835.6 (1494.7–2194.7)	12.6
Guangdong	639.6 (501.8–797.2)	1261.2 (1076.4–1505.2)	97.2	1685.2 (1334.3–2088.1)	1364.1 (1174.2–1600.6)	−19.1
Guangxi	463.9 (368.3–588.2)	1088.1 (885.8–1329.0)	134.5	1787.8 (1435.2–2241.3)	2236.0 (1826.4–2717.6)	25.1
Guizhou	286.4 (226.2–365.5)	667.0 (521.9–858.0)	132.9	1572.3 (1259.6–1972.2)	1922.0 (1513.8–2449.3)	22.3
Hainan	79.8 (63.3–101.6)	123.2 (94.8–159.8)	54.3	2025.2 (1624.4–2519.4)	1398.5 (1085.1–1796.2)	−30.9
Hebei	888.2 (681.8–1137.1)	1822.5 (1485.1–2261.9)	105.2	2138.2 (1665.4–2702.3)	2345.2 (1931.9–2865.0)	9.7
Heilongjiang	737.4 (559.1–930.4)	1270.2 (1045.4–1525.8)	72.2	3686.8 (2866.3–4566.4)	2859.9 (2395.7–3390.3)	−22.4
Henan	1269.1 (1006.0–1574.7)	2242.4 (1832.3–2751.4)	76.7	2249.4 (1800.7–2763.2)	2417.6 (1998.5–2943.1)	7.5
Hong Kong Special Administrative Region of China	69.6 (65.5–76.3)	90.8 (81.5–102.2)	30.6	1369.7 (1290.2–1505.6)	786.0 (705.7–881.4)	−42.6
Hubei	642.7 (514.3–805.1)	1034.8 (853.4–1248.9)	61.0	1909.7 (1551.5–2345.8)	1662.0 (1381.1–1967.2)	−13.0
Hunan	706.9 (554.5–878.8)	1549.0 (1284.5–1859.2)	119.1	1798.3 (1426.3–2218.2)	2084.4 (1741.6–2484.0)	15.9
Inner Mongolia	352.0 (277.0–451.1)	648.1 (526.2–790.8)	84.1	2908.1 (2332.2–3658.3)	2467.7 (2026.8–2961.2)	− 15.1
Jiangsu	489.5 (384.3–618.0)	843.0 (710.1–994.9)	72.2	1000.0 (791.4–1250.3)	875.3 (739.5–1028.2)	− 12.5
Jiangxi	378.3 (299.1–477.3)	656.8 (535.5–790.4)	73.6	1771.3 (1411.3–2196.9)	1564.9 (1289.6–1858.2)	−11.7
Jilin	538.8 (419.2–683.0)	854.0 (667.2–1114.2)	58.5	3666.7 (2915.4–4577.5)	2752.4 (2188.9–3502.6)	−24.9
Liaoning	637.8 (499.8–798.2)	1117.1 (943.8–1341.7)	75.1	2321.8 (1845.0–2863.8)	1979.6 (1681.8–2345.0)	−14.7
Macao Special Administrative Region of China	6.7 (5.9–7.5)	6.6 (5.3–8.3)	−1.1	2679.6 (2355.6–2979.1)	1098.2 (870.6–1364.4)	−59.0
Ningxia	48.6 (36.9–60.3)	148.4 (113.0–191.0)	205.3	2163.5 (1695.5–2641.8)	2649.4 (2069.2–3343.4)	22.5
Qinghai	48.2 (37.1–62.3)	138.9 (103.1–182.5)	187.9	2156.2 (1703.9–2737.8)	2872.5 (2208.7–3675.4)	33.2
Shaanxi	418.8 (332.2–525.8)	899.5 (663.0–1142.5)	114.8	2065.8 (1669.0–2559.3)	2306.1 (1737.2–2879.4)	11.6
Shandong	1114.0 (909.5–1368.5)	2400.2 (1984.6–2879.7)	115.5	1885.6 (1553.7–2303.5)	2138.7 (1787.0–2548.1)	13.4

Table 3 Number of DALYs and age-standardised DALY rates from ischaemic heart disease with percent change, 1990–2015, in provinces of China *(Continued)*

Province	Number of DALY (thousand)			Age-standardized DALY rate per 100,000 people		
	1990	2015	% change	1990	2015	% change
Shanghai	108.1 (87.3–131.2)	161.0 (132.1–196.5)	49.0	881.2 (715.2–1062.1)	524.4 (434.7–638.4)	– 40.5
Shanxi	404.4 (316.4–508.7)	809.3 (600.2–1047.5)	100.1	2168.0 (1724.6–2701.7)	2209.8 (1678.3–2811.7)	1.9
Sichuan	1057.8 (836.1–1326.3)	1117.3 (874.9–1389.6)	5.6	1529.5 (1244.9–1902.9)	1167.6 (923.1–1444.6)	−23.7
Tianjin	155.1 (122.5–194.6)	285.8 (236.6–343.0)	84.3	2296.6 (1845.5–2840.7)	1912.2 (1605.1–2266.2)	−16.7
Tibet	35.3 (26.9–47.0)	50.2 (40.1–63.9)	42.4	2739.3 (2113.4–3645.6)	2328.8 (1890.5–2913.8)	−15.0
Xinjiang	270.9 (210.0–348.0)	602.3 (481.9–754.3)	122.4	3245.9 (2557.4–4111.5)	3040.8 (2488.8–3735.4)	−6.3
Yunnan	346.7 (274.6–439.9)	856.7 (696.1–1062.4)	147.1	1589.4 (1273.6–1993.5)	1962.7 (1614.1–2407.5)	23.5
Zhejiang	278.2 (222.8–342.9)	406.6 (334.2–489.4)	46.2	932.8 (753.9–1133.3)	635.9 (524.2–763.4)	– 31.8

DALYs = disability-adjusted life years

provinces increased before 2005 but declined afterwards. This transition occurred for multiple reasons. The increase before 2005 was mainly caused by the increase in prevalence of IHD risk factors such as hypertension, dyslipidaemia, and ambient particulate matter pollution [15]. The IHD burden declined after 2005 partly due to the implementation of many important strategies related to tobacco use, diet, physical activities, and harmful use of alcohol to prevent and control NCDs [24–26]. In addition, improvement in IHD treatments and the application of

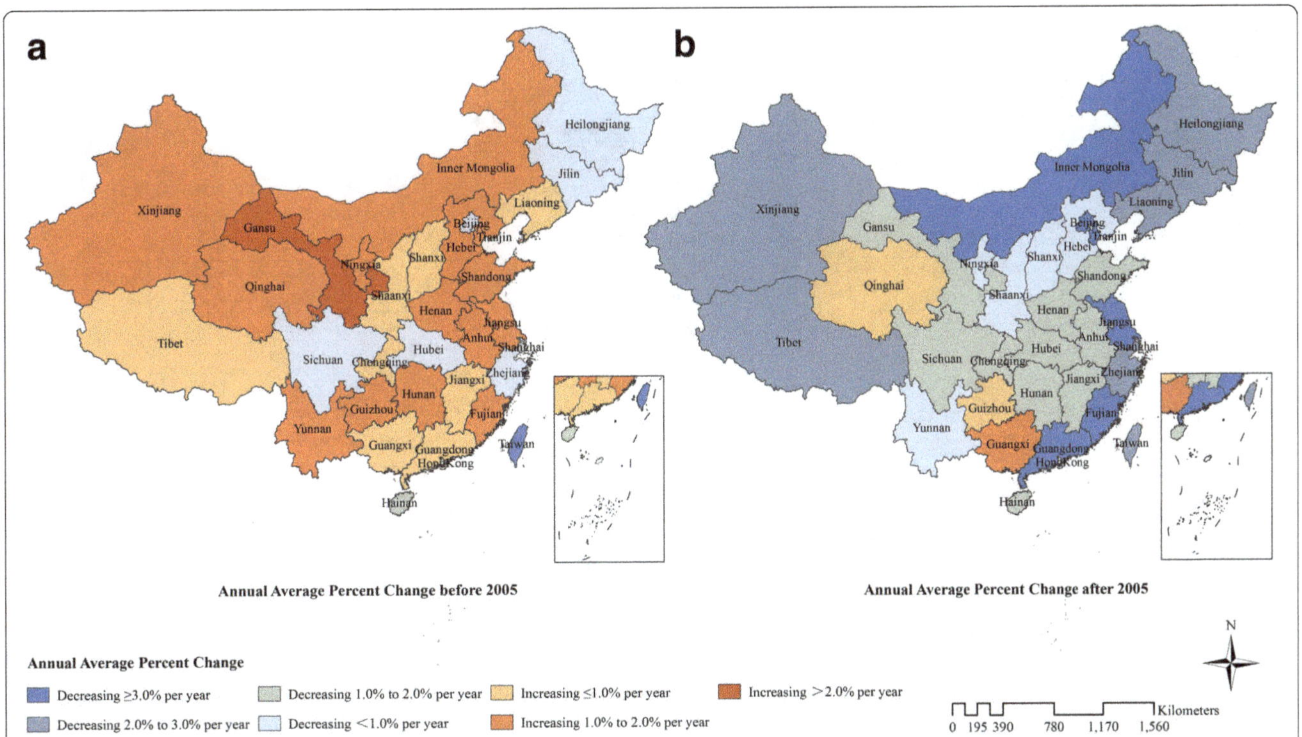

Fig. 2 Annual average percent change of age-standardised DALY rates from ischaemic heart disease for both sexes combined in China before 2005 (**a**) and after 2005 (**b**). DALYs = disability-adjusted life years

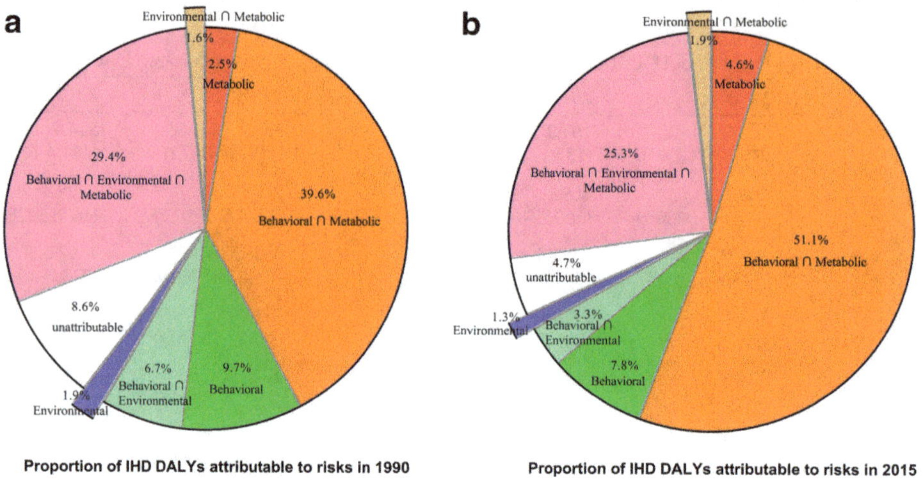

Fig. 3 Proportion of DALYs from ischaemic heart disease attributable to metabolic, environmental and behavioural risk factors and their overlaps, for both sexes combined during 1990 to 2015. DALYs = disability-adjusted life years

cardiac rehabilitation in recent years have led to great advances in reducing the mortality in IHD patients. Regarding the various provinces, the IHD burden was lower among southern provinces than northern provinces, especially in southeastern coastal provinces. These regional disparities are observed partly due to the differences in exposure to metabolic and behavioural risk factors, environmental qualities, meteorological conditions, and household income levels between different regions. Southeastern coastal provinces experienced a lighter IHD burden, as these provinces have been shown to have lower prevalence of hypertension and high total cholesterol [27–29], a lower smoking rate [30], lower air pollution [31], higher household income [32], warm climate conditions and eating habits similar to the Mediterranean diet or Japanese diet [33].

All age DALY rate per 100 000 (95%UI)	1990 leading risks	2015 leading risks	All age DALY rate per 100 000 (95%UI)	% change all-age DALY rate	% change age-standardized DALY rate
519.1 (428.0 – 625.5)	1 High total cholesterol	1 High systolic blood pressure	1080.1 (922.5 – 1226.9)	128.4%	30.2%
472.9 (387.7 – 563.3)	2 High systolic blood pressure	2 High total cholesterol	839.4 (685.0 – 1004.8)	61.7%	-2.0%
468.4 (314.2 – 637.7)	3 Diet high in sodium	3 Diet high in sodium	825.2 (586.6 – 1081.7)	76.2%	4.1%
342.0 (286.1 – 398.9)	4 Smoking	4 Diet low in whole grains	487.3 (302.0 – 682.2)	48.8%	-7.3%
327.6 (204.5 – 458.0)	5 Diet low in whole grains	5 Smoking	487.0 (395.6 – 581.0)	42.4%	-14.3%
316.9 (205.3 – 440.7)	6 Diet low in nuts and seeds	6 Diet low in nuts and seeds	469.5 (302.7 – 655.2)	48.1%	-7.5%
270.2 (211.4 – 331.5)	7 Household air pollution from solid fuels	7 Ambient particulate matter pollution	414.2 (346.9 – 485.9)	56.5%	-3.5%
264.7 (224.6 – 305.6)	8 Ambient particulate matter pollution	8 High fasting plasma glucose	370.1 (261.4 – 505.2)	93.6%	17.7%
250.1 (108.4 – 393.6)	9 Diet low in seafood omega-3 fatty acids	9 Diet low in seafood omega-3 fatty acids	361.5 (156.6 – 579.1)	44.6%	-9.9%
194.2 (71.1 – 318.7)	10 Diet low in fruits	10 Diet low in fruits	282.1 (103.2 – 470.9)	45.3%	-8.8%
191.1 (134.1 – 268.9)	11 High fasting plasma glucose	11 High body-mass index	271.3 (152.0 – 409.9)	160.6%	59.4%
145.5 (53.0 – 260.7)	12 Diet low in vegetables	12 Household air pollution from solid fuels	219.0 (163.7 – 282.2)	-19.0%	-50.3%
108.9 (69.2 – 150.3)	13 Low physical activity	13 Diet low in vegetables	199.5 (73.7 – 362.8)	37.1%	-13.1%
104.1 (44.8 – 179.1)	14 High body-mass index	14 Low physical activity	166.2 (102.6 – 230.7)	52.5%	-6.8%
89.4 (72.2 – 108.7)	15 Secondhand smoke	15 Secondhand smoke	129.5 (101.9 – 159.1)	44.8%	-9.7%
50.2 (2.0 – 98.2)	16 Diet high in processed meat	16 Diet high in processed meat	85.5 (3.6 – 162.4)	70.4%	7.8%
50.0 (35.4 – 65.4)	17 Low glomerular filtration rate	17 Low glomerular filtration rate	81.1 (57.1 – 104.7)	62.0%	-5.5%
47.3 (10.4 – 109.2)	18 Diet high in trans fatty acids	18 Diet high in trans fatty acids	64.3 (13.2 – 153.9)	36.2%	-12.5%
15.8 (4.0 – 34.2)	19 Lead exposure	19 Diet low in polyunsaturated fatty acids	59.9 (20.5 – 121.7)	283.5%	138.4%
15.6 (6.7 – 28.1)	20 Diet low in polyunsaturated fatty acids	20 Lead exposure	25.8 (7.2 – 53.9)	63.3%	-4.4%
11.9 (2.8 – 28.3)	21 Diet low in fiber	21 Diet low in fiber	14.8 (3.3 – 35.8)	24.6%	-19.2%
0.2 (0.1 – 0.3)	22 Diet high in sugar-sweetened beverages	22 Diet high in sugar-sweetened beverages	0.3 (0.2 – 0.4)	50.9%	1.5%

Metabolic · Behavioural · Environmental

Fig. 4 The 22 leading risk factors for DALYs from ischaemic heart disease for both sexes combined in 1990 and 2015 in China. DALYs = disability-adjusted life years

Risk factors

In 2015, over 90% of IHD DALYs were attributable to risk factors that are controllable through reducing and managing related metabolic, behavioural and environmental risk factors. Behavioural risk factors remained the main source of IHD burden in China, but proportion of DALYs attributable to metabolic risk factors has increased previously since 1990, which should be brought to the forefront.

Over the past 30 years, the economy and society in China have undergone rapid improvement with demographic transitions and lifestyle changes with a large impact on population health. Exposure to metabolic and behavioural risk factors has increased to high levels in recent years. A recent report on CVDs in China showed that 25.2% of Chinese adults (approximately 270 million) suffered from hypertension and 33.6% had high-normal blood pressure, but their knowledge rate, treatment rate and control rate for hypertension were only 46.5%, 41.1%, and 13.8%, respectively [33]. Approximately 10% of Chinese adults had high total cholesterol and 25% had high triacylglycerol. The smoking rate was 27.7% in resident aged 15 years and 52.1% in males. A 14.5 g daily average salt intake in Chinese adults was much higher than 5 g recommended by WHO [34]. Moreover, approximately 9.7% of adults had diabetes, and the overweight and obesity rates for adults were 30% and 11.9%, respectively [33]. These findings imply the immense potential of prevention through comprehensive risk factor modification to reduce the IHD burden in China [35, 36].

Study limitations

Our study has several limitations. First, since data for this study were mainly obtained from the GBD 2015 study, all limitations of the GBD 2015 methods outlined elsewhere also apply here [4–7]. The GBD 2015 study used big data analytic technologies to integrate heterogeneous data and estimate burden of diseases and risk factors. Although many methods and processes were used to reduce bias, including misclassification corrections, redistribution of garbage codes, and noise reduction, it was difficult to thoroughly avoid inaccuracy. Therefore, our results on the IHD burden in provinces of China should be interpreted carefully, as the data we used were estimates. Second, accurate data such as follow-up data on non-fatal IHD outcomes and prevalence of IHD risk factors by provinces are very limited. Due to the insufficiency of provincial data regarding risk factors, our study lacked analysis of regional differences in IHD risk factors, which should be conducted in the future.

Implication for policies

Our findings indicate priorities for comprehensive approaches to reduce the IHD burden in China. First, policies should be created to reduce population exposure to major IHD risk factors such as hypertension preventing and curing, cholesterol lowering, advocating healthy diets such as the Mediterranean diet, smoking cessation, controlling ambient particulate matter pollution, etc. Second, it is essential to monitor and manage individuals at high risk for IHD such as those with high blood pressure, dyslipidaemia, high body mass index and hyperglycaemia, especially in males and the elderly, on the community level. Furthermore, improvement in medical care, IHD treatments and social security will help provide more available, affordable, and high quality treatments for IHD patients. Lastly, health education programmes need to be launched to increase awareness of the importance of controlling IHD and personal preventive strategies among the general population.

Conclusion

Although age-standardised DALY rate from IHD declined from 1990 to 2015 in China, population growth and ageing have led to sharp increases in deaths and DALYs from IHD. Regional disparities in IHD burden were observed among provinces of China. The IHD burden in most southern provinces was lower than that of northern provinces, especially in southeastern coastal provinces. Metabolic, behavioural, and environmental risk factors contributed to the majority of the IHD burden. The characteristics of IHD burden and IHD risk factors provide guidance for decision makers to formulate targeted preventive policies and interventions.

Abbreviations

95%UI: 95% uncertainty interval; CVDs: Cardiovascular diseases; DALYs: Disability-adjusted life years; GBD 2015: Global burden of disease, injuries, and risk factors 2015 study; IHD: Ischaemic heart disease; NCDs: Non-communicable diseases.; YLDs: Years lived with disability; YLLs: Years of life lost

Acknowledgements

We wish to thank the Global Burden of Disease Study 2015 collaborators for providing the data.

Funding

This work is supported by the National Natural Science Foundation of China (Grant No. 81773552 and Grant No. 81273179) and the Chinese NSFC International Cooperation and Exchange Program (Grant No. 71661167007).

Authors' contributions

CY and GZ contributed to study conception and design. LW and LL collected the data. GZ, LW, and YZ analysed the data. MZ was the expert from the National CDC of China who helped collect the data and confirm the results. All authors were involved in writing the manuscript and provided final approval of the submitted and published versions.

Competing interest
The authors declare that they have no competing interest.

Author details
[1]Department of Epidemiology and Biostatistics, School of Health Sciences, Wuhan University, #185 Donghu Road, Wuhan, Hubei 430071, China. [2]National Center for Chronic and Non-communicable Disease Control and Prevention, Beijing, China.

References

1. Clark H. NCDs: a challenge to sustainable human development. Lancet. 2013;381(9866):510–1.
2. Roth GA, Johnson C, Abajobir A, Abd-Allah F, Abera SF, Abyu G, Ahmed M, Aksut B, Alam T, Alam K, et al. Global, regional, and National Burden of cardiovascular diseases for 10 causes, 1990 to 2015. J Am Coll Cardiol. 2017; 70(1):1–25.
3. Mathers CD, Loncar D. Projections of global mortality and burden of disease from 2002 to 2030. PLoS Med. 2006;3(11):e442.
4. Wang H, Naghavi M, Allen C, Barber RM, Bhutta ZA, Carter A, Casey DC, Charlson FJ, Chen AZ, Coates MM, et al. Global, regional, and national life expectancy, all-cause mortality, and cause-specific mortality for 249 causes of death, 1980-2015: a systematic analysis for the global burden of disease study 2015. Lancet. 2016;388(10053):1459–544.
5. Kassebaum NJ, Arora M, Barber RM, Bhutta ZA, Brown J, Carter A, Casey DC, Charlson FJ, Coates MM, Coggeshall M, et al. Global, regional, and national disability-adjusted life-years (DALYs) for 315 diseases and injuries and healthy life expectancy (HALE), 1990-2015: a systematic analysis for the global burden of disease study 2015. Lancet. 2016;388(10053):1603–58.
6. Vos T, Allen C, Arora M, Barber RM, Bhutta ZA, Brown A, Carter A, Casey DC, Charlson FJ, Chen AZ, et al. Global, regional, and national incidence, prevalence, and years lived with disability for 310 diseases and injuries, 1990-2015: a systematic analysis for the global burden of disease study 2015. Lancet. 2016;388(10053):1545–602.
7. Forouzanfar MH, Afshin A, Alexander LT, Anderson HR, Bhutta ZA, Biryukov S, Brauer M, Burnett R, Cercy K, Charlson FJ, et al. Global, regional, and national comparative risk assessment of 79 behavioural, environmental and occupational, and metabolic risks or clusters of risks, 1990-2015: a systematic analysis for the global burden of disease study 2015. Lancet. 2016;388(10053):1659–724.
8. Grad C, Zdrenghea D. Heart rate recovery in patients with ischemic heart disease risk factors. Clujul Med. 2014;87(4):220–5.
9. Aalami Harandi S, Sarrafzadegan N, Sadeghi M, Talaei M, Dianatkhah M, Oveisgharan S, Pourmoghaddas A, Salehi A, Sedighifard Z. Do Cardiometabolic risk factors relative risks differ for the occurrence of ischemic heart disease and stroke? Res Cardiovasc Med. 2016; https://doi.org/10.5812/cardiovascmed.30619.
10. Cooper R, Cutler J, Desvigne-Nickens P, Fortmann SP, Friedman L, Havlik R, Hogelin G, Marler J, McGovern P, Morosco G, et al. Trends and disparities in coronary heart disease, stroke, and other cardiovascular diseases in the United States: findings of the national conference on cardiovascular disease prevention. Circulation. 2000;102(25):3137–47.
11. World Health Organization, World Heart Federation, World Stroke Organization. Global atlas on cardiovascular disease prevention and control: policies, strategies and interventions. 2011. http://www.who.int/cardiovascular_diseases/publications/atlas_cvd/en/. Accessed 12 Sept 2016.
12. Nowbar AN, Howard JP, Finegold JA, Asaria P, Francis DP. 2014 global geographic analysis of mortality from ischemic heart disease by country, age and income: Statistics from World Health Organization and United Nations. Int J Cardiol. 2014;174(2):293–8.
13. Barquera S, Pedroza-Tobías A, Medina C, Hernández-Barrera L, Bibbins-Domingo K, Lozano R, Moran AE. Global overview of the epidemiology of atherosclerotic cardiovascular disease. Arch Med Res. 2015;46(5):328–38.
14. Gaziano TA, Bitton A, Anand S, Abrahams-Gessel S, Murphy A. Growing epidemic of coronary heart disease in low- and middle-income countries. Curr Probl Cardiol. 2010;35(2):72–115.
15. Yang G, Wang Y, Zeng Y, Gao GF, Liang X, Zhou M, Wan X, Yu S, Jiang Y, Naghavi M, et al. Rapid health transition in China, 1990-2010: findings from the global burden of disease study 2010. Lancet. 2013;381(9882):1987–2015.
16. National Health and Family Planning Commission of the People's Republic of China. The plan of healthy China 2030. 2016. http://www.nhfpc.gov.cn/xcs/wzbd/201610/21d120c917284007ad9c7aa8e9634bb4.shtml. Accessed 25 Oct 2016.
17. Lim SS, Allen K, Bhutta ZA, Dandona L, Forouzanfar MH, Fullman N, Gething PW, Goldberg EM, Hay SI, Holmberg M, et al. Measuring the health-related sustainable development goals in 188 countries: a baseline analysis from the global burden of disease study 2015. Lancet. 2016;388(10053):1813–50.
18. Zhou M, Wang H, Zhu J, Chen W, Wang L, Liu S, Li Y, Wang L, Liu Y, Yin P, et al. Cause-specific mortality for 240 causes in China during 1990-2013: a systematic subnational analysis for the global burden of disease study 2013. Lancet. 2016;387(10015):251–72.
19. Reddy KS. Global burden of disease study 2015 provides GPS for global health 2030. Lancet. 2016;388(10053):1448–9.
20. Moran AE, Forouzanfar MH, Roth GA, Mensah GA, Ezzati M, Flaxman A, Murray CJ, Naghavi M. The global burden of ischemic heart disease in 1990 and 2010: the global burden of disease 2010 study. Circulation. 2014; 129(14):1493–501.
21. Salomon JA, Haagsma JA, Davis A, de Noordhout CM, Polinder S, Havelaar AH, Cassini A, Devleesschauwer B, Kretzschmar M, Speybroeck N, et al. Disability weights for the global burden of disease 2013 study. Lancet Glob Health. 2015;3(11):e712–23.
22. Wirtz VJ, Kaplan WA, Kwan GF, Laing RO. Access to medications for cardiovascular diseases in low- and middle-income countries. Circulation. 2016;133(21):2076–85.
23. Barker-Collo S, Bennett DA, Krishnamurthi RV, Parmar P, Feigin VL, Naghavi M, Forouzanfar MH, Johnson CO, Nguyen G, Mensah GA, et al. Sex differences in stroke incidence, prevalence, mortality and disability-adjusted life years: results from the global burden of disease study 2013. Neuroepidemiology. 2015;45(3):203–14.
24. World Health Organization. WHO framework convention on tobacco control. World Health Organization. 2003. http://www.who.int/fctc/text_download/en/. Accessed 10 Nov 2017.
25. World Health Organization. Global strategy on diet, physical activity and health. World Health Organization. 2004. http://www.who.int/dietphysicalactivity/goals/en/. Accessed 10 Nov 2017.
26. World Health Organization. Global strategy to reduce the harmful use of alcohol. World Health Organization, 2010. http://www.who.int/substance_abuse/publications/global_strategy_reduce_harmful_use_alcohol/en/. Accessed 9 Nov 2017.
27. Li D, Lv J, Liu F, Liu P, Yang X, Feng Y, Chen G, Hao M. Hypertension burden and control in mainland China: analysis of nationwide data 2003-2012. Int J Cardiol. 2015;184:637–44.
28. Wang J, Zhang L, Wang F, Liu L, Wang H. China National Survey of chronic kidney disease working group. Prevalence, awareness, treatment, and control of hypertension in China: results from a national survey. Am J Hypertens. 2014;27(11):1355–61.
29. Yang J, Wang ZQ, Zhao YF, Li YC, Yin P, Liu SW, You JL, Zhou MG. Burden of disease attributed to high total cholesterol in 2013 in China. Zhonghua Yu Fang Yi Xue Za Zhi. 2016; https://doi.org/10.3760/cma.j.issn.0253-9624.2016.09.004.
30. National Center for Disease Control and Prevention of China. Report on adults tobacco survey in 14 Chinese cities, 2013–2014. http://www.tcrc.org.cn/html/zy/cbw/jc/3192.html. Accessed 20 Aug 2015.
31. Ebenstein A, Fan M, Greenstone M, He G, Yin P, Zhou M. Growth, pollution, and life expectancy: China from 1991-2012. American Economic Review: Papers & Proceedings. 2015;105(5):226–31.
32. National Bureau of Statistics of the People's Republic of China, National data. 2017. http://www.stats.gov.cn. Accessed 9 Nov 2017.
33. Zhang R, Wang Z, Fei Y, Zhou B, Zheng S, Wang L, Huang L, Jiang S, Liu Z, Jiang J, et al. The difference in nutrient intakes between Chinese and Mediterranean. Japanese and American Diets Nutrients. 2015;7(6):4661–88.

Permissions

All chapters in this book were first published in CD, by BioMed Central; hereby published with permission under the Creative Commons Attribution License or equivalent. Every chapter published in this book has been scrutinized by our experts. Their significance has been extensively debated. The topics covered herein carry significant findings which will fuel the growth of the discipline. They may even be implemented as practical applications or may be referred to as a beginning point for another development.

The contributors of this book come from diverse backgrounds, making this book a truly international effort. This book will bring forth new frontiers with its revolutionizing research information and detailed analysis of the nascent developments around the world.

We would like to thank all the contributing authors for lending their expertise to make the book truly unique. They have played a crucial role in the development of this book. Without their invaluable contributions this book wouldn't have been possible. They have made vital efforts to compile up to date information on the varied aspects of this subject to make this book a valuable addition to the collection of many professionals and students.

This book was conceptualized with the vision of imparting up-to-date information and advanced data in this field. To ensure the same, a matchless editorial board was set up. Every individual on the board went through rigorous rounds of assessment to prove their worth. After which they invested a large part of their time researching and compiling the most relevant data for our readers.

The editorial board has been involved in producing this book since its inception. They have spent rigorous hours researching and exploring the diverse topics which have resulted in the successful publishing of this book. They have passed on their knowledge of decades through this book. To expedite this challenging task, the publisher supported the team at every step. A small team of assistant editors was also appointed to further simplify the editing procedure and attain best results for the readers.

Apart from the editorial board, the designing team has also invested a significant amount of their time in understanding the subject and creating the most relevant covers. They scrutinized every image to scout for the most suitable representation of the subject and create an appropriate cover for the book.

The publishing team has been an ardent support to the editorial, designing and production team. Their endless efforts to recruit the best for this project, has resulted in the accomplishment of this book. They are a veteran in the field of academics and their pool of knowledge is as vast as their experience in printing. Their expertise and guidance has proved useful at every step. Their uncompromising quality standards have made this book an exceptional effort. Their encouragement from time to time has been an inspiration for everyone.

The publisher and the editorial board hope that this book will prove to be a valuable piece of knowledge for researchers, students, practitioners and scholars across the globe.

List of Contributors

Derrick Lopez, Judith M Katzenellenbogen, John A Woods and Sandra C Thompson
Western Australian Centre for Rural Health, The University of Western Australia, Crawley, Western Australia, Australia

Judith M Katzenellenbogen, Frank M Sanfilippo, Michael ST Hobbs, Matthew W Knuiman and Tom G Briffa
School of Population Health, The University of Western Australia, Crawley, Western Australia, Australia

Peter L Thompson
School of Medicine and Pharmacology, Sir Charles Gairdner Hospital Unit, The University of Western Australia, Nedlands, Western Australia, Australia

I-Ting Tsai
Department of Emergency, E-Da Hospital, I-Shou University, Kaohsiung 82445, Taiwan

Chao-Ping Wang, Wei-Chin Hung, Cheng-Ching Wu, Fu-Mei Chung and Teng-Hung Yu
Division of Cardiology, E-Da Hospital, I-Shou University, No. 1, Yi-Da Rd, Jiau-Shu Village, Yan-Chao District, Kaohsiung 82445, Taiwan

Yung-Chuan Lu
Division of Endocrinology and Metabolism, E-Da Hospital, I-Shou University, Kaohsiung 82445, Taiwan

Chia-Chang Hsu
Division of Gastroenterology and Hepatology, Department of Internal Medicine, E-Da Hospital, I-Shou University, Kaohsiung 82445, Taiwan

Li-Fen Lu
Division of Cardiac Surgery, Department of Surgery, E-Da Hospital, I-Shou University, Kaohsiung 82445, Taiwan

Yau-Jiunn Lee
Lee's Endocrinology Clinic, Pingtung 90000, Taiwan

Chao-Ping Wang and Yung-Chuan Lu
School of Medicine for International Students, E-Da Hospital, I-Shou University, Kaohsiung 82445, Taiwan

I-Ting Tsai
Department of Nursing, I-Shou University, Kaohsiung 82445, Taiwan

Cheng-Ching Wu
Department of Biomedical Engineering, National Cheng Kung University, Tainan 70101, Taiwan

Harindra C Wijeysundera, Paul Fefer, Maria C Bennell and Dennis T Ko
Schulich Heart Centre, Division of Cardiology, Sunnybrook Health Sciences Centre, University of Toronto, Toronto, Ontario, Canada

Harindra C Wijeysundera, Peter C Austin and Dennis T Ko
Institute of Health Policy, Management and Evaluation, University of Toronto, Toronto, Ontario, Canada

Harindra C Wijeysundera, Feng Qiu, Peter C Austin and Dennis T Ko
Institute for Clinical Evaluative Sciences (ICES), Toronto, Ontario, Canada

Harindra C Wijeysundera
Li Ka Shing Knowledge Institute of St. Michael's Hospital, Toronto, Ontario, Canada

Paul Fefer
Leviev Heart Center, Sheba Medical Center, Tel Hashomer and Tel Aviv University, Ramat Aviv, Israel

Christos Graidis, Dimokritos Dimitriadis, Vasileios Karasavvidis, Georgios Dimitriadis, Efstathia Argyropoulou, Fotios Economou, Dadoush George, Antonios Antoniou and Georgios Karakostas
Department of Interventional Cardiology, Kyanous Stavros Hospital, Vizyis-Vyzantos 1 Street, Thessaloniki 54636, Greece

Christophe Bauters and Gilles Lemesle
Centre Hospitalier Régional et Universitaire de Lille, Lille, France

Christophe Bauters
Inserm U1167, Institut Pasteur de Lille, Université Lille Nord de France, Lille, France

Christophe Bauters and Gilles Lemesle
Faculté de Médecine de Lille, Lille, France

Christophe Bauters and Gilles Lemesle
Hôpital Cardiologique, CHRU de Lille, Boul. Prof. Leclercq, 59037 Lille Cedex, France

Sara Gargiulo, Maria Piera Petretta, Adelaide Greco, Matteo Gramanzini, Gabriele G Schiattarella, Giovanni Esposito, Arturo Brunetti and Alberto Cuocolo
Department of Advanced Biomedical Sciences, University Federico II, Via Pansini 5, 80131 Naples, Italy

Sara Gargiulo, Adelaide Greco, Matteo Gramanzini and Arturo Brunetti
CEINGE Scarl, Naples, Italy

Sara Gargiulo, Mariarosaria Panico, Michele Larobina and Matteo Gramanzini
Institute of Biostructure and Bioimaging, National Council of Research, Naples, Italy

Mario Petretta
Department of Translational Medical Sciences, University Federico II, Naples, Italy

Manal S. Fawzy, Nagwa M. Aly and Dahlia I. Badran
Department of Medical Biochemistry, Faculty of Medicine, Suez Canal University, Ismailia, Egypt

Eman A. Toraih
Department of Histology and Cell Biology (Genetics Unit), Faculty of Medicine, Suez Canal University, Ismailia, Egypt

Abeer Fakhr-Eldeen
Clinical Pathology Department, Faculty of Medicine, Sohag University, Sohag, Egypt

Mohammad H. Hussein
Pulmonologist, Ministry of Health, Cairo, Egypt

M. N. Krishnan
Govt. Medical College, Kozhikode, Kerala, India

G. Zachariah
Mother Hospital, Thrissur, Kerala, India

K. Venugopal
Pushpagiri Hospital, Tiruvalla, Kottayam, Kerala, India

P. P. Mohanan
Westfort High-tech Hospital, Thrissur, Kerala, India

S. Harikrishnan and G. Sanjay
Sree Chitra Tirunal Institute for Medical Sciences and Technology, Trivandrum, Kerala, India

L. Jeyaseelan
Department of Biostatistics, Christian Medical College, Vellore, Tamil Nadu, India

K. R. Thankappan
Achutha Menon Centre for Health Science Studies, Sree Chitra Tirunal Institute for Medical Sciences and Technology, Trivandrum Medical College, Thiruvananthapuram, Kerala, India

Christos Graidis, Dimokritos Dimitriadis, Vasileios Karasavvidis, Georgios Dimitriadis, Efstathia Argyropoulou, Fotios Economou, George Spiromitros, Antonios Antoniou and Georgios Karakostas
Department of Interventional Cardiology, Kyanous Stavros Hospital, Vizyis-Vyzantos 1 Street, Thessaloniki 54636, Greece

Fu-Zong Wu, Kang-Ju Chou, Yi-Luan Huang and Ming-Ting Wu
Department of Radiology, Section of Thoracic and Circulation Imaging, Kaohsiung Veterans General Hospital, Kaohsiung, Taiwan

Fu-Zong Wu and Kang-Ju Chou
Centre for Evidence-Based Medicine, Kaohsiung Veterans General Hospital, Kaohsiung, Taiwan

Fu-Zong Wu, Kang-Ju Chou and Ming-Ting Wu
Faculty of Medicine, School of Medicine, National Yang Ming University, Taipei, Taiwan

Kang-Ju Chou
Department of Internal Medicine, Kaohsiung Veterans General Hospital, Kaohsiung, Taiwan
Raquel Bravo-Escobar, Adela María Gómez-González, Angel Montiel-Trujillo, Rafael Aguilar-Jimenez and Rosa Carrasco-Ruíz
Unidad de Rehabilitación Cardiaca, Hospital universitario Virgen de la Victoria de Málaga, Campus de Teatinos s/n, 29010 Málaga, España

Alicia González-Represas
Facultad de Fisioterapia, Departamento de Biología Funcional y Ciencias de la Salud, Universidad de Vigo, Campus A Xunqueira s/n, 36005 Pontevedra, España

Angel Montiel-Trujillo
Servicio de Cardiología, Hospital universitario Virgen de la Victoria de Málaga, Campus de Teatinos s/n, 29010 Málaga, España

Pablo Salinas-Sánchez
Facultad de Medicina, Departamento de Anatomía Humana, Medicina legal e Historia de la Ciencia, University of Málaga, Campus de Teatinos s/n, 29010 Malaga, España

Joan Duran, Pilar Sánchez Olavarría, Marina Mola, Víctor Götzens, Alex Cordero and Josep Maria de Anta
Unitat d'Anatomia i Embriologia Humanes, Departament de Patologia I Terapèutica Experimental, Facultat de Medicina, Campus de Ciències de la Salut de Bellvitge, Universitat de Barcelona, L'Hospitalet de Llobregat, Barcelona 08907, Spain

Pilar Sánchez Olavarría
Departamento de Estadística, Facultad de Ciencias, Universidad de Valparaíso, Valparaíso, Chile

Marina Mola
Neurovascular Research Group (NEUVAS), Institut Municipal d'Investigació Mèdica. Hospital del Mar, PRBB, Parc de Recerca Biomèdica de Barcelona, Barcelona, Spain

Julio Carballo, Eva Martín Pelegrina and Màrius Petit
Department of Cardiology and Hemodynamics, Centre Cardiovascular Sant Jordi, Barcelona, Spain

Imanol Otaegui, Bruno García del Blanco and David García-Dorado
Department of Cardiology, Hospital Universitari Vall d'Hebron, Barcelona, Spain

Omar Abdul-Jawad
Department of Cardiology, Hospital Mútua de Terrassa, Terrassa, Barcelona, Spain

Josep Reig
Departament of Morphological Sciences, Universitat Autònoma de Barcelona, Bellaterra, Cerdanyola del Vallès, Barcelona, Spain

Alex Cordero
Àrea Epigenetics and Cancer Biology Area, Institut d'Investigació Biomèdica de Bellvitge (IDIBELL), L'Hospitalet de Llobregat, Barcelona, Spain

Yujiao Sun, Xin Yu, Ying Zhi, Song Geng, Hua Li, Ling Chen, Chunwei Wu and Guoxian Qi
Department of Cardiology of Aging, Department of Cardiology, The First Affiliated Hospital of China Medical University, NO.155 Nanjing North Street, Heping Ward, Shenyang 110001, China

Ting Liu and Ke Xu
Department of Radiology, The First Affiliated Hospital of China Medical University, Shenyang, China

Asim Rizvi, Bríain ó. Hartaigh, Donghee Han, Ji Hyun Lee, Jackie Szymonifika, Millie J. Gomez, Quynh A. Truong, Fay Y. Lin and James K. Min
Dalio Institute of Cardiovascular Imaging, NewYork-Presbyterian Hospital, New York, NY, USA

Paul Knaapen
Department of Cardiology, VU University Medical Center, Amsterdam, The Netherlands

Jonathon Leipsic
Department of Medical Imaging, University of British Columbia, St. Paul's Hospital, Vancouver, BC, Canada

Leslee J. Shaw
Emory University School of Medicine, Atlanta, GA, USA

Daniele Andreini
Centro Cardiologico Monzino, IRCCS, Milan, Italy

Gianluca Pontone
Istituto di Ricovero e Cura a Carattere Scientifico, Centro Cardiologico Monzino, Milan, Italy

Subha Raman
Davis Heart and Lung Research Institute and Heart Center, The Ohio State University, Columbus, OH, USA

Muhammad Akram Khan
The Cardiac Center of Texas, McKinney, TX, USA

Michael Ridner
Heart Center Research, LLC, Huntsville, AL, USA

Faisal Nabi
Houston Methodist DeBakey Heart & Vascular Center, Houston Methodist Hospital, Houston, TX, USA

Alessia Gimelli
Fondazione Toscana/CNR Gabriele Monasterio, Pisa, Italy

James Jang
Division of Cardiology, Kaiser Permanente San Jose Medical Center, San Jose, CA, USA

Jason Cole
Mobile Cardiology Associates, Mobile, AL, USA

Ryo Nakazato
Cardiovascular Imaging Lab, St. Luke's International Hospital, Tokyo, Japan

Christopher Zarins
Heart Flow, Inc., Redwood City, CA, USA
Department of Surgery, Stanford University, Stanford, CA, USA

Quynh A. Truong and James K. Min
Department of Medicine, Weill Cornell Medical College, New York, NY, USA

Fay Y. Lin, Quynh A. Truong and James K. Min
Department of Radiology, Weill Cornell Medical College, New York, NY, USA

Hyuk-Jae Chang
Division of Cardiology, Severance Cardiovascular Hospital, Yonsei University Health System, Seoul, South Korea

James K. Min
Radiology and Medicine, New York-Presbyterian Hospital and Weill Cornell Medical College, 413 E. 69th Street, Suite 108, New York, NY 10021, USA

Ki-Bum Won, Hyuk-Jae Chang, Sanghoon Shin, In-Jeong Cho, Chi-Young Shim, Geu-Ru Hong and Namsik Chung
Division of Cardiology, Yonsei Cardiovascular Center, Yonsei University College of Medicine, Seoul, Republic of Korea

Ki-Bum Won
Division of Cardiology, St. Luke's International Hospital, Tokyo, Japan

Jimin Sung
Graduate School of Health and Welfare CHA University, Seongnam, Republic of Korea

Young Jin Kim and Byung-Wook Choi
Division of Radiology, Yonsei Cardiovascular Center, Yonsei University College of Medicine, Seoul, Republic of Korea

Hyuk-Jae Chang
Severance Biomedical Science Institute, Seoul, Republic of Korea

Hyuk-Jae Chang
Yonsei Cardiovascular Center, Yonsei University College of Medicine, 50 Yonsei-ro, Seodaemun-gu, Seoul 120-752, Republic of Korea

Ke-Fei Dou and Xiao-Jin Gao
State Key Laboratory of Cardiovascular Disease, Department of Cardiology, Cardiovascular Institute, Fuwai Hospital and National Center for Cardiovascular Diseases, Chinese Academy of Medical Sciences and Peking Union Medical College, Beijing, China

Xiao-Jin Gao
National Center for Cardiovascular Diseases, Chinese Academy of Medical Sciences and Peking Union Medical College, A 167, Beilishi Road, Xicheng District, Beijing 100037, China

Bo-Qia Xie
Department of Cardiology, Beijing Chaoyang Hospital, Capital Medical University, Beijing, China

Yan Li and Zuo-Xiang He
Department of Nuclear Medicine, Cardiovascular Institute, Fuwai Hospital and National Center for Cardiovascular Diseases, Chinese Academy of Medical Sciences and Peking Union Medical College, Beijing, China

Min-Fu Yang
Department of Nuclear Medicine, Beijing Chaoyang Hospital, Capital Medical University, 8th Gongtinanlu Rd, Chaoyang District, Beijing 100020, China

Boonsub Sakboonyarat and Ram Rangsin
Department of Military and Community Medicine, Phramongkutklao College of Medicine, Bangkok 10400, Thailand

Rosane Paixão Schlatter and Carisi Anne Polanczyk
Graduate Cardiology Program, Universidade Federal do Rio Grande do Sul (UFRGS), Porto Alegre, RS, Brazil

Carisi Anne Polanczyk
Department of Cardiology, Hospital de Clinicas de Porto Alegre (HCPA), Porto Alegre, RS, Brazil

Carisi Anne Polanczyk
Department of Cardiology, School of Medicine, UFRGS, Porto Alegre, RS, Brazil

Carisi Anne Polanczyk and Rosane Paixão Schlatter
National Health Technology Assessment Institute, CNPq, Porto Alegre, RS, Brazil

Vânia Naomi Hirakata
Research and Graduate Studies Department. Hospital de Clinicas de Porto Alegre HCPA, Porto Alegre, RS, Brazil

Rosane Paixão Schlatter
Programa de Pós-graduação em Cardiologia, Hospital de Clínicas de Porto Alegre, Rua Ramiro Barcelos, 2350, CEP, Porto Alegre, RS 90035-903, Brazil

Audrius Alonderis , Nijole Raskauskiene, Vaidute Gelziniene, Narseta Mickuviene and Julija Brozaitiene
Behavioral Medicine Institute, Lithuanian University of Health Sciences, Vyduno 4, 00135 Palanga, Lithuania

Ganshen Zhang, Chuanhua Yu, Lu Wang, Yunquan Zhang and Lisha Luo
Department of Epidemiology and Biostatistics, School of Health Sciences, Wuhan University, #185 Donghu Road, Wuhan, Hubei 430071, China

Maigeng Zhou
National Center for Chronic and Non-communicable Disease Control and Prevention, Beijing, China

Index

www.ingramcontent.com/pod-product-compliance
Lightning Source LLC
LaVergne TN
LVHW080702210926
848485LV00003B/409